The Loss of Sadness

The Loss of Sadness

How Psychiatry Transformed Normal Sorrow
Into Depressive Disorder

Allan V. Horwitz and Jerome C. Wakefield

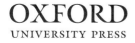

OXFORD
UNIVERSITY PRESS

2007

OXFORD
UNIVERSITY PRESS

Oxford University Press, Inc., publishes works that further
Oxford University's objective of excellence
in research, scholarship, and education.

Oxford New York
Auckland Cape Town Dar es Salaam Hong Kong Karachi
Kuala Lumpur Madrid Melbourne Mexico City Nairobi
New Delhi Shanghai Taipei Toronto

With offices in
Argentina Austria Brazil Chile Czech Republic France Greece
Guatemala Hungary Italy Japan Poland Portugal Singapore
South Korea Switzerland Thailand Turkey Ukraine Vietnam

Published by Oxford University Press, Inc.
198 Madison Avenue, New York, New York 10016

www.oup.com

Oxford is a registered trademark of Oxford University Press

Library of Congress Cataloging-in-Publication Data
Horwitz, Allan V.
The loss of sadness : how psychiatry transformed normal sorrow into depressive disorder / Allan V.
Horwitz and Jerome C. Wakefield.
    p. ; cm.
Includes bibliographical references and index.
ISBN 978-0-19-531304-8
1. Psychiatry—Miscellanea. 2. Depression, Mental—Miscellanea. 3. Mental illness—Miscellanea.
I. Wakefield, Jerome C. II. Title.
[DNLM: 1. Diagnostic and statistical manual of mental disorders. 2. Depression. 3. Depressive Disorder.
WM 171 H824L 2007]
RC480.5.H667 2007
616.89—dc22   2006032581

9 8 7 6 5 4

Printed in the United States of America
on acid-free paper

To David Mechanic
—AVH

To my parents, Helen and Ted Sherman
—JCW

Foreword

The book you are about to read is a brilliant tour de force of scholarship and analysis from two of our leading thinkers about psychiatric diagnosis and the nature of mental disorders. Allan Horwitz and Jerome Wakefield's *The Loss of Sadness* represents the most cogent and compelling "inside" challenge to date to the diagnostic revolution that began almost 30 years ago in the field of psychiatry. The authors begin by arguing for the existence of a universal intuitive understanding that to be human means to naturally react with feelings of sadness to negative events in one's life. In contrast, when the symptoms of sadness (e.g., sad feelings, difficulty sleeping, inability to concentrate, reduced appetite) have no apparent cause or are grossly disproportionate to the apparent cause, the intuitive understanding is that something important in human functioning has gone wrong, indicating the presence of a depressive disorder. Horwitz and Wakefield then persuasively argue, as the book's central thesis, that contemporary psychiatry confuses normal sadness with depressive mental disorder because it ignores the relationship of symptoms to the context in which they emerge. The psychiatric diagnosis of Major Depression is based on the assumption that symptoms alone can indicate that there is a disorder; this assumption allows normal responses to stressors to be mischaracterized as symptoms of disorder. The authors demonstrate that this confusion has important implications not only for psychiatry and its patients but also for society in general.

The book's thesis is of special interest to me, because I was the head of the American Psychiatric Association's task force that in 1980 created the *DSM-III* (i.e., the third edition of the *Diagnostic and Statistical Manual of Mental Disorders*, the Association's official listing of recognized mental disorders and the criteria by which they are diagnosed). This was the first edition of the *Manual* to offer explicit symptomatic criteria for the diagnosis of each mental disorder. Now in its fourth edition, the *DSM* is generally considered to have revolutionized the psychiatric profession. It serves to define how researchers collect their samples, what conditions insurance companies will reimburse, what conditions courts and social agencies treat as illnesses, and how individuals themselves interpret their emotional experiences. The *DSM*'s standardization of psychiatric diagnosis by using explicit rules for making a diagnosis has been critical to the explosion of research and knowledge in the mental health field. It has allowed clinicians and researchers with different theoretical perspectives, and thus different languages, to communicate with each other. It has also addressed doubts about psychiatry's scientific status, such as concerns about the reliability of its diagnoses.

Yet the very success of the *DSM* and its descriptive criteria at a practical level has allowed the field of psychiatry to ignore some basic conceptual issues that have been lurking at the foundation of the *DSM* enterprise, especially the question of how to distinguish disorder from normal suffering. This book will bring increased attention to these conceptual problems.

My involvement in an earlier debate over whether to remove homosexuality from *DSM-II* in 1973 led me to grapple with the question of how to define mental disorder. I formulated the definitions of mental disorder in the introductions to the *DSM-III*, the *DSM-III-R* (the DSM's third edition revised), and the *DSM-IV*, which aim to explain the reasons that certain conditions were included in and other types of problems excluded from the *Manual*. Since then, Dr. Wakefield has critiqued my efforts in ways that I have largely become convinced are valid. His evolution-based "harmful dysfunction" analysis of the concept of mental disorder raises subtle, nuanced questions about mental disorder that challenge one's thinking, no matter where one falls on the issues. It is easily the most widely cited and provocative analysis of the concept of mental disorder that exists today, simultaneously defending the concept as legitimate and providing a framework for this book's critique of current diagnostic standards as too broad. Moreover, Horwitz and Wakefield point out that the *DSM* is not consistent even in applying its own definition of mental disorder to the diagnostic criteria sets for specific disorders. Whereas the *DSM* definition of mental disorder, like the harmful-dysfunction approach, clearly specifies that a disorder involves a dysfunction in the individual and is not an expectable response to a stressor, the formulation of the *DSM*'s diagnostic criteria sets rarely took this into account. In other words, its criteria specified the symptoms that must be present to justify a given diagnosis but ignored any reference to the context in which they developed. In so doing, they allowed normal responses to stressors to be characterized as symptoms of disorder.

Many critiques of the *DSM* have come from the "outside" in that they have been suspicious of the very notion of a mental disorder and thus rejected the idea of a psychiatric diagnostic manual as inappropriately medicalizing social problems. In contrast, Horwitz and Wakefield recognize the *DSM*'s contributions and accept its assumption that there are genuine mental disorders in the strict medical sense. Ironically, it is by taking seriously the *DSM*'s claim to be a manual of mental disorders (and thus to fall within the scope of medicine) that the authors are able to mount a devastating critique of the way the *DSM* operationalizes the diagnosis of depression (and by implication, other diagnostic categories as well) with inadequate attention to context. Because their analysis is anchored in psychiatry's own assumptions, it will be hard for those now constructing the *DSM-V* (expected publication in 2011) to ignore.

Horwitz and Wakefield trace the history of the diagnosis of depression, beginning with Hippocrates and working through to the present, and show with impressive and persuasive scholarship just how consistently their view—rather than the *DSM*'s approach in which symptoms alone can indicate disorder—is reflected in the historical traditions of medicine and psychiatry, even including the work of Emil Kraepelin, the psychiatrist often considered the inspiration for the *DSM-III*. It should be noted that at the time the diagnostic criteria for depression were originally developed, they were intended for research samples in which it was a reasonable assumption that the patients were disordered. The authors argue that, when those same diagnostic criteria that contain no reference to context are used in community epidemiological studies and screening of the general population, large numbers of people who are having normal human responses to various stressors are mistakenly diagnosed as disordered. The researchers who have conducted the major epidemiological studies over the past two decades have totally ignored this problem. The result has been semiofficial prevalence rates that many find unbelievable.

The authors' analysis of disorder itself does not state exactly where the line between dysfunction and normality is to be drawn and allows that the boundary is fuzzy. I have to admit that I would be inclined to draw the boundary so as to include more under "disorder" than they do. Frankly, I remain cautious about the possibility of incorporating context into diagnostic criteria and about the unreliability and false negatives that might result. But it has yet to be tried in a serious way. This book will place this issue on psychiatry's agenda and make it one of the major topics that should be considered in the upcoming revisions that will yield the *DSM-V*. However the problem is resolved, because of this book the question will have to be posed; it can no longer be ignored.

Relentless in its logic, Horwitz and Wakefield's book forces one to confront basic issues that cut to the heart of psychiatry. It has caused me to rethink my own position and to consider how the authors' concerns might best be handled. It will shape future discussion and research on depression, and it will be an indispensable guide to those who are rethinking psychiatric diagnostic criteria in preparation for the *DSM-V*. It would be interesting to look back 100 years from now and see whether context is as crucial to diagnostic criteria as the authors believe it to be or whether the stricter symptom-based approach can somehow rebound from their critique. But either way, psychiatry will rest on firmer logical foundations as a result of their critique, and this book will stand as a watershed in the conceptual development of the field.

Robert L. Spitzer, MD
Professor of Psychiatry
New York State Psychiatric Institute

Preface

This book is the result of an unusually cooperative effort. The order of authors is alphabetical; we are both fully and equally responsible for the intellectual content throughout the book, which has resulted from a tireless and stimulating mutual process of feedback, incremental improvement, and debate at every stage. Our coauthorship, nevertheless, occurred serendipitously. We were each independently planning books about depression, with essentially the same overall message. When we discovered this in discussion one day, we decided to join forces. However, the ways by which we each came to our original ideas of writing such a book were quite different.

Jerome Wakefield, having written extensively about the concept of mental disorder, was scheduled to publish an invited journal article critiquing psychologist Neil Jacobson's behaviorist attack on the medical model of depression. The theme of the article was that neither those who believe in the "disorder" approach to depression expressed in the *Diagnostic and Statistical Manual of Mental Disorders (DSM)* nor those, like Jacobson, who deny that depression is a medical disorder are correct. Instead, they are talking past each other about different kinds of cases. Wakefield intended to argue that instead of trying to decide between these rival views, psychiatry should instead be drawing a distinction between the genuinely disordered and those with normal responses to misfortune whom the *DSM* has misclassified.

Following Jacobson's untimely death, the journal decided not to proceed with the article given that he would be unable to reply to it. Meanwhile, Wakefield realized that the topic was far broader than first conceived and that a balanced consideration of both the disordered and nondisordered forms of depression and sadness called for book-length treatment. The issue itself seemed urgent because, if mental health professionals were talking past each other about it rather than recognizing its complexity, then they would inevitably be talking past some of their patients, as well. We hope that this book will indeed encourage these different factions to talk to each other and to realize the distinctions to be made between those who are depressed and those who are normally sad.

Allan Horwitz had recently completed a book about the new paradigm of "diagnostic psychiatry" introduced in the *DSM-III* in 1980. By then the *DSM* had grown to several hundred diagnoses, with depression becoming the signature diagnosis of contemporary psychiatry. Careful study of this condition in particular thus promised to illuminate broader issues that faced the field. Horwitz's work in the sociology of stress had convinced him that many of the conditions that sociologists studied were similar to those that psychiatry classified as Major Depression yet that they were not disordered but were normal human responses to stressful social circumstances. Like Wakefield, he was also convinced that there were depressive conditions that were truly disordered. A book on depression seemed to him to be a way at once to examine the successes and limitations of psychiatry's new paradigm and to identify conceptual problems in the sociology of medicine, all through the lens of a detailed analysis of this one pivotal diagnostic category.

It also seemed that joining forces with Wakefield might help navigate between the Scylla of social constructionism and the Charybdis of biological essentialism and produce an analysis that grounds the distinction between normality and disorder in biological factors while at the same time maintaining an important role for social factors in making this distinction. We hope that the result of our collaboration is a book that does indeed manage to wend a balanced path between the biological and the social and between normal suffering and mental disorder.

All books are products not just of authors but also of the environments in which they are written. It has been our good fortune to have written this book in exceptionally fine circumstances. For Horwitz, the Institute for Health, Health Care Policy, and Aging Research and the Sociology Department at Rutgers have provided intellectual stimulation, extraordinary colleagues, and ideal working conditions. In particular, David Mechanic, the director of the Health Institute, has been a constant source of inspiration, wisdom, and encouragement. Deborah Carr, Gerald Grob, Ellen Idler, Sarah Rosenfield, and Eviatar Zerubavel have been both careful readers and special friends. For Wakefield, these ideas germinated at the Rutgers Health Institute as well but were pursued for publication in his current home at New York University School of Social Work. The school and its dean, Suzanne England, and stimulating new colleagues, as well as NYU's amazing intellectual energy under the leadership of John Sexton and David McLaughlin, have offered exceptional support, opportunity, and inspiration. We are also grateful to Peter Conrad, Randolph Nesse, Sharon Schwartz, and Robert Spitzer for their comments on particular chapters of this manuscript.

In an ideal world, all authors would have editors with the extraordinary talent and critical skills of Marion Osmun at Oxford University Press. We have been extremely lucky to have her as the editor of this book; we and the book have benefited enormously from her support and wisdom.

Finally, personal indebtedness is owed most of all to our families. Wakefield's wife, Lisa, provided not only consistent support but also a thoughtful and challenging sounding board; his children, Joshua and Zachary, provided a joyful reprieve from work. His parents, Helen and Ted Sherman, provided a background of enduring love and support. Horwitz's father, who died just after the manuscript was completed, was a lifelong model of scientific creativity and achievement. His daughters, Rebecca, Jessica, and Stephanie, provided welcome and delightful diversions during the writing of this book.

Contents

The Loss of Sadness

1

The Concept of Depression

The poet W. H. Auden famously deemed the period after World War II the "age of anxiety."[1] For Auden, the intense anxiety of that era was a normal human response to extraordinary circumstances, such as the devastation of modern warfare, the horrors of the concentration camps, the development of nuclear weapons, and the tensions of the cold war between the United States and the Soviet Union. Were Auden still alive, he might conclude that the era around the turn of the twenty-first century is the "age of depression."[2] There would, however, be a crucial difference between the two characterizations: whereas the age of anxiety was viewed as a natural response to social circumstances that required collective and political solutions, ours is viewed as an age of sadness that is abnormal—an age of depressive psychiatric disorder that requires professional treatment.

Consider Willy Loman, the lead character in Arthur Miller's classic play *Death of a Salesman* and possibly the fictional character most representative of American life during the decades following World War II.[3] As he enters his 60s, despite his fervent belief in the American dream that hard work will lead to success, Willy Loman has never accomplished very much. He has heavy debts, his health is failing, he is barely able to continue working at his job as a traveling salesman, and his sons despise him. When he is finally fired from his job, he is forced to admit to himself that he is a failure. He kills himself in an automobile accident in the hope of getting his family some money from an insurance settlement. The tremendous popularity of *Death of a Salesman* on its introduction on Broadway in 1949 stemmed from Willy Loman's embodiment of the Everyman in American life who embraced the goal of achieving great wealth but found himself destroyed by it.

Death of a Salesman received a very different response during its revival 50 years later.[4] According to a piece in *The New York Times* titled "Get That Man Some Prozac," the director of the revived version sent the script to two psychiatrists, who diagnosed Loman as having a depressive disorder.[5] The playwright, Arthur Miller, objected to this characterization, protesting: "Willy Loman is not a depressive. . . . He is weighed down by life. There are social reasons for why he is where he is." The response of the psychiatrists is as exemplary of our time as Loman was of his. What our culture once viewed as a reaction to failed hopes and aspirations it now regards as a psychiatric illness. The transformation of Willy Loman from a social to a psychiatric casualty represents a fundamental change in the way we view the nature of sadness.

The Ubiquity of Depression

The ascendancy of depressive disorder is a major social trend manifested in a variety of ways:

Amount of depression in the community. Many researchers claim that substantial and growing proportions of the population suffer from depressive disorder. Estimates from epidemiological studies indicate that Major Depression afflicts about 10% of adults in the United States each year and nearly a fifth of the population at some point in their lives.[6] Rates among women are even higher, about twice as high as in men.[7] Depending on the definition employed, depression can afflict as many as half of the members of some groups, such as female adolescents and the elderly.[8] Moreover, these numbers seem to be steadily growing. For the past several decades, each successive birth cohort has reported more depressive disorders than previous generations showed.[9] Although these rising rates are more likely to be an artifact of the way community surveys measure this condition than to reflect an actual increase,[10] there is a widespread perception that depressive disorder is growing at an alarming pace.

Number of patients in treatment for depression. The number of persons treated for depression in the United States has grown explosively in recent years. Most depressed people are treated in outpatient settings, where treatment of depression increased by 300% between 1987 and 1997.[11] By 1997, fully 40% of all psychotherapy patients, double the percentage of a decade before, had diagnoses of a mood disorder, the larger category that comprises mainly depression.[12] The overall percentage of the population in treatment for depression in a particular year grew from 2.1% in the early 1980s to 3.7% in the early 2000s, an increase of 76% in just 20 years.[13] Some groups experienced a much greater increase; for example, in just the period between 1992 and 1998, health care providers diagnosed 107% more elderly persons with depression.[14]

Prescription of antidepressant medication. Although medication has been a common treatment for life problems since the 1950s, its use has undergone a staggering growth in recent years. Antidepressant medications, such as Prozac, Paxil, Zoloft, and Effexor, are now among the largest selling prescription drugs of any sort.[15] Their use among adults nearly tripled between 1988 and 2000.[16] In any given month, 10% of women and 4% of men now use these drugs.[17] During

the 1990s, spending for antidepressants increased by 600% in the United States,
exceeding $7 billion annually by the year 2000.[18]

Estimates of the social cost of depression. Depression is believed to be the source
of huge social costs. The World Health Organization (WHO), the leading international body that deals with health, projects that by 2020 depression will become the second leading cause of worldwide disability, behind only heart disease.
The WHO estimates that depression is already the leading cause of disability for
15- to 44-year-olds.[19] In the United States, economists estimate that depression
is responsible for $43 billion in costs every year.[20]

Scientific publications on depression. Research on depression has become a
major industry.[21] In 1966, 703 articles containing the word *depression* in their
titles were published in medical journals. In 1980, the year in which the American Psychiatric Association (APA) published its landmark third edition of the
Diagnostic and Statistical Manual of Mental Disorders (*DSM-III*) with new definitions of depressive disorder, 2,754 articles on depression were published. This
number steadily increased over the following 15 years, and then exploded in
the mid-1990s. By 2005, there were 8,677 articles about depression published,
more than 12 times the number in 1966. The number of articles concerned with
depression is now far higher than any other psychiatric diagnosis and has grown
far more rapidly than the general growth in psychiatric research publications.

Media attention to depression. Depression has become a central concern in the
culture more generally. Popular television shows, best-selling books, and major
articles in national magazines often feature this illness. Many memoirs about
personal experiences of depression, including William Styron's *Darkness Visible*,
Kay Jamison's *An Unquiet Mind*, Elizabeth Wurtzel's *Prozac Nation*, and Andrew
Solomon's *The Noonday Demon*, have reached the best-seller list. A look at the
new books in the psychology sections of bookstores reveals a virtual tidal wave
of books on how to prevent or cope with depression of all sorts. The acclaimed
television series, *The Sopranos*, features as its central character a Mafia boss who
has—among other psychiatric conditions—depression and whose consump-
tion of antidepressant medications is a major theme of the show. A number
of prominent public personalities, including Tipper Gore, Mike Wallace, and
Brooke Shields, have received massive publicity after disclosing their depressive
conditions.

Normal Versus Disordered Sadness

Although the belief that depression is a widespread phenomenon is new, the
symptoms we now associate with it, including intense sadness and the many
other emotional experiences and physical symptoms that often accompany sadness, have been noted since the beginning of recorded medical history.[22] Yet, in
attempting to understand the recent upsurge in diagnosed depressive disorder,

it is important to recognize that until recently, two broad types of conditions that manifest these same symptoms were sharply distinguished from each other. One, normal sadness, or sadness "with cause," was associated with experiences of loss or other painful circumstances that seemed to be the obvious causes of distress. The response to such normal reactions was to offer support, to help the individual cope and move on despite the loss, and to avoid confusing the person's sadness with illness.

The other kind of condition, traditionally known as *melancholia,* or depression "without cause," was a medical disorder distinguished from normal sadness by the fact that the patient's symptoms occurred despite there being no appropriate reason for them in the patient's circumstances. These conditions were relatively rare but tended to be long lasting and recurrent. Because they were not proportional reactions to actual events, such conditions were assumed to stem from some sort of internal defect or dysfunction that required professional attention. Yet these pathological conditions involve the same sorts of symptoms—such as sadness, insomnia, social withdrawal, loss of appetite, lack of interest in usual activities, and so on—associated with intense normal sadness.

This separation of normal sadness and depressive disorder is a sensible and legitimate, indeed a crucial, one. It is consistent not only with the general distinction between normality and disorder used in medicine and traditional psychiatry but also with common sense, and it has both clinical and scientific importance. Yet contemporary psychiatry has come to largely ignore this distinction.

We argue that the recent explosion of putative depressive disorder, in fact, does not stem primarily from a real rise in this condition. Instead, it is largely a product of conflating the two conceptually distinct categories of normal sadness and depressive disorder and thus classifying many instances of normal sadness as mental disorders. The current "epidemic," although the result of many social factors, has been made possible by a changed psychiatric definition of depressive disorder that often allows the classification of sadness as disease, even when it is not.

The "Age of Depression" Results
From a Faulty Definition of
Depressive Disorder

Unlike Auden's "age of anxiety," which resulted from identifiable social conditions, there are no obvious circumstances that would explain a recent upsurge in depressive disorder. The most commonly heard suggestions—such as that modern life is less socially anchored and involves more alienation or that media constantly expose us to extremes of wealth and beauty that cause us to feel inadequate by comparison—would tend to explain only normal sadness reactions (analogous to the normal anxiety responses to which Auden pointed), not the massive growth of a mental disorder. No environmental pathogen that might

have resulted in a real increase in physiologically, psychologically, or socially induced brain malfunctions has been identified or even theorized. Certainly, progress in effectively treating depressive disorder with psychotropic medication has
resulted in increased treatment of a condition about which physicians believe
they can at least do some good, and perhaps it has motivated diagnosis of formerly ambiguous cases as depression in the hope of offering effective treatment.
But that does not by itself explain the vast growth in the numbers of people who
seemingly have and are treated for this disorder; better treatments do not usually lead to a substantial increase in disease prevalence. Nor would improved
treatments explain the results of epidemiological studies that bypass patients
and directly interview community members not in treatment. Thus the seeming explosion of cases of depressive disorder is puzzling. What has happened to
create the appearance of this epidemic?

What has happened, we argue, is largely diagnostic inflation based on a relatively new definition of depressive disorder that is flawed and that, combined
with other developments in society, has dramatically expanded the domain of
presumed disorder. To understand how this phenomenon has occurred, it is useful to place current psychiatric practices in historical context and to consider
how odd current diagnostic definitions of depressive disorder are by historical
standards. One must also confront the esoterica of modern psychiatric classification presented in successive editions of the American Psychiatric Association's *DSM*. Often called the "bible of psychiatry," the *DSM* provides diagnostic
definitions for all mental disorders.

But how can something as simple and limited as a definition have substantial
consequences for such a field as psychiatry and thus for the media that popular-
ize its claims and findings and for the thinking of society at large that relies on
its expertise? In response to criticisms during the 1960s and 1970s that different
psychiatrists would not diagnose the same person with the same symptoms in the
same way (this problem was known as the "unreliability" of diagnosis), in 1980
the *DSM* began to use lists of symptoms to establish clear definitions for each disorder.[23] Almost all mental health professionals across a variety of settings, from
hospital clinics to private practices, now use these formal definitions for clinical
diagnosis. Moreover, these definitions have percolated out of the mental health
clinical arena and are used in epidemiological studies of disorder in the community, in research studies of treatment outcomes, in marketing of antidepressant medications, in preventive efforts in schools, in screening in general medical
practice, in court proceedings, and in many other settings. In effect, these *DSM*
definitions have become the authoritative arbiter of what is and is not considered
mental disorder throughout our society. What might seem like abstract, distant,
technical issues concerning these definitions in fact have important consequences
for individuals and how their suffering is understood and addressed.

The fact that these symptom-based definitions are the foundation of the entire
mental health research and treatment enterprise makes their validity critically

important. Psychiatric research and treatment are like an upside-down pyramid, and the *DSM* definitions of mental disorders that determine who is counted as disordered are the one small point on which the soundness of the entire pyramid rests. Even the best clinical history taking and diagnostic interviewing or the best research sample selection, experimental design, and statistical analysis of data will not produce meaningful results if they use an invalid definition of disorder that mixes normal and abnormal features. Archimedes famously boasted, "Give me a lever long enough, and a pivot on which to rest it, and I will move the earth." In modern psychiatry, definitions move the treatment and research firmament, and modern clinicians with an invalidly broad definition can move diagnosed disorder to virtually whatever level they desire, especially when they deal with a disorder such as depression that features such symptoms as sadness, insomnia, and fatigue, which are widespread among nondisordered people. Thus the recent focus in psychiatry on reliability of diagnosis based on symptoms has been pursued at some cost to validity—that is, whether the diagnosis represents a correct attribution of disorder.[24] The *DSM*'s criteria for Major Depressive Disorder are one instance in which increased reliability has had the inadvertent side effect of creating substantial new validity problems.

The *DSM*'s Definition of Major Depression

The current official psychiatric definition of depressive disorder that is the basis for clinical diagnosis and research studies is found in the most recent edition (4th ed., text revision) of the *DSM*.[25] The *DSM* definition of Major Depressive Disorder (MDD), the category under which most depressive disorders fall, is lengthy and has several qualifiers and exceptions. We defer full analysis and critique of the *DSM*'s approach to depressive disorder until chapter 5. For purposes of this initial discussion, we consider the most important features of the definition, which consists of symptom and duration requirements and a bereavement exclusion.

DSM diagnosis of MDD requires that five symptoms out of the following nine be present during a 2-week period (the five must include either depressed mood or diminished interest or pleasure): (1) depressed mood; (2) diminished interest or pleasure in activities; (3) weight gain or loss or change in appetite; (4) insomnia or hypersomnia (excessive sleep); (5) psychomotor agitation or retardation (slowing down); (6) fatigue or loss of energy; (7) feelings of worthlessness or excessive or inappropriate guilt; (8) diminished ability to think or concentrate or indecisiveness; and (9) recurrent thoughts of death or suicidal ideation or suicide attempt.[26]

These symptom criteria form the heart of the definition of MDD, but there is one further important clause in the definition: "The symptoms are not better accounted for by Bereavement, i.e., after the loss of a loved one, the symptoms persist for longer than 2 months or are characterized by marked functional impairment, morbid preoccupation with worthlessness, suicidal ideation, psychotic symptoms, or psychomotor retardation."[27] In other words, patients are exempt from diagnosis if their symptoms are due to what the *DSM* defines as a normal period of bereavement after the death of a loved one, lasting no more than 2 months and not including especially serious symptoms, such as psychosis or thoughts about suicide. This limited "bereavement exclusion" is the definition's only acknowledgment that some instances of normal intense sadness might satisfy the symptomatic criteria.

The *DSM* definition of depressive disorder is reasonable in many ways. Its criteria might give rise to disagreements about particular symptoms, but each is widely and consensually believed to be an indicator of depressive disorder, and pre-*DSM* psychiatry recognized them as such. One might also debate the exact number of symptoms needed for diagnosis; some would argue for laxer requirements with fewer symptoms, others for more stringent symptom requirements to ensure that disorder exists, and still others would insist that there should be no sharp cutoff but rather a dimensional continuum of severity.[28] One might also dispute whether the required duration of 2 weeks is sufficient, but it is sometimes clear within 2 weeks of onset that someone has a depressive disorder, and clinicians should not be kept from diagnosing such cases even if the typical duration of depressive disorders is much longer. Likewise, it seems reasonable to exclude people who are recently bereaved. The criteria are also fairly clear and, in most cases, not more difficult to measure than typical psychiatric symptoms in other disorders. The reasonableness, clarity, and efficiency of its use help account for the nearly universal adoption of the *DSM* definition of MDD.

What, then, is the problem with this definition? The essence of the definition is that, aside from a few exceptions, the presence of a particular group of symptoms is sufficient to diagnose the presence of the disorder. Yet symptoms such as depressed mood, loss of interest in usual activities, insomnia, lessened appetite, inability to concentrate, and so on might naturally occur for a period of 2 weeks in the absence of any disorder after any of a wide range of negative events, such as betrayal by romantic partners, being passed over for an anticipated promotion, failing a major test that has serious implications for one's career, discovering a life-threatening illness in oneself or a loved one, or enduring the humiliation that follows revelations of disgraceful behavior. Such reactions, even when quite intense due to the severity of the experience, are surely part of normal human nature. Just as it is obvious why the *DSM* excludes bereavement from diagnosis, by parity of reasoning it seems obvious that it should also exclude these other sorts of reactions to negative circumstances. The diagnosis, however, does not exclude such nongrief responses. Because of the symptom-based nature of the criteria, any sadness response involving enough of the specified symptoms for at least 2 weeks will be misclassified as a disorder, along with genuine psychiatric disturbances. In attempting to characterize the kinds of symptoms suffered in depressive disorders without reference to the context in which the symptoms occur, contemporary psychiatry has also inadvertently characterized intense normal suffering as disease.

Consider, for example, the following cases:

Case 1: Ending of a Passionate Romantic Relationship

A 35-year-old single female professor has sought psychiatric consultation to obtain medicine for insomnia. She must present a paper as part of a job interview and is afraid that she is not able to function adequately enough to do so. She reports that for the past 3 weeks she has experienced depressed mood and extreme feelings of sadness and emptiness, as well as lack of interest in her usual activities (in fact, she has spent much of her time lying in bed or watching television). Her appetite has diminished, and she lies awake long into the night unable to fall asleep due to the pain of her sadness. She is fatigued and lacking in energy during the day and cannot concentrate on her work. Because her painful feelings distract her during work, she is barely able to meet minimal occupational obligations (e.g., she shows up at her classes poorly prepared, has not attended faculty meetings, and has difficulty concentrating on her research). She has also avoided social obligations.

When asked about what might have precipitated these distressing feelings, she reports that about a month before, a married man with whom she had had a passionate 5-year love affair decided he could not leave his wife and ended the affair. The woman had perceived this relationship as a unique, once-in-a-lifetime romance that had an extraordinary combination of emotional and intellectual intimacy.

The woman agrees to check in with the psychiatrist periodically. Subsequently, as weeks go by, her sense of loss subsides gradually and is replaced by a feeling of loneliness and the need to get on with her life and find a partner. Eventually, she starts dating again, and after several more months the woman meets a new love interest, and any residual symptoms disappear.

Case 2: Loss of a Valued Job

A 64-year-old married man has developed feelings of sadness and emptiness, lack of pleasure in activities, insomnia, fatigue and lack of energy, and feelings of worthlessness. He is not interested in seeing friends and seems unable to concentrate on anything. He yells at his wife when she attempts to console him and rejects her efforts to comfort him.

The feelings were triggered 2 weeks before when the company the man worked for unexpectedly fired him as part of a corporate downsizing. The firing came just 6 months before he would have qualified for the company's retirement plan. One of the major reasons the man chose to work for the company and then spend two decades with it had been the prospect of generous retirement benefits. The loss of these benefits means that he and his wife have very little retirement income other than Social Security to look forward to.

Subsequently, the couple is forced to sell their house and move to a small apartment. The man finds part-time work that, along with Social Security, provides barely enough resources to sustain him and his wife. He remains bitter about how he was treated, but his symptoms gradually subside over time.

Case 3: Reaction to a Life-Threatening Medical Diagnosis in a Loved One

A 60-year-old divorced woman who is visiting a medical center distant from her home asks a physician at the center for medication to help her sleep. The woman's daughter, an attorney and her only child, to whom she is very close and who is the pride of her life, was diagnosed just 3 weeks before with a rare and potentially fatal blood disease. After receiving the news of her daughter's diagnosis, the mother was devastated by feelings of sadness and despair and was unable to function at work or socially. Although she kept up a brave front for her daughter and was able to help her child with the arrangements for the medical consultation, the mother has been in a state of great distress since the diagnosis; she cries intermittently, is unable to sleep, lacks the ability to concentrate, and feels fatigued and uninterested in her usual activities as she attempts to come to terms with the news of her daughter's condition.

These symptoms gradually abate over a number of months during her daughter's treatment and struggle with the illness, which eventually stabilizes but remains a threat. The woman continues to periodically feel sad about her daughter's situation, but her other symptoms subside as she adjusts to the new circumstances and limits of her daughter's life.

Each of these people easily meets the symptomatic requirements for MDD and the *DSM* would thus classify them as psychiatrically disordered. Their symptoms persist beyond the 2-week duration criterion, they are experiencing significant role impairment or distress, and the bereavement exclusion does not apply to them. Yet these reactions seem to fall within the normal range for persons who have suffered from the sudden end of a passionate romantic relationship, the loss of a valued job, or the diagnosis of a serious illness in a beloved child. The symptoms that these people report are neither abnormal nor inappropriate in light of their particular situations.

What characteristics tend to suggest that these conditions are not disorders? In each case, symptoms emerge only after the occurrence of a discrete life event involving great loss. Further, the severity of these loss responses, although very intense, is reasonably proportional to the nature of the losses that have been experienced. Finally, the symptoms either end when circumstances change for the better, endure because the stressful situation persists, or eventually go away with the passage of time. We do not believe that most thoughtful clinicians today, if making an independent judgment outside the sway of the *DSM*, would classify such reactions as disorders, any more than their predecessors did.

Stating that the *DSM*'s definition of depressive disorder mistakenly encompasses some normal emotional reactions in no way implies that there are not genuine depressive disorders. Such disorders do exist, they can be devastating, and the *DSM*'s definition does encompass them. However, they look very different from the kinds of normal reactions described here. Popular portrayals of depression uniformly present a picture of profound, immense, and immobilizing suffering that is bewilderingly disengaged from actual life circumstances, and this sort of experience does imply genuine disorder.

For example, consider the case of Deanna Cole-Benjamin, featured in a *New York Times Magazine* story about a new treatment for depression:

> Her youth contained no traumas; her adult life, as she describes it, was blessed. At 22 she joined Gary Benjamin, a career financial officer in the Canadian Army, in a marriage that brought her happiness and, in the 1990's, three children. They lived in a comfortable house in Kingston, a pleasant university town on Lake Ontario's north shore, and Deanna, a public-health nurse, loved her work. But in the last months of 2000, apropos of nothing—no life changes, no losses—she slid into a depression of extraordinary depth and duration.
>
> "It began with a feeling of not really feeling as connected to things as usual," she told me one evening at the family's dining-room table. "Then it was like this wall fell around me. I felt sadder and sadder and then just numb."
>
> Her doctor prescribed progressively stronger antidepressants, but they scarcely touched her. A couple of weeks before Christmas, she stopped going to work. The simplest acts—deciding what to wear, making breakfast—required immense will. Then one day, alone in the house after Gary had taken the kids to school and gone to work, she felt so desperate to escape her pain that she drove to her doctor's office and told him she didn't think she could go on anymore.
>
> "He took one look," she told me later, "and said that he wanted me to stay right there in the office. Then he called Gary, and Gary came to the office, and he told us he wanted Gary to take me straight to the hospital."[29]

Aside from the extraordinary severity and duration of the symptoms, it is noteworthy that the seriousness of this depressive condition has no relation to any events that normally might be expected to trigger such episodes.

Or consider Andrew Solomon's powerful depiction of his depressive illness:

> [My depression] had a life of its own that bit by bit asphyxiated all of my life out of me. At the worst stage of major depression, I had moods that I knew were not my moods: they belonged to the depression . . . I felt myself sagging under what was much stronger than I; first I could not use my ankles, and then I could not control my knees, and then my waist began to break under the strain, and then my shoulders turned in, and in the end I was compacted and fetal, depleted by this thing that was crushing me without holding me. Its tendrils threatened to pulverize my mind and my courage and my stomach, and crack my bones and desiccate my body. It went on glutting itself on me when there seemed nothing left to feed it.[30]

Again, Solomon's profound depression has "a life of its own," in the sense that its seriousness is not related to specific losses or other negative events that might normally lead to such feelings.

In perhaps the most elegant description of depression, *Darkness Visible*, William Styron describes his reaction to learning that he had won a prestigious literary prize:

> The pain persisted during my museum tour and reached a crescendo in the next few hours when, back at the hotel, I fell onto the bed and lay gazing at the ceiling, nearly immobilized and in a trance of supreme discomfort. Rational thought was usually absent from my mind at such times, hence *trance*. I can think of no more apposite word for this state of being, a condition of helpless stupor in which cognition is replaced by that "positive and active anguish."

Styron's condition persists independently of any social context: "In depression . . . the pain is unrelenting, and what makes the condition intolerable is the foreknowledge that no remedy will come—not in a day, an hour, a month, or a minute. If there is mild relief, one knows that it is only temporary; more pain will follow."[31] Styron's debilitating symptoms did not emerge after any stressful experience but actually arose after what would ordinarily be a cause for celebration.

The sociologist David Karp's *Speaking of Sadness* offers another typical depiction:

> By any objective standard I should have been feeling pretty good. I had a solid academic job at Boston College, had just signed my first book contract, and I had a great wife, beautiful son, and a new baby daughter at home. . . . Each sleepless night my head was filled with disturbing ruminations and during the day I felt a sense of intolerable grief as though somebody close to me had died. I was agitated and sensed a melancholy

qualitatively different from anything in the past. . . . I thought for sure that my depression was rooted in these situational demands and that once I got tenure it would go away. I was promoted in 1977 and found that the depression actually deepened.[32]

Just as Styron's depression developed after a positive experience, Karp's dangerously severe condition was isolated from the actual circumstances of his life.

As these examples illustrate, the cases that both popular media and psychiatric texts typically depict are clearly genuine disorders. Yet these descriptions also illustrate that symptoms in themselves do not distinguish depressive disorders from normal sadness; the symptoms are not qualitatively different from what an individual might naturally experience after a devastating loss, as in our earlier case illustrations of normal reactions to major life disruptions. Instead, it is the absence of an appropriate *context* for symptoms that indicates a disorder. These cases either emerged in the absence of any loss event or developed after the occurrence of a positive event, such as winning a prestigious award or obtaining tenure. Their severity was of grossly disproportionate intensity to the sufferer's actual circumstances. Finally, symptoms persisted independently of any stressful contexts, took on a life of their own, and were immune to changes in external conditions. The fact that the literature emphasizes such examples can mislead us into overlooking the fact that the *DSM* diagnostic criteria themselves are not limited to such conditions and invalidly encompass a great range of intense normal reactions.

The basic flaw, then, of the *DSM* definition of MDD, as well as of all efforts that rely on it, is simply that it *fails to take into account the context of the symptoms and thus fails to exclude from the disorder category intense sadness, other than in reaction to the death of a loved one, that arises from the way human beings naturally respond to major losses.* The resultant lumping of nondisordered with dysfunction-caused symptoms of depression, and the classification of both as *disorders,* is a fundamental problem for current research, treatment, and social policy regarding depression. Moreover, as we show, the problem has been getting much worse in recent years, with growing pressure to use a lower number of symptoms, sometimes as few as two, as sufficient criteria for diagnosing a disorder. The potential for false-positive diagnoses—that is, people who meet the *DSM's* diagnostic criteria but do not in fact have a mental disorder—increases exponentially as the number of symptoms required for a diagnosis decreases.

The *DSM's* overinclusive criteria for depressive disorder ultimately compromise psychiatry's own goals and concepts. The *DSM* aims to identify psychological conditions that can be considered genuine medical disorders and to distinguish them from problematic but nondisordered conditions.[33] Thus the error we are pointing to in disorder categories such as MDD is an error in terms of the *DSM's* own stated aspirations.

The Distinction Between Normality and Disorder

Our core argument about the *DSM*'s definition of depressive disorder depends on the assumption that normal sadness can be intense; can be accompanied by sleeplessness, lack of concentration, changed appetite, and so on; can be impairing or distressful; and can last for 2 weeks, as the criteria demand. But what is the implicit understanding of normality and disorder by which one can distinguish painful sadness that is normal from that which is disordered?

Normal functioning is not mere statistical commonality. Some disorders can be statistically "normal" in a population, as are gum disease and atherosclerosis in ours, yet they are disorders nonetheless; and some normal variations can be quite rare. We must also distinguish disorder from social desirability and social values. Even the *DSM* acknowledges that an individual who is socially deviant or whose nature is in conflict with the values of society is not thereby necessarily disordered.[34] Adequate accounts must not only distinguish disorder from social values but also explain in what ways disorders are real medical ailments that represent, at least in part, some objective problem in individual functioning.

The most plausible demarcation point between human normality and disorder in the medical sense is, we believe, that between biologically "designed" functioning (i.e., the result of natural selection) and the failure of such functioning, that is, *dysfunction*.[35] This view comports well with commonsense intuitions and is probably the most widely accepted and defensible view among those who are concerned with the conceptual foundations of psychiatry, as well as medicine more generally.[36] For example, the criterion for normal functioning of bodily organs is what they are biologically designed to do and how they are designed to do it. Thus the heart serves to pump blood, the kidneys to eliminate waste, and the lungs to enable us to breathe, and if these functions are accomplished by the structures designed to accomplish them, functioning is normal. Disorder exists when the organ is unable to accomplish the function for which it is biologically designed.

Similarly, psychological processes that were selected as part of human nature have natural functions, that is, the effects for which they were naturally selected. Considerable neurobiological and psychological research suggests that the mind is made up of many specific modules or mechanisms that are designed to respond to specific environmental challenges.[37] Thus *contextuality* is an inherent aspect of many psychological mechanisms; they are designed to activate in particular contexts and not to activate in others. Fear responses, for example, are biologically designed to arise in dangerous situations but not in safe situations. Likewise, innate mechanisms that regulate reactions of sadness, despair, and withdrawal naturally come into play after humans suffer particular kinds of losses.[38] Conversely, dysfunctions in which sadness mechanisms do not operate as designed constitute disorders. The implication is that only in the light of some account, however provisional or sketchy, of how loss response mechanisms are designed to work and thus of their normal functioning do we have grounds for calling some responses to loss *disordered.*

As with all human traits, there is much variation among individuals in the sensitivity with which they respond to loss with sadness. Culture also influences designed tendencies in various ways, so evaluating whether a response fits within the naturally selected range is sometimes no easy task. Nevertheless, under appropriate conditions, virtually all humans have the capacity to develop nondisordered sadness as a biologically selected adaptation to handling loss. In principle, this biological capacity provides a baseline for judging some cases as clear examples of normality and disorder.

An important caveat: because of our primitive state of knowledge about mental functioning, our understanding of how normal emotions, including sadness, are designed to work remains speculative and open to revision. Yet some fundamental principles, at least in a broad provisional form, seem over-whelmingly plausible and offer a sufficient basis for critically examining the va-lidity of criteria for depressive disorder. These principles allow us to make some general distinctions between cases that clearly seem to indicate normal sadness and cases of depressive disorders, while acknowledging a large domain of bor-derline, ambiguous, and fuzzy cases. We emphasize three essential features of nondisordered loss in chapter 2: they emerge because of specific kinds of envi-ronmental triggers, especially loss; they are roughly proportionate in intensity to the provoking loss; and they end about when the loss situation ends or gradu-ally cease as natural coping mechanisms allow an individual to adjust to the new circumstances and return to psychological and social equilibrium.

Important questions arise because we do not yet know precisely which in-ternal mechanisms produce loss responses or what these mechanisms are ac-tually like. If the mechanisms are inferred to exist but their specific nature is unknown, how can one tell that normal loss responses are indeed part of our biological heritage? And, without knowing the mechanisms, how can we tell what is normal and what is disordered?

The fact is that, although the distinction cannot yet be determined precisely, in the history of medicine and biology scientists have routinely drawn such in-ferences about normal and disordered functioning from circumstantial evidence without knowing the underlying mechanisms. So, for example, Hippocrates knew that blindness and paralysis are disorders and that there are mechanisms that are designed to allow human beings to see via their eyes and move via mus-cular effort, but he knew little of the mechanisms themselves and thus little of the specific causes of most cases of blindness and paralysis (other than gross injury). It took thousands of years to figure out those mechanisms, but during that time it was universally understood from circumstantial evidence that sight and move-ment are parts of human biological design. It is no different in principle with human mental capacities that are part of our biological nature, such as basic emotions.

Another concern might be that, because we do not understand the loss response mechanisms, we cannot with confidence state the function of the loss response and cannot therefore know what is normal and abnormal. Indeed, unlike the functions of the eyes and muscles, the functions of loss responses are not apparent and are subject to dispute.[39] Fortunately, it is often possible from available evidence to infer roughly what responses of a mechanism are normal, even without knowing the reason for the responses. For example, everyone agrees that sleep is an elaborately designed response and that some sleep conditions are normal whereas others are sleep disorders, but there is little scientific consensus on the functions that explain why we sleep. Without an adequate understanding of the function of loss responses to guide us, we too must engage in such admittedly presumptive but, we believe, still plausible inferences.

By depressive disorders, then, we mean sadness that is caused by a harmful dysfunction (HD) of loss response mechanisms.[40] According to the HD definition, a collection of symptoms indicates a mental disorder only when it meets both of two criteria. The first is dysfunction: something has gone wrong with some internal mechanism's ability to perform one of its biologically designed functions. Second, the dysfunction must be harmful. Cultural values inevitably play the primary role in defining what sorts of dysfunctions are considered harmful. In sum, a mental disorder exists when the failure of a person's internal mechanisms to perform their functions as designed by nature impinges harmfully on the person's well-being as defined by social values and meanings.

The HD analysis of disorder does not attempt to yield a precise conceptual boundary because the concepts of normality and disorder, like most concepts, do not themselves have precise boundaries and are subject to indeterminacy, ambiguity, fuzziness, and vagueness and so yield many unclear cases. Despite such fuzzy boundaries, the HD concept of disorder is useful and coherent because it enables us to adequately distinguish a range of clear normal cases from a range of clear disorders. Analogously, there are real distinctions between red and blue, child and adult, and life and death, although there are no sharp boundaries between these pairs. By contrast, current diagnostic criteria for depressive disorder, we argue, substantially fail to distinguish even many clear cases of normal sadness from disorder.

Mechanisms that are biologically designed to generate loss responses may fail to perform their functions in the appropriate contexts in a variety of ways.[41] Loss responses can emerge in situations for which they are not designed, they can be of disproportionate intensity and duration to the situations that evoke them, and in extreme cases they can occur spontaneously, with no trigger at all. For example, depressions such as William Styron's, which arose after the reception of a prestigious award, or David Karp's, which emerged after a successful tenure decision, indicate that loss response mechanisms have gone awry. Dysfunctions of loss responses may also involve distorted cognitive perceptions of the self, the world, and the future that trigger inappropriate sadness.[42] Such distortions may yield inappropriately sensitive mechanisms that magnify the meanings of minor losses beyond the normal range of culturally appropriate stimuli. Someone who becomes deeply depressed after the death of a pet goldfish or a minor perceived slight, for example, displays such overly sensitive, disproportionate loss response mechanisms, unless special circumstances make the loss of much greater importance than is usual.

Yet it is not just the emergence of depression in the absence of appropriate causes that defines a dysfunction. Disorders might arise after an initially normal-level response to actual losses, but the response might then become disengaged from the circumstances of the loss and persist with disproportionate intensity long after the initial provoking conditions have ended. Or, among susceptible individuals, the experience of loss events can sometimes produce biochemical and anatomical vulnerabilities that make recurrences of depressive episodes more likely with less and less provocation.[43] Even if they begin as normal responses, emotional reactions that become detached from a specific time, place, and circumstance indicate dysfunctional loss response mechanisms.

Finally, dysfunctions in loss responses can sometimes cause symptoms that are so extreme that they indicate dysfunction in themselves. Depressive reactions that feature prolonged complete immobilization or loss of contact with reality, such as hallucinations, delusions, and the like, would not stem from appropriately functioning loss mechanisms and have always been recognized as disorders. Such inappropriate and excessive responses are analogous to dangerously high fevers or uncontrolled vomiting, which are design failures of otherwise adaptive responses.

Note that our distinction between sadness due to internal dysfunction versus sadness that is a biologically designed response to external events differs in important respects from the traditional distinction within psychiatry between depressions that are *endogenous* (i.e., spontaneously caused by internal processes, having no external trigger) and *reactive* (i.e., triggered by some external event).[44] Endogenous depressions by definition arise in the absence of real loss, and so are almost always due to internal dysfunctions. In contrast, many reactive depressions are proportionate to environmental events and so are normal responses.

However, not all reactive depressions are normal. External events can so deeply affect individuals that they trigger internal dysfunctions. For example, environmental traumas such as the sudden death of a loved one, forced relocation from one's home, or being the victim of a violent crime can cause designed loss response mechanisms to break down and an enduring disorder to occur.[45] As noted, emotional reactions can be so disproportionate to their triggering events as to suggest dysfunction, or the symptoms can take on a life of their own and fail to extinguish when the stressor ends. Thus, among reactive depressions to losses, some are disorders and some are not. The *presence* of an internal dysfunction, not the *cause* of this dysfunction (which may be endogenous or reactive), defines depressive disorders. Consequently, there is no simple one-to-one relationship between the traditional endogenous-reactive distinction and our distinction between internal dysfunction and biologically designed response.

To address a final point of possible confusion: the evolutionary design approach to distinguishing normal from disordered conditions does not imply that all depressive disorders have physiological causes or that there is always a brain problem when there is a depressive disorder. Although physiological causes do often produce disorders, psychological or social factors can also lead to dysfunctions. Biological design includes the design of various mental mechanisms (e.g., belief, desire, emotion, perception) that work via meanings humans assign to represent reality, and physiological descriptions may not capture how such meanings operate. There might be mental disorders that cannot be described as malfunctions in the underlying physiological machinery but as malfunctions at the mental level of meanings. This is not as mysterious as it might sound; think of the fact that computer software can malfunction in hardware that itself is working properly. The processing of meanings that recent cognitive science envisions as analogous to the "software" of the mind can perhaps similarly go awry without any underlying physiological malfunction. Our discussion is neutral on such issues of etiology, although we generally believe that there can be an array of biological, psychological, and social causes of both normal sadness and depressive disorder; research that resolves the clash of theories about the causes of depression must decide this issue.

One great advantage of our critique based on the HD approach is that it acknowledges that depressive disorders do exist and provides defensible grounds for improving psychiatry's diagnostic criteria. There are other, more radical, critiques of psychiatric diagnosis that dismiss diagnosis in general and that leave no room for constructive engagement with psychiatry. For example, psychiatrist Thomas Szasz's argument that there are no mental disorders because disorders require physical lesions; sociologist Thomas Scheff's labeling theory that reduces diagnosis to social control; behaviorist claims that all behavior is the outcome of learning processes and therefore that no mental disorder can exist; or anthropologists' assertions that distinctions between normal and abnormal functioning are purely cultural and therefore arbitrary all deny the possibility of making a conceptually coherent diagnostic distinction between depressive disorders and normal intense sadness responses.[46] They thus understate the real and distinct problems that genuine depressive disorders pose while at the same time they preclude the prospect of effectively critiquing overexpansive psychiatric definitions of disorder.

The Advantages of Distinguishing Normal Sadness From Depressive Disorder

Even if the *DSM* criteria are flawed in a way that allows the creation of an inflated amount of depressive disorder, why is correcting this error so important? There are some considerable advantages to doing so:

Pathologization of normal conditions may cause harm, and avoidance of such pathologization may decrease such harm. Not only may patients be misled to consider themselves disordered and undertake unnecessary treatment, but also the social responses to nondisordered and to dysfunctional conditions usually differ. Social networks typically respond with social support and sympathy to sadness that appears after stressful life events.[47] Dysfunctional depressions, in contrast, typically elicit hostility, stigma, and rejection and lead to the loss of social support.[48] To subject those with normal sadness to the social prejudice faced by those with mental illness does not serve to combat that prejudice. It remains true, however, that for those who do have a genuine mental disorder, the disadvantages of diagnostic stigma must be balanced against the fact that diagnosis of their abnormal conditions with an official label that offers access to services may come as a welcome relief.

The distinction between disordered and normal sadness should improve assessments of prognosis. An essential purpose of diagnosis is prognosis: predicting the future course of a disorder.[49] The prognoses for people whose symptoms stem from nondisordered sadness usually differ from those for people with disorders. Symptoms of nondisordered conditions are likely to abate over time without intervention, to disappear if precipitating circumstances change, and to be responsive to generic social support. In contrast, symptoms that stem from internal dysfunctions are likely to be chronic and recurrent and to persist independently of stressful life circumstances.[50] An adequate distinction between disorder and nondisorder should provide better prognostic predictions.

Accurate diagnoses point to appropriate treatments. Although medication or therapy can help ease the pain that arises from both normal sadness and depressive disorder, they are often unnecessary in cases of nondisordered sadness, which do not involve internal dysfunctions. In some cases, such as bereavement, treating normal loss responses as diseases can even be counterproductive because it may exacerbate and prolong symptoms.[51] Conversely, the treatment of depressive disorders often involves pharmacotherapies, cognitive and other psychotherapies, or a combination of modalities to overcome dysfunctional conditions. An adequate conceptual distinction between dysfunctions and normal responses may enable us better to specify what sorts of responses can work most effectively for symptomatically similar, but actually distinct, conditions.

Separating normal sadness from depressive disorders can help in recognizing the relationship of sadness to adverse social conditions and thus in identifying appropriate social interventions. Psychiatry now tends to view depression as a major cause of many social problems, including welfare dependence, drug addiction, and poverty.[52] The first course of action would be to treat the illness and then to help depressed individuals to overcome their other challenges. Normal sadness, however, is much more likely to be the result rather than the cause of social problems. Recognizing the impact of social problems on normal human emotions would suggest that correcting these problems would be an appropriate initial response.

The separation of depressive disorder from normal intense sadness should provide a basis for more accurate epidemiological estimates of the prevalence of depressive disorders and the cost of treating it. The failure to distinguish normal from disordered sadness results in large overestimates of people who have mental disorders, misleading policy makers into formulating poor public policy. Prevalence estimates count as diseased all people who have sufficiently intense symptoms, whether disordered or not.[53] They direct the attention of policy makers and mental health professionals toward conditions that may not need intensive expert attention and away from problems that can most benefit from professional help. Conflating normal sadness with depressive disorder also results in greatly overinflated estimates of the economic costs of depression.[54] These overstatements, in turn, have potentially negative policy implications in that they increase the reluctance of elected officials, insurance companies, and other policy makers to develop cost-effective responses to depression. Although no one who is suffering should be denied access to services, separating nondisordered from dysfunctional conditions can focus the expertise of mental health professionals on true mental disorders and lead to a more efficient use of mental health resources.

Distinguishing disorder from normal sadness allows for a better estimate of unmet need for mental health services. Because they fail to distinguish normal sadness from depressive disorder, and because nondisordered individuals are less likely to seek treatment, population surveys make it seem as if only a minority of disordered people are treated for their conditions. This has led social policies to focus on the presumed vast amount of unmet need for treatment.[55] These policies now emphasize widespread screening for depression among people who have not voluntarily sought treatment. Screening instruments likely uncover more normal sadness than depressive disorder but treat both conditions as if they were disorders. The reduction of such overdiagnosis could reduce the needless and potentially harmful overprescription of medication.

Drawing a more careful distinction between disorder and normal sadness allows researchers to select samples that more accurately reflect true disorders. Meaningful research into the causes of depressive disorder and into the best treatments for either depressive disorder or intense normal sadness requires that the groups studied be reasonably homogeneous in nature so that the results can be appropriately understood and generalized. The causes of depressive symptoms that arise from dysfunction are generally different from the causes of normal sadness, so the entire field of depression research remains problematic until the appropriate distinction is made.

Distinguishing nondisordered from dysfunctional loss responses avoids medicalizing our thinking about normal sadness and thus maintains the conceptual integrity of psychiatry. Aside from any other advantages, the long-term credibility of psychiatry and psychiatric diagnosis depends on getting the disorder-nondisorder distinction right by labeling only genuine psychiatric conditions as disorders. The failure to adequately separate naturally designed sadness responses from internal dysfunctions misconstrues as a mental disorder a basic and universal aspect of the human condition and thus inappropriately pathologizes a tremendous range of human behavior, undermining the credibility of psychiatry.

Understanding how psychiatry has blurred a crucial distinction and tends to misclassify intense sadness as a disorder is also useful to the ordinary person. Every time people enter physicians' offices or their children take routine screening instruments in school, the conceptual muddles we identify in this book could lead to unwarranted diagnoses and treatment. To be an effective consumer of medical services, prepared patients should understand both how professionals arrive at the diagnoses to which they are subject and what questions to ask about the problems these diagnoses may entail.

Finally, it should be kept in mind that the truth about whether someone is disordered or normally sad often matters in a practical way because diagnoses of mental disorders influence many consequential decisions. For example, such diagnoses can make it more difficult to obtain life or health insurance or increase the cost of such insurance; they can be negative considerations in divorce proceedings that consider custody of children; and they frequently disqualify individuals from participating in clinical trials for new medications for severe conditions such as cancer. Because of the role that diagnosis has in so many areas of our lives and the assumption that a diagnosis represents a genuine medical condition, confusing depressive disorder with normal sadness should not be taken lightly.

Some Caveats: What About the Disadvantages of Such a Distinction?

Some might object that drawing a distinction between normal and disordered sadness, whatever its intellectual merits, is potentially harmful for various reasons. We can't address all the potential concerns, but it is worth briefly considering a few.

Are we somehow dismissing the suffering of those with normal sadness? By calling certain responses "normal," we in no way intend to minimize, let alone demean, the level of suffering involved; indeed, the extreme pain of normal sadness can often match that of depressive disorder. But just as you would want to distinguish a normal intense pain that results from, say, childbirth or a broken bone (which you would want to manage and treat) from an equally intense pain that results from a pain disorder in which the pain is not a normal response to a bodily lesion (which would have important implications for treatment), these intense forms of sadness need to be distinguished so that they can be understood and optimally managed and treated.

Could our analysis result in insurance barriers that would deny treatment to people who seek it even though they are not truly disordered? Yes, that is possible, but unlikely. The reality is that clinicians always have found and always will find ways of responding to patient needs and of classifying these needs consistent with diagnostic definitions so that they receive reimbursement for treatment. Moreover, as in other medical domains, a strong argument can be made for reimbursement of treatment for nondisordered intense emotional responses because of the disabling effects they can have and as a preventive measure. An accepted distinction between normal and disordered intense sadness might even facilitate a discussion of such changes in the reimbursement system.

Are we moralists who think that people should not generally rely on treatment, and specifically on medication, but should somehow be forced to muddle through their difficulties? We are not arguing for or against using medication to treat normal feelings of sadness. That is a matter for individuals and their physicians to decide. Rather, we are arguing that conceptually illegitimate diagnoses of normal responses to events as disorders could prejudice such decisions by making it seem as though there is an internal malfunction for which medication is the optimal treatment when evidence suggests that other interventions may offer equal or better relief and avoid the possible negative side effects of medication. We are simply saying that such treatment decisions should be based on a correct understanding of the condition. Indeed, once an adequate conceptual distinction is made, clearer research on optimal treatment of intense normal sadness might move forward more effectively.

Doesn't diagnosis with a medical disorder reduce blame, and aren't we therefore encouraging the blaming of sad individuals for being emotionally weak? For example, if intense sadness is not diagnosed as a disorder, won't it then be assumed that experiencing such feelings is a character flaw, and won't people be urged to "shape up" and be strong rather than indulging such feelings? There is in fact scant scientific evidence on whether diagnosis does lead to beneficial relief from personal blame, in contrast to the vast evidence that it leads to harmful stigma. But it must be acknowledged that diagnosing individuals with a medical disorder, even if unjustified, may sometimes protect them from misplaced blame by family members and others for weakness of character. We argue, however, that there are ways to respond to such misplaced blame other than the extreme misuse of medical categories. In particular, our analysis emphasizes that intense sadness is a natural human capacity and not a character weakness; indeed, normal sadness probably has healing and reparative functions that are still not understood.[56] Oddly enough, many cultures actually blame individuals if they are inadequately sad when loss occurs (such as displaying too few or too briefly the signs of mourning after the death of a relative) because it seems to show lack of commitment or caring. The fact that intense sadness may be related characterologically to depth of feeling and may thus be more important for coping with loss in some individuals than in others is hardly a weakness. Our analysis suggests that blaming can easily be addressed without labeling the individual as disordered. It should also be recognized that diagnosis with a disorder is no redoubt against personal contempt and blame.

Isn't it cold-blooded that we focus on conceptual issues and don't spend much time exploring the painful experience of depression itself? There are rafts of books detailing the great impact of depression and vividly documenting the experience of it. Our focus is different because our goal is different, namely, to provide an understanding and critical perspective on how that experience is conceptualized, how it has come to be exploited by a variety of groups, and how its classification has changed in questionable ways over time.

A Note on Terminology

A few terminological clarifications at this point might prevent needless confusion later on. First, although we use *sadness* to describe both the normal human emotion and the experiences described in depressive disorders, the normal responses we consider in fact go beyond sadness and include certain episodes of emotional emptiness, shame, humiliation, and related responses to losses of various kinds, such as loss of self-esteem or loss of standing in a group. So we sometimes use broader, more abstract language such as *loss responses* to refer to such experiences. Even when we do use the word *sadness,* it should be understood that this is shorthand for a broader domain.

Second, when we write of "normal" sadness, we do not mean that everything is statistically normal, or normal in the sense of "okay." Rather, we mean that the sadness is functionally normal or nondisordered, that is, it is the result of the relevant mental processes working as they were biologically designed to work in response to loss. Such "normal" responses can be "abnormal" in a variety of ways: they may be much more intense in some people than in others due to human variation in temperament or different cultural meaning systems; they may be statistically highly unusual because they are responses to a highly unusual environmental circumstance (e.g., someone experiencing extreme grief due to the deaths of several family members within a short time); and they may be abnormal in the sense that they constitute a severe deviation from the individual's usual functioning. None of these forms of statistical abnormality implies disorder.

Third, many of the same kinds of psychological (e.g., blue mood) and physical (e.g., fatigue) phenomena occur in disordered and nondisordered sadness responses. There is no convenient neutral term to describe these phenomena, so we accept the general convention and refer to them as *symptoms.* But it should be kept in mind that this is potentially misleading because of the association of "symptoms" with a medical diagnosis of disorder. The use of the word *symptom* here is intended to be neutral as to whether the phenomenon is a manifestation of disorder or a normal response.

Fourth, as a convenient way to refer to whatever as yet unknown structures in the mind are designed to produce loss responses, we use the phrase *loss response mechanisms.* The term *mechanism* is common in evolutionary discussions and should not be construed as implying anything reductionistic or literally "mechanistic" about the mind. We assume, for example, that complex individual and cultural meanings enter into loss responses. The term *mechanism* simply indicates that, given that loss responses are part of our biological heritage, there are some structures in the person that are biologically designed to produce such responses at appropriate times.

Finally, because we often refer to similar phenomena when we discuss disorders and normal responses, we use several conventions to try to remain clear about what is under discussion at a given time. When we discuss a specific *DSM* category of disorder (which may, according to our argument, actually mistakenly include some normal as well as disordered conditions), we adopt the *DSM* convention of capitalizing a category, and so write, for example, of Major Depressive Disorder or, more simply, Major Depression. In addition, because the term "depression" is ambiguous as to normal or disordered conditions, we specifically use the term *disorder* when discussing depressive pathology—referring to it usually as "depressive disorder." We do not capitalize this phrase because we are not referring to a *DSM* category—which, we argue, confuses disorder and normality—but to just those conditions that are genuine disorders. (We refrain from using the common phrase *clinical depression* to refer specifically to disorders because many instances of normal sadness are now seen in clinics.) When we want to refer to all sadness conditions, whether normal or disordered, we use generic phrases such as "depressive condition" or, simply, "depression."

What We Hope to Accomplish

Depression has gained an iconic status in both the contemporary mental health professions and the culture at large. Many experts claim it is a dire public health problem that afflicts a large proportion of the population. The seeming massiveness of the problem simultaneously calls for urgent policy responses and yet paralyzes the will to respond.

While recognizing the reality of depressive disorder and the enormous suffering it causes, this book strives to bring perspective into discussions of depression. It shows how an inadequate conceptual distinction between disorder and nondisorder is a crucial weakness in the entire clinical and research industry devoted to this condition and demonstrates that the problems amplify as the erroneous definition echoes through various social institutions. In particular, virtually all discussions of this condition ignore the critical question of when depressive symptoms indicate a mental disorder and when they are nondisordered responses to loss. Answers to this question would affect our understanding of how many people have mental disorders, to what degree we can prevent depression, whom we should treat for this condition, and what sort of policies we should develop. Exploring the current misdefinition of depression is a way of showing how seemingly esoteric technical issues can inadvertently influence broader social movements and how various constituencies are motivated to exploit and perpetuate conceptual errors once they are made.

2

The Anatomy of Normal Sadness

S adness traditionally has been viewed as humanity's natural response to deaths of intimates, losses in love, reversals of fortune,
and the like. It arises, as Shelley says, because "the world's wrong!"[1] And, when
the losses and strains that evoke the sadness are profound, the resulting emotions
can also be severe, seeming to defy expression. In Samuel Coleridge's words:

> A grief without a pang, void, dark, and drear,
> A stifled, drowsy, unimpassioned grief,
> Which finds no natural outlet, no relief,
> In word, or sigh, or tear.[2]

The potential intensity of what appears to be normal sadness poses some difficult questions for psychiatric diagnosis. How is it possible to separate experiences of normal sadness from depressive disorders? How, after all, do we know
that intense sadness is within the bounds of human nature and therefore can
be psychiatrically normal, as common experience, as well as literature, would
suggest? How can the known variations in the expression of sadness across cultures be consistent with a biologically designed and universal human capacity
for sadness? And, if sadness is indeed a normal part of human nature, what is
it for, that is, for what function could this painful and often debilitating emotion possibly have been naturally selected? To lay a foundation for the argument
that modern psychiatry confuses sadness with depressive disorder, this chapter
considers the characteristics and evolutionary enigma of normal sadness and
presents evidence that it is a designed aspect of human nature.

Components of Normal Sadness

Normal sadness, or nondisordered responses to loss, has three essential components important to our argument: it is context-specific; it is of roughly

proportionate intensity to the provoking loss; and it tends to end about when the loss situation ends, or else it gradually ceases as coping mechanisms adjust individuals to new circumstances and bring them back into psychological and social equilibrium.

First, loss responses are inherently context specific in the sense that they respond to a specific range of the "right" stimuli and do not respond outside that range to the "wrong" stimuli.[3] Nevertheless, the kinds of losses that fall within the range that can trigger normal sadness vary considerably. Some are losses of valued intimate attachments involving closeness, love, and friendship. Others derive from the hierarchical aspects of social relationships, such as losses of power, status, resources, respect, or prestige. A third kind of loss relates to the failure to achieve valued goals and ideals that provide coherence and purpose to life.[4] Any of these types of losses that are unexpected, humiliating, threatening to long-term well-being, and seemingly without remedy and in which the lost object cannot easily be replaced are especially likely to evoke intense sadness responses.[5]

Although many sadness responses emerge after distinct losses, others stem from persistent and chronically stressful social situations, such as long-standing economic hardships that seem unjustified, enduring conflicts within interpersonal relationships, or continuing inability to achieve important goals.[6] As hopes for change wane, these persistent strains can produce long-standing states of sadness that may disappear only when the chronic stressors are over or when people are able to change their evaluative criteria.

The fact that sadness follows acute losses or is simultaneous with chronic strains, however, does not in itself mean that its symptoms are normal. Environmental stresses may trigger depressive disorders in people who are predisposed to depression, or the stresses may be of such unusual severity as to produce a breakdown of normal loss response mechanisms in those not predisposed. For example, many combat pilots develop symptoms that suggest disorder if they engage in enough wartime sorties.[7] In other cases, the presence of a disorder precedes and itself provokes the stressful event that might mistakenly be thought to be its cause, as when preexisting depressions lead people to be fired from jobs or rejected by romantic partners.[8] Emergence under appropriate circumstances is a necessary but not a sufficient condition for the presence of normal sadness.

The second component of nondisordered sadness is that it is of roughly proportionate intensity to the magnitude and permanency of the loss itself, which involves two factors. The first is cognitive: nondisordered loss responses involve reasonably *accurate* perceptions of the negative circumstances, rather than gross distortions.[9] For example, the belief that one's spouse has been sexually unfaithful may cause intense sadness proportional to the perceived loss, but if the belief is delusional to begin with, then the sadness is not normal. The normality of such perceptions of the magnitude of the loss must be judged in the context of the life, values, and meaning system of the individual.

The other factor in proportionality is affective: the emotional and symptomatic severity of the response should be of roughly proportionate intensity to the seriousness of the loss that has been experienced. Minor setbacks should generally be minimally disturbing, leading to relatively mild reactions in which people are disappointed, discouraged, downcast, or dispirited. Moderate loss events should generally trigger relatively medium-intensity reactions of dismay, resignation, and gloominess. Serious and highly threatening situations should generally evoke reactions of greater severity, including intense states of deep sorrow, despondency, anguish, pain, numbness, and dejection.[10] It bears emphasis that under the proportionality requirement designed responses to severe losses can also be quite severe—indeed, as severe as some depressive disorders—and can potentially satisfy *DSM* diagnostic criteria for Major Depressive Disorder despite not being disordered. Individual differences in temperament as well as cultural differences in expressiveness may also influence responses to be more or less intense. However, evolutionary processes should provide some limits to the severity of depressed moods after a loss, because responses of disproportionately high intensity and long duration would not allow people to disengage from inhibited states and return to more productive activities. Nondisordered loss responses cannot encompass gross breakdowns in basic psychological systems, such as delusional and psychotic symptoms, if the individual is to be able to adapt to the new circumstances.

The third and final component of nondisordered loss responses is that they not only emerge but also persist in accordance with external contexts and internal coping processes. Normal sadness remits when the context changes for the better or as people adapt to their losses. Some loss events, such as the death of an intimate, are irreversible, and the duration of normal sadness after these losses is highly variable but gradually desists over time. Other loss events, such as breakups of important romantic relationships or losses of valued jobs, naturally lead to sadness that is time limited and that quickly improves after the emergence of positive changes, such as entering a new relationship after a marriage dissolves or finding a new job after a period of unemployment.[11]

The sensitivity of designed sadness responses to external contexts does not necessarily mean that they will be transient. As long as stressful environments persist, symptoms can also be long-standing. Sadness endures in contexts such as troubled marriages, oppressive jobs, persistent poverty, or chronic illness because the stressful circumstances that produced it remain unchanged. Ordinary sadness, therefore, is not necessarily of shorter duration than dysfunctional depression.

Examples of Normal Sadness

Grief as a Prototype of Normal Sadness

As long as emotions have been recorded, experiences of grief have been central to portrayals of basic human nature. Few depictions match the intensity of Achilles' reaction on hearing of the death of his friend Patroclus:

> A black cloud of grief came shrouding over Achilles.
> Both hands clawing the ground for soot and filth,
> He poured it over his head, fouled his handsome face
> And black ashes settled into his fresh clean war-shirt.
> Overpowered in all his power, sprawled in the dust,
> Achilles lay there, fallen
> Tearing his hair, defiling it with his own hands.[12]

Such descriptions are common across cultures and historical epochs. The oldest literary depiction of grief occurs in the epic poems about the king Gilgamesh, initially composed in Babylonia in the third millennium B.C., almost 1500 years before Homer's *Iliad* and in an alien culture. Yet the severe grief of the king Gilgamesh over the death of his close friend Enkidu is portrayed in terms strikingly similar to that of Achilles over his friend Patroclus:

> Hear me, O Elders of Uruk, hear me, O men! I mourn for Enkidu, my friend,
> I shriek in anguish like a mourner. . . . And after you (died) I let a filthy mat
> of hair grow over my body, and donned the skin of a lion and roamed the
> wilderness. . . . Like a lioness deprived of her cubs he keeps pacing to and
> fro. He shears off his curls and heaps them onto the ground, ripping off his
> finery and casting it away as an abomination.

Gilgamesh experiences enormous sadness, cries bitterly, is possessed by restless agitation, and suffers from a sense of worthlessness leads him to cast aside finery and cover himself with filth. Unable to bear his ordinary social activities, he wanders alone in the desert. In his travels mourning Enkidu and seeking immortality (thoughts about one's own death are another common symptom of grief), Gilgamesh comes upon a tavern to which he wishes entry. He boasts of his achievements to establish his identity, but the tavern-keeper notices most the dramatic symptoms of grief, and he challenges Gilgamesh. In a moving description of grief's expectable effects, Gilgamesh answers:

> Tavern-keeper, should not my cheeks be emaciated? Should my heart
> not be wretched, my features not haggard? Should there not be sadness

deep within me! Should I not look like one who has been traveling a long distance, and should ice and heat not have seared my face!.... Should I not roam the wilderness? My friend, Enkidu, the wild ass who chased the wild donkey, panther of the wilderness, we joined together, and went up into the mountain. We grappled with and killed the Bull of Heaven, we destroyed Humbaba who lived in the Cedar Forest, we slew lions in the mountain passes! My friend, Enkidu, whom I love deeply, who went through every hardship with me, the fate of mankind has overtaken him. Six days and seven nights I mourned over him and would not allow him to be buried until a maggot fell out of his nose.[13]

Such grief after the death of an intimate provides a model for the way that sadness responses are designed to work. It arises in circumstances of loss, its intensity is proportionate to the importance and centrality to one's life of the lost individual, and it persists for some time and then gradually subsides as one adapts to the changed circumstances.

The *DSM* definition of Major Depressive Disorder (MDD) excludes conditions that arise from bereavement because these normal responses often meet its symptomatic criteria and could be incorrectly diagnosed as disorders. Bereaved people commonly develop symptoms, including depressed mood, inability to feel pleasure, loss of appetite, inability to concentrate, insomnia, and so forth, which can be identical to those of depressive disorders.[14] Although normal bereaved individuals in our culture rarely show some of the common symptoms of depressive disorder, such as lowered self-esteem, they nevertheless often report enough depressive symptoms to meet *DSM* criteria for MDD, and nearly all individuals report at least some symptoms. Over three-quarters of the bereaved report crying, sleep disturbance, and low mood, and over half also indicate loss of appetite in the month following the loss.[15] Without the bereavement exclusion, between one-third and one-half of bereaved people could be classified as having a depressive disorder during the first month after the death.[16] Among people who have lost spouses, most studies find that between 20 and 40%—and some find that more than half—experience symptoms comparable in severity to MDD criteria over the first few months.[17] Rates of depressive symptoms in parents' reactions to the deaths of their children[18] or of adolescents' reactions to the deaths of their parents[19] are even higher, more intense, and longer lasting than those that follow the deaths of spouses.[20]

The intensity of grief generally varies in a roughly proportionate manner with the context and the circumstances that determine the magnitude of the loss, and it also varies greatly from individual to individual according to temperament. Despite the high proportions of bereaved people who develop symptoms comparable to those of depressive disorder, most do not develop such symptoms, and a substantial number experience no distress at all after their losses.[21] Although individual differences in sensitivity to loss certainly play a role, the nature and context of the loss also shape the intensity of the response. For example, expected deaths that occur after chronic illnesses produce fewer depression-like symptoms than sudden and traumatic or otherwise unexpected deaths.[22] Because people who become bereaved at younger ages are more likely to experience one or more of these circumstances, they report more symptoms than older people do.[23]

The quality of the relationship with the lost intimate also strongly affects the intensity of the subsequent bereavement. Losses of long-standing, close, and intense relationships produce more distress than losses of more distant ties.[24] This is the reason that spouses who report good relationships before the deaths of their husbands or wives report more depressive symptoms.[25] Conversely, spouses who had more negative and ambivalent feelings toward their partners before the death experience fewer depressive symptoms after it than people with more positive feelings do.[26] Likewise, bereaved elderly people with high levels of caregiving strain prior to the deaths of their partners report declining levels of distress following the deaths.[27] Indeed, death can bring relief and escape from stressful situations among those who had felt trapped in bad marriages with seriously ill spouses.[28]

The persistence, as well as the intensity, of the loss response also depends on the enduring circumstances that follow the loss. Whether grief persists or not is a function of the degree of social and economic upheaval the loss produces and of the resources available to cope with these upheavals.[29] In the long run, economic deprivation that follows the death of a husband is more strongly associated with the intensity of sadness than is widowhood in itself.[30] The presence or absence of social support that provides resources to cope with the loss is also a good predictor of the duration of sadness.[31] Longer duration of the loss response, therefore, need not indicate the presence of a disorder, but it can mark the persistence of the stressful situation that accompanies the loss and thus the correspondingly greater negative meaning of the loss.

Normal grief also appears naturally designed to desist with the passage of time. Relatively few bereaved individuals show serious symptoms for long periods, and most gradually adapt to their losses and recover their preloss levels of functioning.[32] In one major study, 42% of the bereaved met criteria for depressive disorder after 1 month, but only 16% remained in this state after a year.[33] Other studies confirm that about 10–20% of bereaved persons fulfill *DSM* diagnostic criteria for depressive disorder a year after the death, and even for many of these, psychological functioning returns to preloss levels by 2 years.[34] The evidence thus supports the conclusion that, although large numbers of grief reactions satisfy *DSM* symptomatic and duration diagnostic criteria for depressive disorder, the vast majority are transient normal responses to loss, with only a small proportion becoming chronic conditions that are likely disorders.

However, grief can sometimes trigger mental dysfunction of a more severe or persistent nature than is consistent with a normal response. When grief involves extreme immobilization, pronounced psychotic ideation, or severe symptoms that persist despite the passage of time and changing circumstances, then it can be presumed that an individual's reaction to the death of an intimate has caused a breakdown in his or her psychological functioning. In general, about 10% of the bereaved come to suffer from chronic depressive conditions that may well be disorders.[35] For some in this group, the death of an intimate intensifies to a pathological level depressive symptoms that existed prior to the death.[36] For others, the reaction to the death itself triggers a failure in normal coping functions. Such pathological states constitute Complicated Grief, which the *DSM* correctly recognizes as a form of depressive disorder, and such transformations of grief into enduring depressive disorder have been recognized since antiquity.[37]

For most people, however, bereavement is a normal feature of human experience that will naturally dissipate with the passage of time, not a mental disorder, as the *DSM* recognizes. Mistakenly labeling such normal responses as depressive disorders can have a variety of negative consequences. Interventions such as grief counseling and efforts that force people to acknowledge their grief have not been shown to be very effective and can be harmful.[38] Indeed, an alarmingly high number of grieving people worsen after receiving treatment.[39]

The problem is that the *DSM* contains no comparable recognition of the many circumstances other than bereavement that can lead to intense, but normal, sadness. Yet, with respect to these other circumstances of loss, the same sort of evidence exists that sadness responses are as normal as most cases of bereavement.

Loss Responses to Profound Threats in Relationships

Although the permanency of the loss associated with grief distinguishes it from most other losses, grief need be no different in principle from intense sadness that arises, for example, after the unsought end of a love affair, the news that one's spouse has been unfaithful, the dissolution of a marriage, the failure to achieve one's cherished life goals, the loss of financial resources, the loss of social supports and relationships, or the diagnosis of a serious illness in oneself or a loved one.[40] Even the death of beloved pets or celebrities whom one does not personally know can create periods of low mood, low initiative, and pessimism as normal reactions to loss.[41] The *DSM*'s own general definition of mental disorder provided in its introduction excludes all "expectable and culturally sanctioned response(s) to a particular event, *for example*, the death of a loved one" from its definition of mental disorder, using grief as the prototypical excluded category.[42] Yet, emotionally painful responses to other particular loss events such as marital, romantic, health, or financial reversals plainly can be just as "expectable and culturally sanctioned" responses as those of bereavement and should therefore fall under the definition's exclusion as well. The criteria for MDD, however, do not follow out this logic, and they contain no exclusions for other loss responses comparable to the one for bereavement.

Marital dissolution is perhaps the most common trigger of intense normal sadness that can be severe enough to meet *DSM* symptomatic criteria for depressive disorder.[43] The intense sadness that follows the loss of romantic attachments has long been a central literary theme. The double suicides of Romeo and Juliet, for example, do not result from mental disorder but from a tragic misunderstanding after the perceived loss of a lover. Other literary suicides, such as Emma Bovary's or Anna Karenina's, stem from realizations that the consequences of stigmatized romantic entanglements are inescapable.

Current research supports the intuition that severe losses of intimate attachments naturally lead to sadness responses: in many studies marital dissolution is more consistently and powerfully associated with depression than any other variable.[44] Indeed, rates of depressive episodes that meet *DSM* criteria are comparable for persons who experience marital dissolution and those who experience bereavement.[45] People who undergo marital dissolution are far more likely to develop first onsets of MDD over a 1-year period than people who do not.[46] "Adjusting for age, sex, and baseline history of other psychiatric disorders," writes sociologist Martha Bruce, "the effect of marital separation and divorce on first-onset major depression is very large (Odds ratio) = 18.1."[47] Studies indicate that from 30 to 50% of people undergoing the process of marital dissolution experience symptoms comparable in intensity to those of depressive disorder.[48] Given that as many as 60% of marriages are expected to end in divorce or separation, a huge proportion of the population should experience nondisordered sadness with symptoms comparable to those of MDD at some point in their lives from this cause alone.

As with bereavement, whether or not people develop symptoms of intense sadness during periods of marital dissolution largely varies as a function of the social context before and after the separation. At one extreme, symptoms can decline when marital stress was high before the period of dissolution.[49] In some cases, marital dissolutions can even lead to better mental states when they involve leaving unwanted marriages and entering new partnerships. At the other extreme, marital dissolutions that are unwanted or that involve features that are degrading, shameful, threatening to future well-being, entrapping, or devaluing of the person who is experiencing the loss are especially prone to produce intense depressive symptoms.[50] For example, wives who have suffered humiliation due to the unexpected infidelity of their husbands have three times more depressive symptoms than those who have suffered losses that do not involve such humiliation.[51]

Just as the intensity of normal sadness after marital dissolutions varies as a function of social circumstances, its persistence also depends on the stressfulness of the context. In contrast to the highly stressful period of marital separation, the divorce itself often indicates the resolution of a stressful situation.[52] By 2 years following the divorce, divorced people have comparable rates of depression to married people.[53] The huge rates of nondisordered sadness that arise during periods of marital dissolution are associated with severe symptoms that rarely persist far beyond the divorce.[54]

In addition to the loss of an intimate partner, marital dissolutions often negatively affect many aspects of life, including social status, personal identity, financial resources, friendship networks, living situations, and relationships with children, in ways that can intensify the associated loss response. People undergoing marital dissolution who face the secondary stressors of falling standards of living, weakening of support networks, downward residential mobility, and problems in dealing with children all report more symptoms of distress than those who do not face these additional stressors.[55] Conversely, sadness after marital dissolution is particularly likely to remit in response to positive environmental changes or "fresh start" events such as remarriage or forming new relationships.[56]

In a minority of cases, a depressive disorder might have preceded and been one cause of the marital dissolution.[57] In another small group of people, the experience of marital dissolution is severe enough to lead to breakdowns of loss response mechanisms that are pathologically immobilizing or that persist long after the period of the breakup. The preceding evidence suggests, however, that most people who develop symptoms comparable to those of depressive disorder during periods of marital dissolution do not have mental disorders. They are responding to situations that naturally lead people to be intensely sad.

Other Examples: Job or Status Loss, Chronic Stress, Disasters

In addition to losses of intimate attachments, losses of status and resources often evoke normal sadness. The loss of a valued job is one common situation that produces high rates of intense sadness. Such losses, as well as financial strain, underemployment, demotions, and failures to achieve promotions, are associated with declining status, prestige, and resources and consequent sadness that cannot be explained by depressive states that existed before the economic adversity.[58] Becoming unemployed has a particularly strong relationship with elevated levels of depression-like symptoms; indeed, about a quarter of people who become unemployed develop symptoms severe enough to resemble *DSM* clinical criteria.[59] But any serious loss of financial resources or a continuing state of economic strain can yield such experiences.[60] For example, about a third of the people who suffered severe loss of retirement savings as a result of a bank fraud developed symptoms comparable to those of MDD.[61]

The context in which the job loss occurs, and thus its meaning to the individual, predicts which unemployed persons are likely to develop symptoms equivalent to those of *DSM* depressive disorder. People who lose valued and rewarding jobs are especially likely to become symptomatic, whereas those who previously held highly stressful jobs are less likely to become sad.[62] Also, sadness is more likely to emerge when people unexpectedly lose jobs than when the loss was anticipated.[63] Job loss is particularly likely to lead to normal sadness when it is associated with many secondary stressors such as economic and interpersonal strains.[64]

Just as distress from loss of intimate attachments ends when new attachments form, studies indicate that levels of distress become elevated shortly before or immediately after becoming unemployed but dramatically decline after reemployment, a sign of a normally functioning loss response.[65] This is the reason that workers who lose jobs during prosperous periods when opportunities for reemployment are plentiful are not likely to become distressed.[66]

Especially humiliating status losses can sometimes be intense enough to produce outcomes as extreme as suicide among individuals who were normal in all respects before the loss. Examples include executives who are responsible for profound business failures or persons indicted in corruption scandals.[67] Consider the case of Hajimu Asada and his wife Chisako: "The chairman of a Japanese poultry company blamed for failing to alert the authorities about an outbreak of avian influenza committed suicide with his wife, as the disease showed signs of spreading in Japan."[68] Failures to uphold social norms, especially in intensely collectivist social settings, can lead to shame of enough intensity to provoke suicide.[69] For example, suicide rates were extraordinarily high during the Chinese Cultural Revolution, especially among persons accused of being landlords, wealthy peasants, intellectuals, and dissidents.[70]

Other losses that lead to nondisordered sadness arise when large discrepancies exist between the goals to which people aspire and their actual accomplishments.[71] Undergraduates who are denied admittance to long-desired professional schools or graduate students who cannot find jobs in their academic fields understandably often show signs of sadness.[72] Indeed, the failure to achieve valued goals is the most powerful predictor of low mood among undergraduates.[73] Likewise, adults who do not attain goals they set for themselves earlier in life report more distress than people whose attainments more closely match their former aspirations.[74] Similarly, women who strongly desire to bear children but who are infertile often experience intense distress.[75] Such symptoms disappear when the discrepancy between aspirations and accomplishments narrows: for example, the depressive symptoms of women who have suffered miscarriages do not persist when they subsequently become pregnant and give birth.[76]

Enormous proportions of populations who experience disasters that entail massive losses develop depressive feelings. For example, from 40 to 70% of civilian refugees displaced from their homes by mass violence display symptoms of Major Depression.[77] In most cases, however, symptoms do not endure.

For example, 5 weeks after the terrorist attack of September 11, 2001, one of every five residents of New York City reported enough symptoms to qualify for a diagnosis of MDD. During this period, about three-quarters of New York City residents cried, over 60% felt very nervous or tense, about 60% had trouble getting to sleep, and nearly half felt more tired than usual and didn't feel like eating. Very few people who experienced such understandable depressive symptoms immediately after the attack, however, remained depressed 6 months later, although not many were treated for their conditions.[78] Likewise, immediately after natural disasters such as earthquakes, tornadoes, or floods nearly all affected individuals report some distress, which quickly dissipates as living conditions normalize.[79]

Some of the most consistent associations between social context and sadness do not stem from such acute situations of loss but instead from chronic social stressors such as long-term joblessness, persistent debt, living in unsafe and threatening neighborhoods, chronic physical illnesses, troubled marriages, or oppressive work conditions. Unlike a typical episode of designed sadness that remits when the conditions that gave rise to it end, ongoing stressors can lead to persistent states of sadness that nonetheless are normal reactions to chronically problematic circumstances. Such chronic and persistent strains can be even more strongly related than the number of time-limited stressful life events to depressive symptoms.[80] The relationship between long-term financial and social disadvantage and experiences of sadness is strong enough that persons in the lowest socioeconomic quintile are up to seven times more likely than those in the highest quintile to satisfy symptomatic criteria for MDD.[81] Some have claimed that such individuals have depressive disorders that caused them to sink into the conditions they are in, but many careful studies have established that disadvantageous social conditions are far more likely to precede the development of symptoms of depression than they are to result from preexisting depressive conditions.[82]

Supporting the idea that much of this suffering is normal sadness, some evidence shows that when people move from chronic impoverished conditions to relatively more prosperous ones their levels of distress fall. In the course of one large study of rural children, a casino opened, providing the quarter of the sample who were American Indian with substantial income supplements. Depression-like symptoms of children whose families rose out of poverty fell about 30% over the 4-year period before and after the casino opened, whereas symptom levels of the persistently poor remained stable.[83] Rates of symptoms among the group that experienced improved financial conditions were no different from those among participants who were never poor. Other studies find that rising incomes lead to declining numbers of depressive conditions among impoverished people.[84] These findings suggest that a large proportion of apparent depressive disorders among indigent people are not internal dysfunctions and would not persist if conditions of deprivation improved.

We are reminded here of an anecdote that a colleague told us. An eminent researcher presented a paper on women who he claimed were suffering from chronic depressive disorder. One woman with children had been abandoned by her husband and was facing an enormous and chronic challenge in dealing with her impoverished circumstances. Her symptoms of sadness, worry, sleeplessness, and so on were indeed severe. Then, the woman won a lottery, yielding her a considerable amount of money. Strikingly, her chronic symptoms disappeared, leading our colleague to doubt that she had ever had a genuine disorder but instead had been understandably distressed by the overwhelming challenges that faced her.

We conclude that grief reactions are indeed a model for responses to numerous kinds of loss situations. A fairly high proportion of people develop symptoms in response to various losses, including symptoms sufficient in kind, number, severity, and duration to satisfy *DSM* criteria for MDD; these symptoms are proportionate in severity to the meaning of the situation that evoked them; and their persistence stems from the persistence of the original stressor or from additional stressors that follow the initial loss. Leaving aside the death of a loved one, the kinds of acute and chronic losses that lead to intense sadness among some nondisordered people—romantic breakups, losses of jobs or failure to gain anticipated promotions, disasters, illness, and so forth—are common. When these losses are serious, people who suffer them unsurprisingly report the experience of sadness-related depressive symptoms. Neither traditional psychiatry (as we show in chapters 3 and 4) nor common sense considered such reactions to be psychiatric disorders, and they do seem to qualify as normal for all the very same reasons that intense grief is considered normal. Given the number of people who experience the described kinds of losses, we expect that substantial numbers of people with normal sadness would satisfy *DSM* criteria for depressive disorder at some point in their lives, thus yielding a potentially significant number of false-positive diagnoses.

Evidence That Sadness Is a Normal, Designed Response

How do we know that the kind of sadness described in this chapter is indeed normal, that is, a result of human species-typical biological design? Although it may seem obvious that negative emotions such as sadness, anger, and fear in response to certain situations are results of natural selection, some social scientists believe instead that such emotional responses reflect learned, socially constructed scripts.[85] We consider three lines of evidence relevant to the question of whether the emotion of sadness and its attendant symptoms substantially result from innate mechanisms or from cultural scripts: loss responses among human and nonhuman primates, human infant loss responses that occur developmentally prior to socialization into a culture's emotional scripts, and the cross-cultural universality of loss responses.

Continuities Across Species

Nonhuman primates show a clear resemblance to humans in the way they respond to loss—that is, in their observable features of expression, behavior, and brain functioning. As Darwin noted, apes and humans show similar facial expressions in situations that are associated with sadness, including elevated eyebrows, drooping eyelids, horizontal wrinkles across the forehead, and outward extension and drawing down of the lips.[86] In addition, displays of sadness among apes, like human responses, include decreased locomotor activity, agitation, slouched or fetal-like posture, cessation of play behavior, and social withdrawal.[87] Most important, the loss situations that commonly lead to depressive responses are similar in primates and in humans. Nonhuman primates react to separations from intimates—for example, an infant monkey separating from its mother—with physiological responses similar to those that correlate with sadness in humans, including elevated levels of cortisol and ACTH hormones and impairments of the hypothalamic-pituitary-adrenal (HPA) axis.[88] Adult nonhuman primates that are separated from sexual partners or peers show similar reactions.[89]

Primate studies also show that symptoms of depression that develop after separations rapidly disappear when the situation of loss is resolved, such as when an infant monkey is reunited with its mother.[90] Also, primates in environments that feature readily available mother substitutes rarely exhibit severe or enduring reactions in response to maternal separations.[91] Such transient sadness responses to separation are part of innate coping mechanisms among many species.[92] However, prolonged separations and separations marked by profound isolation can produce neuroanatomical changes that permanently affect nonhuman primate brain functioning, analogous to the triggering of genuine depressive disorder in humans.[93]

Nonhuman primates also share with humans social hierarchies with high and low status positions and situations of chronic social subordination that lead to behavioral and brain reactions similar to the normal depressive responses in their human counterparts.[94] Subordinate nonhuman primates have higher levels than dominants of stress hormones and lower levels of blood serotonin, the neurochemical linked to depression among humans.[95] The loss of rank in nonhuman primate social hierarchies also triggers the production of the neurochemical correlates of depression.[96]

Experimental studies of nonhuman primates show how normal depressive symptoms can be a function of social situations. Psychiatrist Michael McGuire and his colleagues studied vervet monkeys, who possess strong and enduring hierarchical status relationships with one dominant male in each group.[97]

The highest ranking males have serotonin levels that are twice as high as those of other males in the group. When experimenters withdrew the dominant males from the group, their serotonin levels fell, and they refused food, showed diminished activity, and appeared to human observers to be depressed. Conversely, the serotonin levels of previously dependent monkeys who gained high status after the removal of the previously dominant male rose to values that characterized dominant males. Similar results have been obtained with female monkeys.[98]

Studies of nonhuman primates in natural settings confirm the findings of laboratory research.[99] Neuroendocrinologist Robert Sapolsky's studies of wild baboons living freely in East Africa show that chronic social subordination is associated with high stress hormones consistent with depressive symptoms in humans and that when rank in status hierarchies changes, these physiological profiles change as well.[100] Moreover, they depend on the social context: the behavioral and neurochemical advantages of high rank are found only in stable dominance hierarchies, whereas in unstable hierarchies in which the position of the dominant is precarious, high rank is not associated with fewer stress hormones.[101] Thus humans appear to have inherited from their primate ancestors a natural tendency to become sad in particular contexts of status and relationship loss.

Loss Responses in Presocialized Infants

The human tendency to become sad in certain contexts appears early—in infancy. Indeed, it appears before the infant has even learned culturally appropriate ways of expressing sadness. The British child psychiatrist John Bowlby has conducted the most influential studies demonstrating how attachment losses lead to depressive reactions among infants.[102] Bowlby persuasively argued that human infants are designed to need strong attachments and that they develop certain types of sadness responses as a coping mechanism when they are separated from their primary caregivers. He observed that healthy infants who were separated from their mothers initially reacted by crying and displaying other expressions of despair. They protested the separation and searched for their mothers. These responses usually evoked sympathy from the mothers, who responded by attending to their infants' needs. When separations were prolonged, however, the infants withdrew and became inactive and apathetic, similar to the symptoms of an intense adult loss response. Prolonged separations resulted in a state of detachment in which young children ceased to respond to parental figures even after they were restored to their lives.

Bowlby's work indicates that sadness naturally arises in presocialized infants after the loss of close attachments. The liability to experience separation anxiety and grief results from involvement in intense, loving relationships. Sadness that develops after losses of these relationships seems to be an aspect of normal, presocialized human nature. When these losses are prolonged and without compensating remedies, however, they can lead to responses that go beyond normal sadness to become depressive disorders.[103]

Cross-Cultural Uniformity

The capacity for intense sadness in response to loss appears to be a universal feature found in all human groups. Loss responses with the characteristics we have described are found not only throughout Western history (see chapter 3) but also in non-Western societies. Charles Darwin was perhaps the first to comment on the universality of sadness responses: "The expression of grief due to the contraction of the grief-muscles, is by no means confined to Europeans, but appears to be common to all the races of mankind."[104] Darwin provided a description of grief among the Australian aborigines that was comparable to the expression of this emotion among Europeans:

> After prolonged suffering the eyes become dull and lack expression, and are often slightly suffused with tears. The eyebrows not rarely are rendered oblique, which is due to their inner ends being raised. This produces peculiarly-formed wrinkles on the forehead which are very different from those of a simple frown; though in some cases a frown alone may be present. The corners of the mouth are drawn downwards, which is so universally recognized as a sign of being out of spirits, that it is almost proverbial.[105]

Considerable subsequent research confirms Darwin's observations that such expressions, especially the contraction of the muscles at the corners of the mouth, are recognized across cultures as representing grief. The most important studies stem from psychologist Paul Ekman's research on basic human emotions, including sadness. In particular, to test the universality of emotions, Ekman studies facial expressions because they are less susceptible to cultural influences than are verbal reports of emotions.

In one type of study, Ekman asked people to show how their faces would look if they felt sad "because your child died."[106] The resulting facial expressions were photographed. Expressions of sadness in these pictures were marked by eyes that are downcast with drooping or tense upper lids, eyebrows that are drawn together, jaws that are closed or slightly open, and lower lips that are drawn down. The photographs were then shown to people in different cultures, and they were asked to select from among several choices of narratives about the situation that triggered the pictured emotion (the loss of a child is used for sadness). Ekman's results indicate overwhelming agreement among persons in different countries about the emotion each photograph expresses. Very high rates of concurrence, ranging from 73 to 90%, existed across five different cultures (Japan, Brazil, Chile, Argentina, and the United States); the concurrence was even higher within each particular culture in ratings of sadness photographs.[107]

Another study of 10 cultures (Estonia, Germany, Greece, Hong Kong, Italy, Japan, Scotland, Sumatra, Turkey, and the United States) indicated between 76 and 92% agreement on facial expressions of sadness.[108]

In response to objections that his findings actually demonstrate the impact of common learning experiences because of the influence of worldwide media, Ekman studied the Fore culture in Papua, New Guinea, which had not been exposed to any kind of media or had contact with outside cultures.[109] He showed Fore participants photographs of three faces that expressed three different emotions—sadness, anger, and surprise. He then told a story involving only one of these emotions and asked which of the photographs best matched the story. For example, he asked his participants which picture best depicted a man whose child had died. He found that 79% of the Fore—a preliterate, isolated people—agreed with members of literate cultures on the face that most corresponded to sadness in the story that was read to them. Because Ekman's research in this culture did not rely on the use of Western words, it is immune to critiques that Western preconceptions account for the findings.

Ekman and his colleague Wallace Friesen also asked the Fore to show the facial expressions they would have if they were the persons described in the emotion stories (e.g., if their children had died). American college students could accurately judge what emotions videotaped responses of the New Guineans represented. In addition, Ekman's voluminous filming of this culture, as well as of others in Papua New Guinea, showed the same expressions of sadness that were found elsewhere in the world. Ekman's findings indicate that some innate features of the expression of sadness are present in all cultures, presumably because they stem from the evolution of humans as a species.

Cultural Variation and Normal Sadness

The findings that emerge from studies of primates and very young children and across cultures all indicate that sadness responses are biologically based and not due to social scripts alone. In particular, humans appear biologically designed to become sad in certain kinds of situations, especially those involving losses of close attachments, social status, or meaning systems. However, the biological roots of normal sadness in no way preclude important social influences on when or how sadness is expressed. Given that meanings mediate sadness responses and that cultures shape meanings, normal sadness is inherently a joint product of biology and culture (as well as individual variation and learning).

Cultural Meanings and Biological Mechanisms as Complementary

Culture and biological design are not always antithetical to each other; when it comes to emotions, they are complementary. Culture itself is an evolved human capacity; humans are designed to be capable of a degree of socialization and internalization of social values, meanings, and rules. As the sociologist Jonathan Turner has emphasized, people are hardwired to pay attention to cultural symbols, social roles, and interactional needs.[110] Some evolved mechanisms, such as emotions, involve responses to such meanings. Thus cultural meaning plays an essential and perhaps even designed role in shaping the final expression of emotion.

Indeed, many mental features are biologically selected to be capable of cultural variation. For example, the capacity for language appears to be a designed human trait, but the details of grammar and of course the specific sounds that comprise the words of a language, as well as the way those sounds are associated with concepts, vary from culture to culture. Similarly, sexual jealousy is a universal biologically selected emotion that occurs in all human societies, but the specific targets of jealousy vary widely. In some monogamous cultures, anyone who attempts to have sex with another's spouse is a target of such feeling; in some cultures, certain honored strangers are exempt; and in other cultures, a substantial proportion of the community is not subject to jealousy. Language and sexual jealousy, however, are naturally selected capacities.[111] As linguists suggest, the mechanisms that underlie such features may be designed to allow for "parameter setting," in which culture establishes the specific form that the expression of the general, evolved structure will take.

Culture and Definitions of Loss

The categories that trigger sadness—losses of attachment, status, and meaning—are common across all societies.[112] "Sickness of liver," a metaphor for sadness among the Malay, is illustrative: "A Malay loses something he values; he has a bad night in the gambling houses; some of his property is wantonly damaged; he has a quarrel with one whom he loves; his father dies; or his mistress proves unfaithful; any one of these things causes him 'sickness of liver.'"[113]

Nonetheless, culture influences evolutionarily shaped loss responses in a variety of ways. First, cultural meanings influence which *particular* events count as losses. These meanings also influence contextual factors, such as humiliation and entrapment, which determine the severity of loss. For example, in most social groups within the United States, the failure of a woman to give birth to a male child would not be a reason for intense sadness. But in Zimbabwe, the meaning of such failure includes a serious decline in social status, undesirability as a marriage partner, and potential divorce. Consequently, failure to have a male child is a source of serious depressive reactions in Zimbabwean women.[114] Or, in India, among the leading causes of suicide in 1990 were quarrels with in-laws and dowry disputes, which represent major losses in India but would not necessarily bring about such extreme responses in other societies.[115] The fact that such cultural meanings affect to what extent an event falls under a naturally given category does not in the least conflict with the fact that the basic categories themselves are given biologically. Nature supplies the template for triggers of loss responses, but culture provides the content for this template.

Cultural Shaping of Loss Responses

Cultural values also set the parameters for what are considered proportionate responses to loss. They set the scale of intensity and duration of appropriate responses, shape how emotionally expressive people are, and influence which aspects of the response public expressions of the emotion emphasize. Emotional experiences themselves are to some degree malleable; some cultures socialize their members to be highly emotional, whereas others encourage suppression and minimalization of emotion.

All cultures have display norms or "scripts" that guide the overt expression of emotion. Many non-Western cultures encourage the expression of sadness in public ceremonies and organized rituals that shape the nature of the display. For example, among the Kaluli of New Guinea, losses result not in self-blame or guilt but in anger that is turned outward into feelings that one is owed compensation for the loss.[116] Public ceremonies allow for the expression of these feelings in weeping, songs, and the payment of compensation. Other cultures, such as the Navaho, strongly discourage displays of extreme sadness.[117]

Cultural norms also affect what is viewed as the appropriate duration of loss responses. Among the Navaho, outward expressions of grief are limited to 4 days.[118] The bereaved person is not expected to show grief or refer to the dead person beyond this short period. Conversely, Mediterranean societies traditionally dictated long periods of mourning for bereaved widows that could last for many years.[119]

It is, however, important to separate cultural norms for expressing emotions from the experienced emotions themselves. For example, among Iranians: "If someone in your family dies, you have to really act like you are sorry, to wail and kick, otherwise you'll be accused of having ill feelings toward that person, regardless of what your inner feelings are, especially if you stand to inherit something."[120] At the extreme, cultural norms can even transform expressions of grief into cheerfulness. The Balinese, for example, respond to bereavement with laughter.[121] The Irish wake is another, well-known example. But even when cultural norms dictate expressive responses incompatible with sadness, they recognize sadness as the characteristic underlying feeling; thus the Balinese believe that sadness is the natural response to loss but that its expression should be combated because it is detrimental to health and leads others to be sad.[122]

Anthropologists routinely contrast the psychological expression of depression in the West with its somatic presentation in non-Western cultures.[123] For example, Chinese populations tend to focus, after loss, on bodily feelings of distress that often go along with intense sadness, such as back pain, stomachaches, headaches, and the like.[124] Despite the different outward manifestations, however, common underlying emotions appear to be universal. Chinese patients are aware of the psychological aspects of their feelings, but social norms mandate that they express their problems in somatic terms when they seek help from physicians.[125] Members of these cultures express intense sadness facially and behaviorally as do Westerners, and when specifically asked, they report the same psychological and emotional experiences. Moreover, their symptoms are responsive to the same medications that are prescribed for depression in Western societies.[126]

The highly varying cultural expressions of sadness are consistent with the existence of a common underlying emotional state. Indeed, the study of cultural variation in depression cannot even proceed without some underlying notion of what is universal, because it is incoherent to claim that some cultures express depression through physiological symptoms and others through psychological symptoms without having some underlying conception of depression that transcends its cultural symptomatic expression.

Culture and Rates of Depression

Some writers suggest that if depressive symptoms are a result of biological design, then there should not be the substantial amount of social variation that exists in rates of depressive symptoms.[127] This argument mistakenly sees sadness as occurring independently of actual triggering events and their interpretations. But cultural contexts influence the frequency with which people are exposed to the kinds of losses that can trigger sadness, the availability of social support, and the interpretation of those losses; consequently, cultures also differ in rates of normal sadness.[128]

British sociologist George Brown's cross-cultural studies, in which rates of depressive responses vary tenfold across societies, show how this variation is in large part due to varying exposure to the kinds of loss events that naturally cause depression, such as the loss of intimate attachments due to death or separation, the occurrence of chronic stressors, and the inability to achieve goals central to the culture's meaning system. There is a nearly perfect correlation between the number of severe loss events that befall members of different societies and resulting rates of depressive symptoms.[129] At the lowest rate, only 3% of women in a Basque-speaking rural area of Spain feel depressed; these women experience almost no serious events over the course of a year.[130] At the highest rate, over 30% of women in an urban township in Zimbabwe report feeling depressed; women in this area frequently suffer severe loss events.[131]

Also, social reactions to those who experience loss influence rates of sadness. Strong interpersonal ties and networks of social support, as well as powerful collective religious rituals and belief systems, help make people less vulnerable to loss.[132] The Kaluli, for example, feature ritualized group ceremonies after definable loss events, which might account for the apparent rarity of chronic sadness in this society.[133] Some societies mandate the replacement of deceased spouses with a new partner, often a relative—the Bible, for example, refers to the Hebrew practice of widows marrying their dead husbands' brothers—and grief seems to be relatively short-lived in such societies.[134]

Cultural Relativity of the Threshold Between Normality and Disorder

Some also argue that, because culture determines the proportionality of a sadness response, it also determines the threshold between normal and disordered sadness, and thus there is no objective transcultural biological distinction between normality and dysfunction.[135] They claim that the same response may be normal in one culture and disordered in another, implying the cultural relativity of normality.

It is true that such thresholds will vary, but the reason is not that cultures directly or arbitrarily define normality and disorder. Rather, through socialization, cultures shape how normal sadness responses will occur in their members by setting the parameters of the loss response. That is, different thresholds for diagnosis of disorder exist in different cultures because different cultures induce different intensities and durations of response to specific triggers of sadness. In judging whether or not an individual is responding normally, such varying meanings must be taken into account.

For example, a modern American woman who becomes depressed because she has had no further contact with a man she has recently met and with whom she has held hands has not suffered a sufficient loss to explain these symptoms. Cultural values neither define this situation as humiliating nor lead to further social stigmatization, and so the woman's depressive response in the absence of any special personal meanings might be seen as pathological. In contrast, in many Islamic cultures, a young woman who has physical contact with a man whom she does not marry can face social stigmatization and degradation; any touching, however innocuous by Western standards, can lead to serious social consequences.[136] In this case, the woman's sadness response might be seen as normal.

Therefore, it is not simply that what might represent a dysfunction in the case of the Western woman can indicate the normal working of loss response mechanisms in the Muslim woman. Rather, this difference in cultural judgments about normality is based on the proportionality of response to severity of loss; the difference in diagnosis arises precisely because local meanings imply that a given response is likely a result of normal, designed mechanisms in one case and of dysfunction in another. Cultural norms are part of the basis for inferring whether the best explanation for a response is in terms of design or dysfunction. Culture and biology are not two opposing explanations but complementary parts of one explanation; each requires the other for comprehensive and coherent explanations of depressive responses.

Adaptive Functions of Nondisordered Loss Responses

The preceding evidence suggests that sadness after loss is a designed feature of human nature and answers the most common objections to that thesis. But the deepest and most puzzling question about sadness has not been touched: Why does sadness exist? What sort of survival value did this painful and debilitating emotion provide that caused it to be naturally selected?

This topic remains controversial, and there is no easy or generally accepted answer at present to the question of the biological function of sadness. In some cases, a mechanism's biological function is immediately obvious; for example, it cannot be accidental that the eyes see, the hands grasp, the feet walk, or the teeth chew, and it is clear that these beneficial effects explain the existence via natural selection of the respective mechanisms. However, in other cases, although it is obvious that a feature is biologically designed, we have little conclusive knowledge of its function. For example, before physician William Harvey's famous experiments in the 1620s demonstrated circulation of the blood, no one fully understood the function of the heart, even though everyone assumed it was designed for something. Even today, we have little understanding of the function of sleep, although sleep clearly is a designed part of human functioning. Sadness is somewhat like sleep in this respect; the function is not obvious, yet the designed nature is. However, some plausible hypotheses about the functions of sadness do exist, and they suggest how, despite its painful nature, sadness can have a designed biological role.

The puzzle is that depressive experiences seem on their face to be harmful to reproductive fitness. Intensely sad people experience decreased initiative, find less pleasure in life to motivate them, and tend to withdraw from everyday activities. Positive mood, in contrast, encourages activities required to obtain sexual partners, food, shelter, and other resources that increase survival and reproduction. Thus, under ordinary circumstances, consistent levels of negative mood should be selectively disadvantageous. For intense sadness responses to have been naturally selected, there must have been some special circumstances in which the benefits of temporarily experiencing such symptoms outweighed the obvious costs. In those particular contexts, and only in those contexts, states of low mood must have increased fitness precisely *because* they made people less active, less motivated, and so on.[137] The best analogy is to acute pain from an injury, which stops activity but is adaptive because it helps people avoid further damage to tissue. In contrast, chronic pain unrelated to any underlying physiological damage would be harmful in the way that depressive disorder is certainly harmful.[138]

In considering the function of sadness, it is important to keep in mind that the function of a biological mechanism need not be beneficial in the current environment, although it often is. It must have been beneficial in the past, however, and must thus explain why the underlying mechanism was selected and now exists. What evolutionary psychologists John Tooby and Leda Cosmides call the environment of evolutionary adaptation (EEA), probably occurring at the time when humans lived in hunter-gatherer societies on the African plains before or during the Pleistocene era between 2 million to 10,000 years ago, was responsible for shaping many of the genetic traits that humans up to the present still hold.[139] Sadness is designed to cope with contexts that arose in these ancestral conditions but that may be less apparent in current environments. Analogously, human cravings for sweets, salt, and fats may seem puzzling now, when there are plentiful sources of calories and those cravings can lead to obesity and disease, but they were biologically designed when human environments were marked by scarcity of calories. Consequently, it is now part of normal human nature to enjoy these tastes, whatever else wise nutrition may dictate.

Keeping these cautionary points in mind, we can ask: When compared with alternative responses to loss, what benefits might depressive symptoms have conferred that led to their natural selection over the course of human evolution?

Attraction of Social Support

One explanation of the adaptive function of depressive feelings focuses on how emotional behavior communicates inner states to other people so that depressed people attract social support after attachment losses. The Australian psychiatrist Aubrey Lewis was the first to propose that depressive reactions could function as a "cry for help" that calls attention to needy states and elicits social support.[140] The withdrawal, inhibition, and vegetative aspects of depression mimic illness and signal others to draw the suffering individual back into the group.[141] States of social isolation would have been especially threatening in the tightly knit, interdependent human social groups that existed during the EEA, making a positive social response likely. Similarly, some recent evidence indicates that postpartum depression, for example, arises under circumstances, such as poor infant health and a lack of social support, in which it might function as a signal that mothers will reduce their child care efforts until they receive more support from others.[142]

Some reject the idea that depression was designed to attract social support because of empirical evidence that people typically avoid and reject, rather than support, depressed people.[143] Perhaps, instead, only nondisordered sadness that arises in appropriate situations attracts social support. Indeed, intense mobilization of ritual expressions of sympathy universally emerges after bereavements and other serious losses.[144] In contrast, dysfunctional depressions involving severe and sustained states of despondency without sufficient situational cause tend to alienate or anger other people and diminish social support, leading to isolation and rejection of the afflicted people and to fitness disadvantages.

In addition to the attraction-of-support hypothesis, which makes particular sense in understanding sadness after loss of intimate attachments, other theories about the functions of sadness have been advanced. One is that depressive symptoms of despair may have served to protect infants in the immediate aftermath of parental loss. The despair of infants that succeeds the protest at their mother's departure activates an inhibitory, quiet state that, during precivilization, might have prevented the abandoned offspring from drawing the attention of predators to itself.[145] But another theory emphasizes the initial period of loud protest, leading to a very different conclusion; Darwin, for example, explained infant reactions to separation—that is, their screaming—in terms of their attention-getting aspects.[146] Presumably both strategies have their purpose at different times after separation.

John Bowlby proposed another influential account of the adaptive nature of depression after attachment losses.[147] For Bowlby, the prospect of the pain of depressive feelings following attachment loss motivates people to vigorously seek reunion with the lost loved one and not to give up the lost tie. Grief at thoughts of loss allowed social bonds to persist during the frequent, temporary absences of one party in the EEA and thus promoted the maintenance of social relationships. From this viewpoint, grief after the death of a loved one was a by-product of adaptive responses to attachment losses that were not permanent, an explanation that has been widely adopted.[148]

Protection From Aggression After Status Losses

Ethological studies indicate that the capacity to become depressed, as indicated by lowered testosterone, elevated cortisol, and retardation in behavior, is deeply rooted in the reptilian brain and is present in most vertebrates and all mammals.[149] Such depressive responses might have arisen widely as signals of acceptance of defeat in status contests that are ubiquitous in the animal world. The British psychiatrist John Price and his colleagues have developed the most elaborate explanation of this sort of adaptive function. They theorize that negative behavior, mood, and thought arose as adaptive responses to circumstances of defeat and subordination.[150] Indeed, Price views depression as part of an involuntary subordinate strategy (ISS), which refers to a state of inhibited action marked by withdrawal, lack of self-assertion, nervousness, and anxiety (in other works, Price calls the ISS *ritual agonistic behavior*).[151] Price connects ISS responses to primeval brain algorithms that assess relative strengths, weaknesses, power, and rank of organisms and adjust actions accordingly to produce responses of flight, fight, or submission in confrontations with other animals. Depressive feeling is one way that behavior is regulated as a consequence of such assessments. Animals develop ISS responses when they judge themselves to be weaker than their competitors. They cease competing with the dominant animal, accept their defeated status, and signal their submission to the winning party. The inhibited aspects of depressive reactions are adaptive responses to subordinate positions from which there is no possibility of escape.[152]

The defeated party who has failed to defend territory or lost a status contest could respond with renewed anger and aggression rather than concede to the winner. However, the open expression of aggressive emotions and behaviors can lead to the serious injury or death of the defeated party. Many of the symptoms of the ISS involve behaviors that communicate that the loser will not confront the winner, will not attempt to gain dominance, and will give up the struggle. Submissive responses protect the loser from further aggression by showing the dominant animal it is safe from additional challenges and thus need not feel threatened by the continued presence of the loser. Subordinates that make submissive responses are more likely to survive and reproduce than those who respond more aggressively.

The ISS theory explains several aspects of depressive responses. First, it explains the situation-specific qualities of depressive responses; they are adaptive only when facing potential defeat by stronger adversaries. Thus the inhibition of self-assertion that is at the core of ISS would be naturally selected to occur in those contexts. It is also compatible with the widespread finding that depression is more common among people and other animals at the bottom of status hierarchies and explains the persistence of depressive feelings among those who are in enduring states of subordination. Almost universally, women are more likely than men to be in such subordinate positions, which could partially explain their higher rates of depression.[153] Finally, the theory is consistent with the studies reported earlier that show sadness in response to reductions in status.

Promotion of Disengagement From Nonproductive Activities

Another common situation that produces sadness arises when people cannot obtain a crucial resource that is important to them.[154] Depressive experiences also might be adaptive when they disengage people from their investments in unproductive efforts, in unreachable goals, or in goals with low probability of success. They thus help to make possible the eventual reengagement with new, more productive activities.[155] The suspension of current activity, accompanied by the intense ruminative activity that is characteristic of depression, may facilitate the difficult shift of energy to new projects or attachments.[156]

Sadness responses are especially likely to emerge after life crises, when people are forced to reevaluate their futures, and in this context they may be adaptive in helping individuals to avoid rash decisions, to take all possible dangers into account, and not to overestimate the chances of success in new activities. "In this situation," according to psychiatrist Randolph Nesse, "pessimism, lack of energy, and fearfulness can prevent calamity even when they perpetuate misery."[157] The transient nature of most normal sadness allows the individual to emerge properly motivated by newly selected goals. In contrast, depressive disorders involve such severe loss of motivation that efforts cannot be channeled toward new pursuits.

Depressive responses that arise after losses of attachment, defeats in status contests, or the collapse of meaning systems or goal strivings thus could have a variety of functions that would explain why such responses were naturally selected. The communication of low affect after losses of attachment can attract support and sympathy from others, and its anticipation can sustain relationships. The submission of depressed people in subordinate positions can prevent punishment from dominants and promote survival. Lowered motivation and physiological slowness can disengage people from unproductive forms of activity and allow them to reengage in more productive endeavors. Some recent evidence indicates that different situations produce particular types of symptoms: social losses are followed by crying and emotional pain, whereas failure to achieve goals is associated with pessimism, fatigue, and anhedonia.[158] Therefore, the explanations considered here are not mutually exclusive; different types of situations can tend to produce distinct reactions that meet specific adaptive challenges. Although none of these explanations is proven, the existence of plausible reasons for the adaptive functions of sadness supports the thesis that contextually proportionate sadness responses are a designed aspect of human nature.

Conclusion

In contrast to the otherwise universal recognition that it is natural for people to become sad after a great variety of losses, the *DSM* diagnoses all loss responses that meet its symptomatic criteria as disorders, with bereavement as the only acknowledged instance of normal intense sadness. However, a wealth of evidence supports the commonsense judgment that many people who develop symptoms of depression after a loss, even when they meet *DSM* criteria for a disorder, are not disordered but are experiencing a biologically designed response. Sadness after loss is found in all societies, among infants, and in our closest primate cousins; it is clearly biologically rooted and not merely a creation of social scripts.

The differences between the possible advantages of depressive responses in the EEA versus those experiences today deserve special emphasis. Loss response mechanisms would have been formed within environments that featured interaction within small, tightly knit groups, strong rituals of social support after loss, clear social hierarchies, and well-defined goals. In contrast, humans now confront novel environments that pose challenges that inherited loss responses were not designed to meet.[159] Modern societies feature many shifting and changeable interactions that are often being lost, multiple status hierarchies that constantly test one's worth, mobility away from close kin who are less able to provide social support after losses, and few common rituals of solidarity to deal with loss. In addition, ideologies that emphasize personal responsibility rather than fate, a deity, or collective liability enhance the chances that people will blame themselves for their failures. Exposure to the mass media allows status comparisons not just within well-defined local groups but also with innumerable others, many of whom will always seem to be of higher status than oneself.[160] This exposure also can motivate the pursuit of goals that are unreachable because few people have the means to achieve the ideals of beauty, wealth, fame, and success that are promoted to much of the public on a daily basis.[161] In such cases, loss response mechanisms might be functioning appropriately within environments that natural selection did not anticipate. Although therapy may help people cope with such feelings, there is nothing medically wrong with individuals who become transiently sad in these situations.

In contrast to normal sadness, depression that is truly disordered was not naturally selected but instead indicates that something has gone wrong with mechanisms that were designed to respond to loss. Such dysfunction-caused conditions tend to be recurrent, chronic, and not proportionately related to real losses rather than context specific and time limited. Such conditions were never adaptive in the past and certainly are not useful in the present.

The distinction between normal sadness and depressive disorder has been part of Western literature and science since the earliest recorded documents. Only in recent times has the distinction been greatly eroded and in danger of being substantially lost. The following chapters trace this transformation and explore the steps by which large domains of intense normal sadness came to be incorporated within depressive disorder in contemporary psychiatric diagnosis.

3

Sadness With and Without Cause

*Depression From Ancient Times Through
the Nineteenth Century*

D epression has been an omnipresent phenomenon over several
millennia of human history. For virtually all of that time, from
the earliest writings of the ancient Greek physicians to the late twentieth century, Western diagnosticians routinely distinguished depressive disorders, as a
form of madness, from symptomatically similar but nondisordered, normal sadness responses to a wide range of painful circumstances. Then, in 1980, seeking a more scientific foundation for diagnosis by focusing on decontextualized
criteria based on symptoms, the *DSM-III* inadvertently abandoned this critical
traditional distinction, which is now essentially lost in current thinking about
depression. This chapter and the next trace the history leading up to this momentous and, we argue, ultimately detrimental conceptual shift.

Why is reviewing this history important? Current diagnostic practices may
seem obviously right and sensible just because they are accepted, and they are
all that many of us have ever known. To understand the problems with the current diagnostic approach to depressive disorder and to recognize the choices
it represents, it helps to place it in historical context. This history reveals that
the way we think about depressive disorder now is quite new—and radically di-
verges from what has traditionally been considered appropriate.

But the importance of history is more than simply providing context and
contrast. It is easy to assume that current practices, if they are different, must
have emerged from a process in which the traditional alternatives were found to
be flawed and were superseded by a superior approach. The history of thinking
about depression specifically in regard to the role of context in diagnosing disorder dispels such beliefs and reveals instead the contingency and even arbitrariness
of some aspects of current diagnostic practices. It shows that the reasons for the
recent divergence from the traditional approach, although well intentioned and
shaped by admirable scientific aspirations, are anchored neither in evidence nor

in logic, which in fact support the older tradition. Despite the many virtues of the new approach, it is in certain important respects weaker than those it replaced.

Depressive disorder, unlike many other disorders, has an identifiable and lengthy history. Indeed, depression is probably the psychological disorder that is most easily recognizable throughout history; similar symptomatic descriptions occur over a 2,500-year span, representing what historian Stanley Jackson calls a "remarkable consistency."[1] From the earliest medical texts in ancient Greece to the present *DSM*, deep sadness and its variants—hopelessness, sorrow, dejection, despondency, emptiness, despair, discouragement—were often mentioned as core features of depressive disorder, along with related symptoms such as aversion to food, sleeplessness, irritability, restlessness, feelings of hopelessness or worthlessness, suicidal ideation and attempts, fear of death, repetitive focus on a few negative ideas, lack of pleasure or lack of interest in usual activities, fatigue, and social detachment.

Yet traditional diagnostic treatises also agreed in distinguishing depression as a disorder from a nondisordered type of deep sadness or fear that could have many of the same symptoms but that was a normal, proportionate reaction to serious losses. Such losses included the death of intimates, reversals in fortune, disappointments in attaining valued life goals, romantic disappointments, and the like. In addition, it was traditionally acknowledged that variations in temperament predispose some people to more readily or intensely experience sadness or fear but that these variations could be within a normal range of reasonably proportionate responses that did not represent a disorder.

Depressive disorders differed from these normal reactions, according to tradition, because they either arose in the absence of situations that would normally produce sadness or were of disproportionate magnitude or duration relative to their provoking causes. Such conditions indicated that something was wrong in the individual, not in the environment. In essence, then, traditional psychiatry took a *contextual* approach to the diagnosis of depressive disorder; whether a condition was diagnosed as disordered depended not just on the symptoms, which might be similar in normal sadness, and not just on the condition's severity, for normal sadness can be severe and disordered sadness moderate, but on the degree to which the symptoms were an understandable response to circumstances. In this and the following chapters, we elaborate the history of this contextual approach to depression and how the *DSM-III*, overturning thousands of years of thinking, replaced it with relatively precise and communicable symptomatic criteria that largely ignored the complexities of context, with detrimental side effects for psychiatric diagnosis.

Preliminary Caveats

From ancient Greek medical writings until the early twentieth century, what is now termed *depressive disorder* was generally referred to as *melancholia*, which literally means "black bile disorder." Although the name stuck into modern times, it originally reflected the ancient belief that health and disease depend on the balance or imbalance between four bodily fluids, or "humors," and that an excess of black bile—a humor often thought to be produced in the spleen—was responsible for depressive symptoms. Ancient physicians thought that black bile had a natural function in regulating mood and that melancholia represented a failure of this natural functioning. As belief in black bile's role in mental life waned, *depression* eventually arose as the dominant term in the nineteenth and twentieth centuries.

In recognizing the strikingly similar clinical descriptions of depressive disorder across the millennia, several cautions are necessary. First, one must consider the context of each discussion to tell whether a disorder is being described at all. Like today's confusingly overused term *depression,* the terms *melancholy* and *melancholia* also tended to do double duty in referring both to a disorder and to normal emotions, moods, and temperaments.

Second, classic texts were written before most of today's refined distinctions among mental disorders were recognized, and thus the category of melancholia often encompassed what in hindsight can be seen to be quite different disorders. These included psychotic disorders that ranged from schizophrenia to paranoid and other delusional states. For example, what may initially appear to be a description of the cycling of mania and depression in what we would now recognize as bipolar disorder may, on closer inspection, turn out to be more likely a description of the alternating agitation and withdrawal of a schizophrenic patient who was mistakenly classified as melancholic.[2] Because psychotically depressed individuals sometimes have mood-congruent delusions that provide the content for their sadness, early psychiatrists sometimes extended the category of melancholia to others with circumscribed delusions that caused negative emotions. Also, the withdrawal associated with such current diagnoses as avoidant personality disorder and social phobia appears to sometimes have been mistaken for the withdrawal associated with melancholia. However, the predominant picture of those classified as melancholics clearly indicates depressive disorder as we know it.

Third, because melancholia was an etiological description that classified conditions based on their believed cause in excess black bile, older descriptions often placed other conditions that were considered to have a similar etiology in black-bile imbalance together with depressive disorders as "melancholic disorders" in a broad sense, even if they had nothing to do with depression. In ancient times, these "melancholic disorders" included, for example, epilepsy and boils. Melancholia itself as a disorder was just one distinct instance of this broader category.

Fourth, classic descriptions generally, though not always, focused on what we would now call *psychotic depression,* which includes delusions or hallucinations. Indeed, these descriptions often defined melancholy as a form of "delirium without a fever" to distinguish melancholic delusions and hallucinations from those that occurred during a high fever caused by various physical diseases. Melancholia of this kind distinctively involved fixed ideas on specific topics linked to depressive affect, which distinguished melancholia from general cognitive malfunction or psychosis. Nonpsychotic depressive disorders were recognized as well but were not emphasized as constituting the bulk of cases until recent times.

Fifth, there is an ambiguity about the referent of *melancholia* that continues to exist in our own time and that can sometimes cause confusion. The exact extent of the meaning of *melancholia* has varied, sometimes referring to an overall disease, sometimes to sadness as a specific symptom, and sometimes to a syndromal set of coexisting symptoms, of which sadness is just one.[3]

Sixth, contrary to current practice, ancient and many subsequent texts routinely grouped sadness and fear together as symptoms of melancholia. Despondency was thought to be related to fear because melancholics were generally worried or morose not only about actual events but also about negative possibilities in the future that caused apprehension. Contemporary criteria emphasize sadness as an exclusive dominant affect, yet recent studies confirm that anxiety and sadness tend to go together in depression and that it is difficult to distinguish these states, just as tradition would have it.[4] But it is also clear from clinical descriptions that, then as now, sadness alone could be sufficient for melancholia.

A final caveat about our methodology: It is important to look past many differences and confusions in the history of depression to find an underlying coherence and similarity to current judgments. In particular, what are now considered genuine depressive disorders were clearly included within traditional melancholia and were distinguished from normal sadness. No doubt an alternative, postmodernist history of depression might emphasize the social construction of depression, including variations in definitions and in ranges of behavior that were pathologized and the social control correlates of these variations. Although the history of depression certainly contains such elements, the historical record also recognized a common core condition that has been of concern for several millennia.

Indeed, from the earliest times, this record displays what might be considered an "essentialist" view of the classification of melancholia—that is, it involves an inference, common to different writers who may have disagreed in their specific theories, that in melancholia something is going wrong with the internal functioning of mechanisms usually responsible for normal sadness in a way that leads to certain standard symptoms. This view is not an artifact of changing social responses to madness but a considered and plausible judgment. Moreover, it is impossible to analyze responsibly the ways groups have exploited the concept of depression for purposes of social power until one understands the logic of the concept of depression itself. It is the history of this common concept, and especially attempts to distinguish disordered sadness from normal sadness, that we attempt to understand.

The Ancients

Writing in the fifth century B.C., Hippocrates (460–377 B.C.) provided the first known definition of melancholia as a distinct disorder: "If fear or sadness last for a long time it is melancholia."[5] Although theories of depressive disorder have changed, the symptoms that indicate the disorder have not. In addition to fear and sadness, Hippocrates mentioned as possible symptoms "aversion to food, despondency, sleeplessness, irritability, restlessness," much like today's criteria.[6] But Hippocrates' definition indicated that it is not such symptoms alone but symptoms of unexpected duration that indicate disorder. Hippocrates' insistence that the sadness or fear must be prolonged is a first attempt to capture the notion that disproportion to circumstances is an essential aspect of depressive disorder.

Indeed, an ancient, possibly apocryphal, story about Hippocrates illustrates the distinction between disordered sadness without cause and normal sadness with cause.[7] He was asked to diagnose the problem of Perdiccas II, King of Macedonia from 454 to 413 B.C., who had fallen into a morbid condition and displayed a total lack of concern for matters of state. Hippocrates learned that the king's condition stemmed from his secret love for a concubine of his recently deceased father's. He suggested that the king acknowledge his love for the concubine and secure her love in return. In essence, Hippocrates recognized that the king suffered not from a melancholic disease that warranted medical treatment but from a problem stemming from romantic longing.

A century after Hippocrates, Aristotle (384–322 B.C.; or one of his students) in the *Problemata* elaborated the distinction between a variety of normal mood states of sadness on the one hand and pathological disease states on the other. Aristotle clearly expressed the idea that disordered sadness is disproportionate to events. He noted that, if the black bile "be cold beyond due measure, it produces groundless despondency."[8] Here "beyond due measure" refers to what is disproportionate to the circumstances, making the resultant sadness "groundless." Such despondency, for example, "accounts for the prevalence of suicide by hanging amongst the young and sometimes amongst older men too."[9]

Aristotle, the master typologist, suggested several distinctions among types of melancholy. One distinction was between melancholic temperament and melancholic disorder. In this regard, Aristotle inaugurated the tradition that has lasted to our own day of associating depressive temperament with exceptional artistic and intellectual ability: "Why is it that all men who have become outstanding in philosophy, statesmanship, poetry or the arts are melancholic, and some to such an extent that they are infected by the diseases arising from black bile. . . . They are all, as has been said, naturally of this character."[10] Aristotle recognized not only melancholic temperament as a normal variant but also an abnormal degree of melancholy that gifted individuals may possess—and may be possessed by. He did not consider this abnormal degree to be disordered because it contributed to their creativity, although it did leave them vulnerable to melancholic disorder. "We are often," Aristotle noted, "in the condition of feeling grief without being able to ascribe any cause to it; such feelings occur to a slight degree in everyone, but those who are thoroughly possessed by them acquire them as a permanent part of their nature."[11] In Aristotle's view, such extreme melancholic temperaments were generally disorders except in the rare instances in which they were an integral part of a gifted individual's creativity.

As in Aristotle's passage, the key distinction in ancient definitions of mel-ancholia was between states of sadness *without cause* and those with similar symptoms that arose from actual losses; only the former were mental disorders. But "without cause" did not mean uncaused, for throughout history depression has been attributed to postulated physical or psychological causes such as exces-sive black bile, disturbances in the circulation of blood, or depletion of energy. Rather, "without cause" meant that the symptoms of depression were not pro-portional to environmental events that would *appropriately* lead to sadness, such as bereavement, rejection in love, economic failure, and the like.[12] Conversely, ancient Greek and Roman physicians did *not* consider symptoms of depression that occurred "with cause" as signs of a mental disorder because they were nor-mal reactions within their contexts.

Aristotle also grappled with the basic problem of how to define "proportionate" sadness. The puzzle he confronted is this: If the level of sadness or fear varies due to circumstances and has no constant "set point" at which health is defined, how can we define health? Aristotle's answer was that there can be relational definitions of health in which the appropriate amount of sadness varies at any given time in pro-portion to the circumstances that surround it. That is, Aristotle had the insight to recognize that the relational property of the proportionality between sadness and circumstances can remain present even as the actual amount of sadness and the circumstances vary: "It is possible that even a varying state may be well attempered, and in a sense be a good condition, . . . since the condition may be warmer when necessary and then cold again, or conversely." With such proportionate variation as the baseline, Aristotle went on to conceptualize his notion of the abnormally melancholic—but not strictly disordered—temperament or personality as the ten-dency of such variation to be extreme on the high end and thus to some degree to overshoot the mark emotionally: "owing to the presence of excess, all melancholic persons are abnormal, not owing to disease but by nature."[13] A similar test would reveal disordered states not due to temperament, as well.

In sum, Aristotle distinguished (1) a melancholic component in all people that gives rise to normal sadness reactions and varying normal moods; (2) a nor-mal-range melancholic temperament in people with a preponderance of black bile and thus an inherent inclination to sadness; (3) an extreme variant of such temperament that often occurs in the gifted and may be considered at least sta-tistically abnormal but is not yet a disease, especially when it is a handmaiden to creativity; and (4) a pathological, harmful, disordered state of disproportionate sadness or sadness without adequate cause that is without a redemptive part in a creative process. Several of these distinctions can be discerned, for example, in the following passage, which also interestingly anticipates the modern notion that in bipolar disorder melancholic despondency and manic over-confidence can be etiologically linked:

> Those who have a small share of this temperament are normal, but those who have much are unlike the majority. If the characteristic is very intense, such men are very melancholic, and if the mixture is of a certain kind, they are abnormal. But if they neglect it, they incline towards melancholic diseases, different people in different parts of the body; with some the symptoms are epileptic, with others apoplectic, others again are given to deep despondency or to fear, others are over-confident.[14]

Ancient Roman physicians followed their Greek predecessors in distinguishing melancholic states that arose with and without cause, associating only the latter with disease. Thus, for example, the Roman physician Celsus (ca. A.D. 30) echoed Hippocrates in defining melancholia as "prolonged despondency and prolonged fear and sleeplessness"[15] that "consists in depression which seems caused by black bile."[16] He advised that, as part of the treatment, the patient's "depression should be gently reproved as being without cause."[17] Soranus of Ephesus, writing in the late first or early second century A.D., described the melancholic as "downcast and prone to anger and . . . practically never cheerful and relaxed," with "the signs of melancholy . . . as follows: mental anguish and distress, dejection, silence, animosity toward members of the household, sometimes a desire to live and at other times a longing for death, suspicion on the part of the patient that a plot is being hatched against him, weeping without reason, meaningless muttering, and, again, occasional joviality," as well as various, mostly gastrointestinal, symptoms.[18] The reference to "weeping without reason" makes explicit the notion that the emotions of intense sadness are to some extent without cause.

Aretaeus of Cappadocia (ca. A.D. 150–200) made the "without cause" criterion more explicit, noting that melancholic "patients are dull or stern, dejected or unreasonably torpid, without any manifest cause; such is the commencement of melancholy. And they also become peevish, dispirited, sleepless, and start up from a disturbed sleep. Unreasonable fear also seizes them."[19] To further distinguish the disordered from the normal who experience, as Aretaeus put it, "mere anger and grief, and sad dejection of mind,"[20] he presented a case (clearly modeled after the story told of Hippocrates) of extreme but normal sadness that featured symptoms identical to those occurring in melancholia and that, consequently, was mistaken for a disorder:

> A story is told, that a certain person, incurably affected, fell in love with a girl; and when the physician could bring him no relief, love cured him. But

I think that he was originally in love, and that he was dejected and spiritless from being unsuccessful with the girl, and appeared to the common people to be melancholic. He then did not know that it was love; but when he imparted the love to the girl, he ceased from his dejection, and dispelled his passion and sorrow; and with joy he awoke from his lowness of spirits, and he became restored to understanding, love being his physician.[21]

Aretaeus thus illustrated how the "without cause" criterion differentiates normal sadness from melancholic disorder, and he pointed to the possibility that normal conditions can be misdiagnosed if symptoms alone are considered.

Like other writers before him, Aretaeus emphasized the delusions of what we would term psychotic depression: "a lowness of spirits from a single phantasy, without fever . . . the understanding is turned . . . in the melancholics to sorrow and despondency only. . . . Those affected with melancholy are not every one of them affected according to one particular form; but they are either suspicious of poisoning, or flee to the desert from misanthropy, or turn superstitious, or contract a hatred of life."[22] Clearly, such delusions, which the literature through to the twentieth century emphasized, provide an alternative to disproportionality as a way of recognizing disorder due to clear cognitive dysfunction.

In the late second century A.D., Claudius Galenus (131–201), known as Galen, like Aretaeus a Greek physician living in Rome, unified and synthesized the psychiatric knowledge that had accumulated over the previous 600 years. Galen simply repeated the Hippocratic definition of melancholia: "Fear or a depressive mood (dysthamia) which lasts for a long time."[23] His description again emphasized psychotic phenomena but also described well the basic symptoms:

Fear generally befalls the melancholic patients, but the same type of abnormal sensory images do not always present themselves. As for instance, one patient believes he has been turned into a kind of snail and therefore runs away from everyone he meets lest [its shell] should get crushed. . . . Again, another patient is afraid that Atlas who supports the world will become tired and will throw it away and we all will be crushed and pushed together. And there are a thousand other imaginary ideas. . . . Although each melancholic patient acts quite differently than the others, all of them exhibit fear or despondency. They find fault with life and hate people; but not all want to die. For some the fear of death is of principal concern during melancholy. Others again will appear to you quite bizarre because they dread death and desire to die at the same time.[24]

In an implicit acknowledgment of the "without cause" criterion, Galen presented a vivid analogy in which he used the color of black bile to characterize the fear that the melancholic was generating from his or her own brain, a fear that would normally be generated from external circumstances:

> Because of this despondency patients hate everyone whom they see, are constantly sullen and appear terrified, like children or adults in deepest darkness. As external darkness renders almost all persons fearful, with the exception of a few naturally audacious ones or those who were specially trained, thus the color of the black humor induces fear when its darkness throws a shadow over the area of thought [in the brain].[25]

The doctrine that emerged in the period between Hippocrates and Galen, distinguishing melancholic states that stemmed from internal dysfunctions in which emotion is "without cause" from those that were proportional reactions to external circumstances, persisted for thousands of years.[26] Explicit sources regarding melancholia are, however, sparse in the following period. Alexander of Tralles (525–605) included "sadness without reason" among the symptoms of melancholia and recommended that, especially in nonchronic cases, the ideas underlying "groundless sadness" should be addressed.[27] The early tenth-century Arabic physician Ishaq ibn Imran reiterated the "without cause" notion when he defined melancholia partly as "irrational, constant sadness and dejection"; yet he also recognized that real losses could trigger true disorder: "The loss of a beloved child or an irreplaceable library can release such sadness and dejection that melancholy is the result."[28] Similarly, Constantinus Africanus (1020?–1087) defined melancholia partly as "fear of things that were not frightening" and noted that the loss of a loved one or of specially beloved possessions, such as a scholar's loss of his books, could trigger melancholia.[29] Avicenna (980–1037) emphasized "fear without cause," including "the appearance of fear of things which do or do not exist; and a greatness of fear of things which are not customarily feared."[30] Often, the "without cause" requirement was implicit in the explanation that an internal process caused the sadness, as in Hildegard of Bingen's (ca. 1151–1158) description: "Melancholy as a Disease. Bile is black, bitter, and releases every evil, sometimes even a brain sickness. It causes the veins in the heart to overflow; it causes depression and doubt in every consolation so that the person can find no joy in heavenly life and no consolation in his earthly existence."[31] Not until the Renaissance, however, did melancholia return to the central place it had had in ancient Greek and Roman psychiatric medicine.

Depression From the Renaissance to the Nineteenth Century

In the late sixteenth and early seventeenth centuries, authors placed even greater emphasis on the "without cause" criterion for disorder. The French physician Andre Du Laurens (1560–1609), known widely as "Laurentius," wrote *Discourse de la melancholie*, which became known throughout Europe and which heavily influenced later thought. Du Laurens summarized the approach of his time as the "without cause" approach: "A kinde of dotage without any fever, having for his ordinarie companions, feare and sadnes, without any apparent occasion."[32]

On the English side of the Channel, Timothie Bright (1550–1615), a Cambridge-trained doctor of medicine contemporary with Du Laurens, was also much concerned with religious guilt. In his *Treatise of Melancholy* (1568), Bright developed at length the distinction between sorrow with and without cause to allow differential diagnosis between true melancholic disorder and nondisordered states of intense sadness and despair due to the belief that one had sinned and would be the object of God's wrath. He noted that melancholic sadness is such "whereof no occasion was at any time before, nor like to be given hereafter"[33] and argued that "the affliction of soule through conscience of sinne" is "quite another thing than melancholy."[34] Consciousness of sin was "a sorrow and feare upon cause, & that the greatest cause that worketh misery unto man" because of fear of God's wrath, whereas melancholy was "a meere fancy & hath no ground of true and just object." Bright explained in lucid detail how the "Particular difference betwixt melancholy, & the distressed conscience in the same person" which is "the soules proper anguish" could be distinguished based on a contextual understanding of whether the sadness had adequate environmental reasons:

> Whatsoever molestation riseth directly as a proper object of the mind, that in that respect is not melancholicke, but hath a farther ground than fancie, and riseth from conscience, condemning the guylty soule of those ingraven lawes of nature, which no man is voyde of, be he never so barbarous. . . . On the contrarie part, when any conceite troubleth you that hath no sufficient ground of reason, but riseth onely upon the frame of your brayne, which is subject (as hath bene before shewed) unto the humour, that is right melancholicke and so to be accounted of you. These are false points of reason deceaved by the melancholie brayne. . . . Thus I conclude this point of difference, & marke betwixt melancholy and the soules proper anguish. . . . [T]he sense of those that are under this crosse feele an anguish far beyond all affliction of naturall passion, coupled with that organicall feare and heavinesse of heart. The melancholie disposeth to feare, doubt, distrust and heavines, but all either without cause, or where there is cause above it inforceth the passion.

Bright goes on to vividly characterize what the phrase "without cause" means, firmly anchoring the notion in an understanding of the context of the feelings:

> We do see by experience certaine persons which enjoy all the comfortes of this life whatsoever wealth can procure, and whatsoever friendship

offereth of kindnes, and whatsoever security may assure them: yet to be overwhelmed with heavines, and dismaide with such feare, as they can neither receive consolation, nor hope of assurance, notwithstanding ther be neither matter of feare, or discontentment, nor yet cause of daunger, but contrarily of great comfort, and gratulation. This passion being not moved by any adversity present or imminent, is attributed to melancholie.[35]

Bright's assumption, which formed the background for the literature from ancient to modern times, was that there exists a "natural passion" or emotion of sadness that was designed to operate a certain way but that had gone wrong in disorder.

Subsequent works followed suit. For example, Felix Platter (1536–1614) in *Praxeos Medicae* (1602) defined melancholy as a state in which "imagination and judgment are so perverted that without any cause the victims become very sad and fearful. For they cannot adduce any certain cause of grief or fear except a trivial one or a false opinion which they have conceived as a result of disturbed apprehension."[36] Like other authors, Platter encompassed within the "without cause" category both cases lacking any actual situational cause (in cases of delusion or endogenous depression) and cases without proportionate cause (in which the cause exists but is too trivial to justify the reaction).

Robert Burton's classic work, *The Anatomy of Melancholy,* published in 1621, is the most renowned of all Renaissance discussions on the topic. It is founded squarely on the "without cause" tradition. Burton described three major components of depression—mood, cognition, and physical symptoms—that are still viewed as the distinguishing features of the condition. However, he insisted that melancholic symptoms are not in themselves sufficient evidence of disorder; only symptoms that are without cause provided such evidence, as he explained in this codicil to his definition: "*without a cause* is lastly inserted, to specify it from all other ordinary passions of Fear and Sorrow." And, he noted, "signs in the mind" of melancholia included "Sorrow . . . without any evident cause; grieving still, but why they cannot tell."[37]

Burton emphasized that a propensity to melancholy was present in all men, and was a normal and ubiquitous aspect of the human condition:

Melancholy . . . is either in disposition or habit. In disposition, it is that transitory melancholy which goes and comes upon every small occasion of sorrow, need, sickness, trouble, fear, grief, passion, or perturbation of the mind, any manner of care, discontent, or thought, which causeth anguish, dullness, heaviness, and vexation of spirit. . . . And from these melancholy dispositions, no man living is free, no Stoic, none so wise, none so happy, none so patient, so generous, so godly, so divine, that can vindicate himself; so well composed, but more or less, some time or other, he feels the smart of it. Melancholy, in this sense is the character of mortality.[38]

In contrast to normal melancholy that arises naturally in people who have suffered loss and disappointment and that is part of the "character of mortality," Burton held that melancholic afflictions are "contrary to nature."[39] This latter condition, the disorder of melancholy, he defined (following Du Laurens) as "a kind of dotage without a fever, having for his ordinary companions fear and sadness, *without any apparent occasion.*"[40]

Burton was sensitive to the wide individual variation in the nature of loss responses, and he allowed a quite broad range of temperamental reactions to loss to be considered nondisordered as long as they did not become chronic and self-perpetuating:

> For that which is but a flea-biting to one, causeth insufferable torment to another, & which one by his singular moderation, & well composed carriage can happily overcome, a second is no whit able to sustaine, but upon every small occasion of misconceived abuse, injurie, griefe, disgrace, losse, crosse, rumor, &c. (if solitary, or idle) yields so farre to passion, that his complexion is altered, his digestion hindred, his sleepe gone, his spirits obscured, and his heart heavy, his Hypocondries misaffected . . . and he himselfe over come with Melancholy. . . . But all these Melancholy fits . . . are but improperly so called, because they continue not; but come & goe, as by some objects they are moved.[41]

It is only when such normal reactions to specific events become established as an ongoing condition independent of events that Burton sees disorder:

> (I)t falleth out oftentimes that these Dispositions become Habits, and . . . make a disease. Even as one Distillation, not yet growne to custome, makes a cough; but continuall and inveterate causeth a consumption of the lungs: so doe these our Melancholy provocations. . . . This Melancholy of which we are to treat . . . a Chronicke or continuate disease, setled humor . . . not errant but fixed . . . growne to an habit, it will hardly be removed.[42]

In addition to noting normal variation in temperament, Burton was an astute observer of the extremes to which normal reactions to loss could go. He noted that the most extremely painful losses included separation from friends and bereavement following loss of a loved one ("in this Labyrinth of accidental causes [of melancholy] . . . loss and death of friends may challenge first place"[43]) and compellingly described the extremes that nondisordered grief can reach:

> If parting of friends, absence alone, can work such violent effects, what shall death do, when they must eternally be separated, never in this world to meet again? This is so grievous a torment for the time, that it takes

away their appetite, desire of life, extinguisheth all delights, it causeth deep sighs and groans, tears, exclamations . . . howling, roaring, many bitter pangs, and by frequent mediation extends so far sometimes, they think they see their dead friends continually in their eyes. . . . Still, still, still, that good father, that good son, that good wife, that dear friend runs in their minds; a single thought fills all their mind all year long. . . . They that are most staid and patient are so furiously carried headlong by the passion of sorrow in this case, that brave discreet men otherwise often-times forget themselves, and weep like children many months together.[44]

It was not only renowned writers such as Burton but also ordinary medical practitioners who distinguished between melancholic states that arose without cause and those that were proportionate in intensity to their provoking causes. The work of Richard Napier (1559–1634), a physician in rural England whose notebooks have been closely analyzed by the historian Michael MacDonald, illustrates how general physicians of the period classified depressive conditions into three general sorts. The first stemmed from universal experiences of sorrow and grief, rejection in love, loss of fortune, severe illness, and conflicts with spouses, lovers, or parents. Napier explicitly separated these sorts of ubiquitous adverse states from melancholic diseases so that "not every gloomy person suffered from the disease of melancholy."[45]

Two kinds of melancholic states were considered disorders. First, Napier used the term "baseless sorrow" for some of his disordered patients.[46] This referred to cases that were unprovoked or delusional, thus wholly unexplained by external circumstances. The second type of disordered conditions stemmed from sources such as "legitimate occasions in the death of loved ones and were revealed to be the sign of melancholy delusion by their unusual intensity and duration."[47] As MacDonald notes, "Contemporaries believed that the feelings experienced by melancholy and troubled people were exaggerations of normal states of mind. The sheer intensity of their moods was abnormal."[48] Napier's records clearly show that melancholia often arose without situational provocations but sometimes stemmed from a disproportionate response to actual losses. Many diagnoses of melancholia, for example, resulted from bereavement, usually after the loss of a spouse or a child,[49] in which the sadness was of such intensity and duration that it led to states of madness. Judgments of disease consequently required the physician to obtain knowledge of the relationship of the symptoms to the context of the situations in which they arose and persisted.

Writers who followed Burton continued to separate depressions that were with and without cause. For example, toward the end of the seventeenth century, Timothy Rogers (1658–1728) considered the difference between bereavement as normal response to loss and as a triggering cause of depressive disorder. He observed that many people can have a melancholic disorder triggered "by the loss of Children, by some sudden and unlooked for disappointment that ruines all their former Projects and Designs."[50] But Rogers made it clear that such horrible losses do not usually lead to melancholic disorder. He specifically contrasts such a disordered reaction with that of one Lady Mary Lane, to whom his book is dedicated, who experienced intense but normal grief and sorrow at the loss of her father, mother, and several children.[51]

In the eighteenth century the explicit use of the "without cause" criterion became less common, perhaps because writers in this period focused on psychotic forms of depression in which this description seemed unnecessary.[52] Nevertheless, during this period, madness, according to historian Stanley Jackson, "still usually involved a state of dejection and fearfulness *without an apparent cause,* and some particular circumscribed delusion was still a common feature. Sleeplessness, irritability, restlessness, and constipation continued to be usual elements."[53] Samuel Johnson's famous dictionary, for example, contained three meanings for *melancholia;* two refer to mental disorders and one to common, normal emotions.[54] Incidentally, Johnson was partially responsible for beginning the trend to gradually replace the term *melancholia* with *depression.*

Subsequent medical definitions continued to explicitly use the ancient, contextual definition of melancholia. Friedrich Hoffmann (1660–1742) characterized melancholy as "associated with sadness and fear not having any manifest cause."[55] William Cullen (1710–1790), the preeminent authority on melancholy during the latter part of the eighteenth century, noted that melancholy is "always attended with some seemingly groundless, but very anxious, fear."[56] And in the United States, the famed clergyman Cotton Mather (1663–1728) emphasized the lack of sufficient external justification for sadness in melancholic disorder: "These Melancholicks, do sufficiently *Afflict themselves,* and are Enough their *own Tormentors.* As if this *present Evil World,* would not *Really* afford Sad Things Enough, they create a World of *Imaginary Ones,* and by *Mediating Terror,* they make themselves as Miserable, as they could be from the most *Real Miseries.*"[57] Even the philosopher Immanuel Kant (1724–1804) broadly defined melancholia as "unjustified . . . grief" and carefully distinguished a variety of nondisordered conditions, such as individuals who fashionably immerse themselves in melancholic feelings or the supposed "melancholy mathematician" who in fact is merely introverted and thoughtful, from true mental disorder.[58]

The Nineteenth Century

At the beginning of the nineteenth century, the eminent psychiatrist Philippe Pinel (1745–1826) continued to maintain the fundamental separation between melancholic disorders and the consequences of real misfortunes. In his 1801 book on mental disorder, *Traite Medico-Philosophique Sur l'Alienation Mentale,* Pinel noted that melancholia afflicted "some men otherwise in good health, and frequently in prosperous circumstances. Nothing, however, can be more hideous than the figure of a melancholic, brooding over his imaginary misfortunes."[59] Pinel also provided a particularly important application of the proportionality thesis when he distinguished possible nondisordered from disordered causes of suicide. Observing that the French philosopher Montesquieu, in a sophisticated cross-Channel putdown, distinguished nondisordered culturally shaped Roman suicides ("the effect of education; it depended upon their customs and manner of thinking") from disordered English self-destruction ("The English frequently destroy themselves without any apparent cause to determine them to such an act, and even in the midst of prosperity"), Pinel endorses Montesquieu's distinction. He elaborates by saying that normal triggers for suicide might include severe social humiliation or financial reversal, and he performs an act of medical diplomacy regarding disordered sources of suicide by asserting that this is not just an English disease: "The propensity to this horrid deed as existing independent of the ordinary powerful motives to it, such as the loss of honour or fortune is by no means a disease peculiar to England: it is far from being of rare occurrence in France."[60]

A notable student of Pinel's, Jean-Etienne-Dominique Esquirol (1772–1840), continued to embrace the contextual tradition, noting that the disparity between reality and the intensity of sadness may be apparent even to the sufferer: "Some . . . possess a knowledge of their condition, have a consciousness of its falsity, and of the absurdity of the fears in which they are tormented. They perceive clearly that they are irrational, and often confess it, with grief and even despair."[61] Benjamin Rush (1745–1813), known as "the father of American psychiatry," similarly allowed for melancholia to be characterized by false beliefs or disproportionate responses to beliefs:

> Partial derangement consists in error in opinion, and conduct, upon some one subject only, with soundness of mind upon all, or nearly all other subjects. The error in this case is two-fold. It is directly contrary to truth, or it is disproportioned in its effects, or expected consequences, to the causes which induce them.[62]

The prominent British psychiatrist, Henry Maudsley (1835–1918), also noted the misdirection of the melancholic's response in that "impressions which should be agreeable or indifferent are painful."[63] He offered some extreme examples of disproportion:

> In some cases it is striking how disproportionate the delusion is to the extreme mental anguish, the patient assigning some most ridiculously inadequate cause for his gloom: one man under my care, whose suffering was very great, said that it was because he had drunk a glass of beer which he ought not to have done, and another man was, as he thought, lost for ever because he had muttered a curse when he ought to have uttered a prayer.[64]

Maudsley insisted that any delusional ideas are a result, not a cause, of the affective intensification that comes with the disorder.

The influential German psychiatrist Wilhelm Griesinger (1817–1868) also used the disproportionality of melancholic symptoms to their context to define when they indicated a disorder:

> The melancholia which precedes insanity sometimes appears externally as the direct continuation of some painful emotion dependent upon some objective cause . . . e.g., grief, jealousy; and it is distinguished from the mental pain experienced by healthy persons by its excessive degree, by its more than ordinary protraction, by its becoming more and more independent of external influences, and by the other accessory affections which accompany it. In other cases the melancholia originates without any moral cause.[65]

Greisinger called melancholia "a state of profound emotional perversion, of a depressing and sorrowful character";[66] the intended notion of "perversion" is the turning away of a feeling from the objects at which it would be naturally and proportionately aimed. He noted that melancholia involves the same feelings as in nondisordered responses such as grief and jealousy but that it is distinguished by excessive intensity, duration, and, most of all, its "objective groundlessness" in relation to actual external events.[67] But he acknowledged that "the boundary betwixt the physiological state of emotion and insanity is often difficult to trace" because the disorder "may appear as the immediate continuation of a physiological state of the established emotion." He asserts that "the essential difference" between the disorder of melancholia and a nondisordered "gloomy disposition" is that "in the former the patient cannot withdraw himself from his ill-humour."[68]

Simultaneously with the further elaboration and acceptance of the contextual understanding of depressive disorder, another momentous development was occurring in medical thought. As physicians branched out of the asylum and began to see more patients in private practice, they confronted a much larger proportion of patients coming in for help with intense sadness who had no delusions or other psychotic symptoms. Such forms of melancholia had been recognized since antiquity, but the emphasis had always been on the delusional cases ("dotage without a fever"). But now the form without delusion became singled out as "simple" melancholia, the forerunner of today's nonpsychotic unipolar major depression.

For example, the British psychiatrist D. Hack Tuke (1827–1895) explicitly rejected the idea that melancholia must involve delusion and identified the "simple" form that is purely a matter of symptoms of sadness without cognitive impairment, embracing a category of "melancholia, without delusion" along with a melancholic form of "delusional insanity."[69] He insisted that in simple melancholia there is "no disorder of the intellect . . . no delusion or hallucination."[70] But nonetheless he detected "a cerebral malady . . . sustained by a passion of a sad, debilitiating, or oppressive character."[71] Such definitions became broadly accepted and anticipated the contemporary focus on the kind of depressive disorder that is easiest to confuse with normal emotional responses.

The greater attention to simple melancholia implied an even more exclusive focus on contextual criteria in the general definition of melancholia. For example, psychiatrist John Charles Bucknill (1817–1897), the author of the chapter on diagnosing insanity in a well-known manual, separated normal from disordered symptoms using the "without cause" criterion but with no reference to delusion:

> The symptoms of melancholia are sorrow, despondency, fear, and despair, existing in a degree far beyond the intensity in which these emotions usually affect the sane mind, even under circumstances most capable of producing them; and in numerous instances existing without any commensurate moral cause, and often without any moral cause whatever.[72]

Due to the nervous system's responses, "proportioned excitement of function disappears."[73] Bucknill also held that symptoms of "uncomplicated melancholia . . . vary in degree, but not in kind, from that normal and healthy grief and sorrow, of which all men have their share in this chequered existence."[74] As to precipitating causes, he noted: "it is occasioned by all the moral causes of mental disease; especially by griefs, disappointments, reverses, and anxieties of every kind. It is also caused by long-continued ill-health."[75] However, Bucknill insisted that disorder that was triggered by normal grief generally required a hereditary disposition as well.[76]

Likewise, psychiatrist Charles Mercier (1852–1918), in his entry on melancholia in Tuke's influential *Dictionary of Psychological Medicine*, relied exclusively on proportionality to actual events in defining melancholia as "a disorder characterized by a feeling of misery which is in excess of what is justified by the circumstances in which the individual is placed."[77] He noted the possible gradual onset until an excessive, disproportionate level of symptoms is reached and the possible interaction between stress and heredity: "At length the degree of misery and the other symptoms reach such a grade at which the limits of the normal are unmistakably exceeded, and it becomes manifest that the patient is suffering from a morbid depression."[78] Mercier recognized that the causes of normal intense sadness could be risk factors for the development of disorder:

> Untoward circumstances, the loss of friends, or of fortune, or of character; any circumstance which is calculated to produce sorrow, grief, uneasiness, anxiety, in an ordinarily constituted person, may, if it acts upon a person of less than ordinary stamina, produce melancholia. . . . The

more severe the stress, the greater, naturally, is the chance of melancholia occurring.[79]

French physician Maurice de Fleury (1860–1931), in *Medicine and the Mind*, characterized the illness simply as "causeless melancholy."[80] He also offered an explanation of how normal grief over time may transform into disorder, analogous to what is these days known as the "kindling hypothesis": "Grief is a special, lower pitch of brain activity. The mind, if it stays there for a certain time, will form the habit, and henceforward everything will appear to it in a painful, melancholy, pessimistic light."[81]

Another psychiatrist, George H. Savage (1842–1921), emphasized the internal causes of melancholic states that were disordered. He defined melancholia as "a state of mental depression, in which the misery is unreasonable either in relation to its apparent cause, or in the peculiar form it assumes, the mental pain depending on physical and bodily changes, and not directly on the *environment*."[82] Like most other writers, he accepted the category of simple melancholia: "Simple melancholia, i.e., those in whom the misery and its expression are simply slight exaggerations of natural states, those cases in whom there is no real delusion, no fiction such as that they are ruined or damned . . . frequently, the misery gives rise to the delusion."[83]

The most popular psychiatric text of the late nineteenth century, Richard von Krafft-Ebing's (1840–1902) *Text-Book of Insanity*, continued to define melancholia in terms of proportionality of response: "The fundamental phenomenon in melancholia consists of the painful emotional depression, which has no external, or an insufficient external, cause, and general inhibition of the mental activities, which may be entirely arrested."[84]

For Krafft-Ebing:

A painful, depressed state of feeling . . . that has arisen spontaneously and exists independently, is the fundamental phenomenon in the melancholic states of insanity. . . . Even objects which under other conditions would give rise to pleasant impressions seem now, in the mirror of his abnormally changed sense of self, to be worthy of aversion.[85]

Krafft-Ebing observed the challenge of distinguishing normal from abnormal depressive states, especially in cases of simple melancholia:

The content of the melancholic consciousness is psychic pain, distress, and depression. . . . This painful depression in its content does not differ from the painful depression due to efficient causes. . . . The content of melancholic delusions is extremely varied, for they include all varieties of human trouble, care, and fear. . . . The common character of all melancholic delusions is that of suffering. . . . Simple melancholia is decidedly the most frequent form of mental disease . . . only exceptionally observed in institutions for the insane, but it is extremely frequent in private practice (with) innumerable slight cases that do not reach the hospital.[86]

Conclusion

What is striking about this brief overview of conceptualizations of depressive disorder from Hippocrates to Krafft-Ebing is, first, the remarkable consistency of the symptoms that are mentioned—by and large the same kinds of symptoms that current diagnostic manuals emphasize. And, second, there is a remarkably solid and well-elaborated tradition of distinguishing disorder from normal emotion via various versions of the "with cause" versus "without cause" criterion that goes back to ancient times. The entire 2,500-year record indicates an understanding that pathological depression is an exaggerated form of a normal human emotional response and thus that the first step in diagnostic logic must be to use the relation to triggering causes to distinguish the normal from the disordered. A third point is the recent move toward greater focus on "simple melancholia" without delusion, yielding even more reliance on the contextual "without cause" criterion in defining the distinction between normal-range and disordered sadness and presaging our contemporary focus on nonpsychotic unipolar disorder. The power, consistency, and rationale of the "without cause" medical understanding of depressive disorder form the backdrop for the next century's radical departures in diagnostic approach. The following chapter traces the fate of this tradition during the twentieth century.

4

Depression in the Twentieth Century

U ntil the end of the nineteenth century, psychiatry generally used the relationship of symptoms to their provoking causes as an essential part of definitions of melancholic disorder. Although some kinds of cases, such as psychotic depressions, almost always displayed symptoms that implied disorder, diagnosticians understood that they had to consider context, because depressive disorder could often be symptomatically indistinguishable from profound normal sadness. In the late 1800s, the traditional contextual approach to diagnosis of depressive disorder began to divide into two distinct schools. On one side, Sigmund Freud and his followers emphasized the psychological etiology of all mental disorders, including depression, and their continuity with normal functioning. Adherents of this school studied and interpreted the patient's reported thoughts to surmise the existence of underlying unconscious pathogenic meanings and wishes. On the other side, Emil Kraepelin applied a classical medical model that examined the symptoms, course, and prognosis of depression and other disorders to define distinct physical pathologies. Kraepelin's approach inspired a cadre of researchers to translate it into a research program that often used statistical techniques to infer discrete disorders from manifest symptoms.

Many psychiatrists viewed the publication of the *DSM-III* in 1980 as finally resolving the struggle between the Freudian and Kraepelinian schools for the domination of psychiatric nosology largely in favor of Kraepelin's approach.[1] We will see, however, that such a judgment is overly simplistic in many ways. Specifically with respect to depressive disorder, the *DSM-III* criteria in fact represented a rejection of key assumptions underlying both Freud's and Kraepelin's systems and an affirmation of a quite different research tradition that ignored the prior emphasis on contextual criteria.

Continuation of the "With" and "Without" Cause Tradition in the Twentieth Century

Psychodynamic Approaches to Disordered and Normal Sadness

At the beginning of the twentieth century, the Austrian neurologist-turned-psychoanalyst Sigmund Freud (1856–1939) and his disciples developed a revolutionary approach to the study of mental disorders. The heart of this approach was the effort to understand pathological symptoms in terms of unconscious mental processes, rather than in terms of biological predispositions and organic etiologies. Although he acknowledged that the intensity of specific desires involved in pathogenesis could be indirectly due to constitution, Freud focused on postulating immediate causes that were often purely psychogenic, such as repressed desires, psychological conflicts, or the transformation of repressed motivational energy into anxiety, all of which had little to do with hereditary or other direct physical causes. Psychoanalysts paid relatively little direct attention to treating symptoms themselves and focused instead on identifying the underlying, and presumably unconscious, dynamics of mental disorders, which they thought maintained the symptoms. In addition, given the sorts of conflicts and other psychological processes they postulated as etiologies, psychoanalysts viewed the psychodynamics that underlie mental disorders as generally continuous with, not discrete from, the psychodynamics present in normality, thus blurring the boundary between normality and disorder.

For psychoanalysts, depression was one major mechanism underlying symptom formation that, to some degree, was present in nearly every neurosis. They postulated a continuum between ordinary states of sadness, neurotic states of depression, and psychotic states of melancholia. Analysts, for example, considered manic depression an extremely exaggerated expression of the same psychological processes that underlie the universal heightening and reduction of self-esteem that all people experience.[2]

Analytic attempts to explain depression were based on traditional assumptions about the differences between depressive conditions that arose with and without expectable environmental causes. Karl Abraham (1877–1925), a disciple of Freud's, provided the first psychoanalytic explanation of depression, grounding his theory in the distinction between normal grief and depression.[3] Abraham considered outwardly similar states, such as grief and depression, as in fact distinct because they involved different underlying etiological dynamics. The mourner's grief, Abraham explained, stemmed from a conscious preoccupation with the lost person. In contrast, the depressed person was preoccupied with guilt and low self-esteem. Moreover, symptoms of depression resulted from the depressed person's unconscious turning inward of hostility toward another person; hence the common psychoanalytic description of depression as "anger turned inward" and resultant therapeutic strategies aimed at having the patient express the repressed anger.

Freud elaborated on Abraham's distinction between normal grief and depression in his central article on depression, "Mourning and Melancholia." Freud began his essay by noting the differences between normal grief and melancholia and explaining that

> Although grief involves grave departures from the normal attitude to life, it never occurs to us to regard it as a morbid condition and hand the mourner over to medical treatment. We rest assured that after a lapse of time it will be overcome, and we look upon any interference with it as inadvisable or even harmful.[4]

Freud distinguished between the normality of grief and the disorder of melancholia. He asserted that symptoms associated with mourning are intense and are "grave departures from the normal," in the sense that grief is greatly different from usual functioning. Nevertheless, grief is not a "morbid" condition; that is, it is not a medical disorder that represents the breakdown of a biologically normal response. Thus it does not require medical treatment; indeed, Freud emphasized that it would "never occur to us" to provide medical treatment to the bereaved. In addition, he stressed that grief is naturally self-healing, so that with time the mourner would return to a normal psychological state. Medical intervention, he suggested, could actually harm the grieving person through interfering with this natural process.

While noting that mourners did not suffer from the same unwarranted decline in self-esteem that characterized melancholics, Freud emphasized that their symptoms were otherwise similar. Both mourning and melancholia featured profound dejection, loss of interest in the outside world, an inability to feel pleasure, and an inhibition of activity. The distinction between mourning and melancholia lay not so much in their symptoms but in the fact that the former state was a normal reaction to loss, whereas the latter state was pathological.

Freud's version of the distinction between depressions with cause (mourning) and without cause (melancholia) allowed him to elucidate the different psychodynamics that underlay the two conditions. For mourners, the world came to feel empty and without meaning due to conscious losses, whereas melancholics experienced the ego as impoverished due to unconscious losses. The self-reproaches of melancholics pathologically redirected their internalized hostility from earlier love objects onto the self. Therapy, therefore, should teach them to express their inward anger toward the objects that are its actual targets. In contrast, people who experience normal sadness are going through a natural and necessary process that it was "inadvisable or even harmful" to disrupt with medical treatment.

Freud rejected the 2,500-year tradition that postulated physiological causes of pathological depression and adopted a psychogenic theory of causation. Nonetheless, Freud and other psychoanalysts largely accepted as self-evident the traditional distinction between normal intense sadness resulting from loss and symptomatically quite similar pathological depression disproportionate to loss.

Kraepelin and Depressive Disorder

Emil Kraepelin (1856–1926), a German psychiatrist and a contemporary of Freud, attempted to place psychiatry within a strictly biomedical framework that considered mental disorders as manifestations of physical brain pathologies. He used the symptoms and course of disorders to create categories that, he claimed, represented distinct underlying pathological conditions, which he hoped would eventually be confirmed by the identification of anatomical lesions. He built on earlier work that attempted to separate asylum patients into those who might be restored to the community versus those likely to deteriorate. Kraepelin famously used prognosis to distinguish between manic-depressive insanity (now bipolar disorder), which tended to occur in episodes and remit, and dementia praecox (now schizophrenia), which tended to have a deteriorating course, as two fundamental forms of psychotic disorder.

Kraepelin's contributions to psychiatric diagnosis, especially his efforts at categorization based on careful attention to symptoms, are now generally seen as the forerunner of the later *DSM-III* transformation of psychiatric diagnosis. Indeed, the recent *DSMs* are now often referred to as "neo-Kraepelinian."[5] Some prominent historians of medicine, prompted by his perceived relationship to the *DSM-III* approach, see Kraepelin as the major figure in modern psychiatry, surpassing even Freud: "It is Kraepelin," asserts Edward Shorter, "not Freud, who is the central figure in the history of psychiatry."[6] Because Kraepelin's diagnostic approach has become linked to that of the *DSM*, it is pertinent to consider his views at some length.

Kraepelin began his career as a physician in a Munich asylum and maintained his almost exclusive interest in psychotic disorders as a professor at Heidelberg and as the director of the Psychiatric Clinic at Munich.[7] He developed his classification system using descriptions of inpatient cases. Inpatient mental institutions had become a common setting for treating the seriously mentally ill during the nineteenth century.[8] Before this time, most depressed patients, such as those of Richard Napier, would have visited community-based physicians who treated a great variety of severe and less severe conditions. Persons whose sadness stemmed from life problems would have typically handled the problem themselves, sought help from friends and family, or consulted general physicians or clergy.[9]

The effect of the mental hospital was to concentrate the most seriously disturbed, and only this group, within a single location. Those who entered asylums would typically have had such severe conditions that the issue of whether or not their current symptoms were proportionate responses to their circumstances would not have arisen. The pressing question for Kraepelin, therefore, was not whether asylum patients had disorders or normal unhappiness but rather what particular types of disorders they had.

Kraepelin confronted a field in intellectual chaos, with no consensual diagnostic system. Everyone since Greek times had used symptoms to individuate disorders. But without any commonly shared principle for how to divide up the varied symptomatic presentations that physicians and psychiatrists saw, the use of symptoms allowed for many different classification schemes. At one extreme were those who classified virtually any symptom presentation as a separate disorder, leading to disorder proliferation that could reach hundreds of categories. At the other extreme were those who, focusing on psychosis, considered all mental disorders to be variants of a single disorder.[10] For example, the first U.S. census survey to ask about mental disorder in 1840 reflected the latter approach and contained just one category of mental disorder, "insanity."[11]

Kraepelin's careful attention to symptoms and their course in inferring distinct pathological states that caused the symptoms followed a tradition in physical medicine started by the eighteenth-century English physician Thomas Sydenham and developed by the nineteenth-century German pathologist Rudolph Virchow. This approach had been highly successful in helping to distinguish physical diseases, especially as knowledge of infectious agents and physical pathology rapidly grew.[12]

Kraepelin was no doubt also greatly influenced by the growing realization that one of the most dreadful mental disorders of his time, general paresis (about which he wrote a book), resulted from the syphilitic infection of the nervous system. This startling discovery seemed to impart two lessons. First, mental disorders, like physical disorders, could be due to underlying physical pathology of some kind and thus fit directly within traditional diagnostic theory. Second, diagnosticians identified general paresis as a specific syndrome based on its symptoms and its horrific and rapid course and poor prognosis; like syphilis itself, the symptoms changed over time and could differ markedly at different stages of the disease, yet the same underlying disorder was present and simply unfolding. The moral seemed clear; it is not just symptoms at any particular time but symptoms over the course of an illness that served to identify the illness.

Kraepelin's descriptions of the depressive symptoms that occur in the course of various affective or mood disorders—which included psychic symptoms, such as slowness of thinking, sense of hopelessness, inner torment, inhibited activity, and inability to feel pleasure, as well as physical symptoms, such as sleep and appetite disorders and fatigue—remain the basis of current diagnostic classifications of depressive disorders. A cornerstone of Kraepelin's thinking was that a great variety of symptomatic presentations of affective disorders in fact represented one underlying pathology. Based on this hypothetical underlying unity of various symptom presentations, he classified even individuals who were only depressed and had no manic symptoms as having manic-depressive disorder. "In the course of the years," Kraepelin emphasized, "I have become more and more convinced that all (melancholic) states only represent manifestations of a *single morbid process.*"[13] Kraepelin's belief that unipolar depressive states represented variations of the same underlying illness condition as did manic-depressive states was based on the evidence of their overlapping symptoms and the frequent appearance of manic symptoms during recurrences later in the course of disorders that initially displayed only depressive symptoms. Over time, many affective patients had depressive states, manic states, and mixed states. Kraepelin also included within the manic-depressive category even "slight" mood disorders that pass "without sharp boundary into the domain of personal predisposition," under the assumption that these mild conditions were rudiments of and often developed into more severe disorders.[14]

Kraepelin also maintained that most affective disorders stemmed from hereditary predispositions; consequently, "attacks of manic-depressive insanity may be to an astonishing degree *independent of external influences.*"[15] Even many cases that seemed to arise normally from external influences such as deaths, quarrels, unrequited love, infidelity, or financial difficulties actually were manifestations of disorders that stemmed from innate dispositions. "The real cause," Kraepelin wrote, "of the malady must be sought in *permanent internal changes,* which at least very often, perhaps always, are innate."[16] These conditions could be distinguished from normality by telltale evidence such as manic symptoms, inexplicable recurrence, psychotic ideation, or duration well beyond the cessation of the trigger.

The relationship between Kraepelin's work and the *DSM-III* revolution is complex and less clear than is often maintained. The major developer of the *DSM-III,* psychiatrist Robert Spitzer, denies being a "neo-Kraepelinian" on the grounds that he assumes neither that there must be distinct categorical pathologies that underlie different syndromes nor that mental disorders are largely due to physical brain diseases, both basic tenets of Kraepelin's approach.[17] Most fundamentally, Kraepelin rejected the use of any rigid system of symptoms as necessary and sufficient indicators of disorder. Instead, he used all the available evidence, including the prognosis of symptoms, to infer whether various conditions were likely due to the same pathology. He was, contrary to common belief, *against* the sole use of symptomatic criteria to infer which disorder was present. Of course, diagnosticians have to use symptoms as their main resource, but Kraepelin did this in a way that was intended to transcend symptoms and get at underlying pathology, an approach in tension with the *DSM-III*'s heavy reliance on operational definitions solely via symptom syndromes.

Kraepelin's approach to diagnosing distinct pathologies obviously depended on the prior identification of conditions as pathologies, distinct from nonpathological states that do not involve any underlying pathological etiology. How, then, did Kraepelin deal with the distinction between normal sadness and disorder?

Kraepelin and Normal Sadness

Previous commentators have not examined Kraepelin's approach to distinguishing normal sadness from disorder. Admittedly, his works contain little explicitly about this distinction. As noted, the asylum context in which he worked tended to make this distinction irrelevant, as all his patients likely had disorders. Moreover, Kraepelin, like many psychiatrists, was more worried about false negatives and the harm that missing a true case could do than about false positives that mislabel a normal person as disordered.

Nonetheless, Kraepelin required such a distinction, and he embraced the same doctrine as had the medical tradition that preceded him, namely, that nondisordered intense sadness occurs in response to a variety of losses and can symptomatically resemble depressive disorder. Kraepelin thus accepted the traditional principle that the way to distinguish pathological depressive disorder from normal sadness was to determine whether the sadness was without cause (or without proportional cause). Although he did not explicitly state the "without cause" principle directly in his diagnostic criteria, he did make his position on normal sadness clear in scattered remarks:

> Morbid emotions are distinguished from healthy emotions chiefly through the lack of a sufficient cause, as well as by their intensity and persistence. . . . Even in normal life moods come and go in an unaccountable way, but we are always able to control and dispel them, while morbid moods defy all attempts at control. Again, morbid emotions sometimes attach themselves to some certain external occasions, but they do not vanish with the cause like normal feelings, and they acquire a certain independence.[18]

Here, Kraepelin emphasized that either morbid states were without "sufficient cause" in circumstances or, when they initially seem to be with cause, they became independent of circumstances and continued even after circumstances changed. Such cases include conditions that were initially disorders, as well as conditions that began as normal responses but subsequently became morbid.

Kraepelin addressed the issue of differentiating between disorder and normal sadness in some of his case presentations, such as the following:

> I will first place before you a farmer, aged fifty-nine, who was admitted to the hospital a year ago. . . . On being questioned about his illness, he breaks into lamentations, saying that he did not tell the whole truth on his

admission, but concealed the fact that he had fallen into sin in his youth and practiced uncleanness with himself; everything he did was wrong. "I am so apprehensive, so wretched; I cannot lie still for anxiety. O God, if I had only not transgressed so grievously!" . . . The illness began gradually seven or eight months before his admission, without any assignable cause. Loss of appetite and dyspepsia appeared first, and then ideas of sin. . . . The most striking feature of this clinical picture is the *apprehensive depression.* At first sight, it resembles the anxieties of a healthy person, and the patient says that he was always rather apprehensive, and has only grown worse. But there is not the least external cause for the apprehension, and yet it has lasted for months, with increasing severity. This is the diagnostic sign of its morbidity.[19]

Kraepelin noted that even the extreme emotional and physiological symptoms of this patient were consistent with intense normal sadness, especially in a person with a dispositional tendency toward the melancholic side. But, he observed, the patient's symptoms started "without any assignable cause." Moreover, in addition to the fact that "there is not the least external cause for the apprehension," the condition had lasted months (and thus has a prolonged and seemingly inordinate duration) and had not, as normal sadness episodes do, displayed a trajectory of decreasing symptoms; far from it, it has shown "increasing severity" over time even though nothing new occurred in the circumstances to warrant such changes. This disconnection of the patient's condition from external events, and especially the lack of a trajectory showing normal coping and mastery, "is the diagnostic sign of its morbidity."

Kraepelin diagnosed this patient as depressively disordered, and the patient would surely also qualify for the *DSM* diagnosis of Major Depressive Disorder on the basis of the duration and symptoms of the depressive episode, including sleep problems, appetite problems, depressive mood, and intense unjustified guilt and self-reproach. But Kraepelin's comments on differential diagnosis of this depressive disorder from normal sadness imply a divergence from the *DSM*, not in the case of this patient but in the cases of normal responses that might resemble this patient's in manifest symptomatology. What is critical in Kraepelin's discussion is that, after reciting the duration and the symptoms, he noted that "at first sight, it resembles the anxieties of a healthy person," especially one with somewhat melancholic (but normal range) temperament. (Indeed, the patient's lamentations and guilt remind one of Timothie Bright's descriptions, reviewed in the last chapter, of cases of intense normal guilt due to believing one has sinned against God's law.) That is, Kraepelin recognized that symptoms of this duration and severity can be a normal response to events. It is, according to Kraepelin, not the duration or symptoms in themselves but their lack of proportional relation to any plausible external cause that allowed him to see that this condition was a disorder. In contrast, based on its symptom and 2-week duration criteria, the *DSM* would automatically diagnose such an individual as depressively disordered without the kind of assessment Kraepelin performed. From the *DSM*'s perspective, Kraepelin's painstaking discussion is pointless because the possibility of normal response does not exist given the symptoms, so there is no differential diagnosis to be made.

In another passage in which he reiterated the "without cause" criterion as central to diagnosis, Kraepelin made it clear that, even in his day when more severe cases were the rule among psychiatric patients, there was a real possibility of misclassifying a normal person as disordered because the symptoms could be identical:

> Under certain circumstances it may become very difficult to distinguish an attack of manic-depressive insanity from a *psychogenic* state of depression. Several times patients have been brought to me, whose deep dejection, poverty of expression, and anxious tension tempt to the assumption of a circular depression, while it came out afterwards, that they were cases of moodiness, which had for their cause serious delinquencies and threatened legal proceedings. As the slighter depressions of manic-depressive insanity, as far as we are able to make a survey, may wholly resemble the well-founded moodiness of health, with the essential difference that they arise without occasion, it will sometimes not be possible straightway to arrive at a correct interpretation without knowledge of the previous history in cases of the kind mentioned.[20]

Although Kraepelin recognized some psychogenic depressions (i.e., those caused by strictly psychological factors that do not include whatever biological pathology underlies manic-depressive conditions) as disorders, he also used the term *psychogenic* to refer to normal sadness states with sufficient external cause. The crucial point, which Kraepelin derived from his experience, is that "the slighter depressions of manic-depressive insanity, as far as we are able to make a survey, may wholly resemble the well-founded moodiness of health, with the essential difference that they arise without occasion."

Kraepelin acknowledged that he initially believed that the patients in question were disordered, noting that the facts about the context that reversed his judgment only "came out afterwards." This confirms that Kraepelin understood that the symptomatic presentation of normal and disordered cases could be the same, and it explains why he emphasized that the causal context was the essential differentiating criterion. It is also worth noting that none of the normal cases he reported encountering involved bereavement, the one contextual consideration the *DSM* allows, but rather "had for their cause serious delinquencies and threatened legal proceedings." Thus, as we shall see, the *DSM* would likely classify as disordered these cases that Kraepelin diagnosed as normal because it ignores the "essential difference" of context.

Consider another of Kraepelin's cases that raises the issue of the distinction between disorder and normality:

> I will now show you a widow, aged fifty-four, who has made very serious efforts to take her own life. This patient has no insane history. She married at the age of thirty, and has four healthy children. She says that her husband died two years ago, and since then she has slept badly. Being obliged to sell her home at that time, because the inheritance was to be divided, she grew apprehensive, and thought that she would come to want, although, on quiet consideration, she saw that her fears were groundless. . . . This patient, too, is quite clear as to her surroundings, and gives connected information about her condition. She has no real delusions, apart from fear that she will never be well again. Indeed, we find that the real meaning of the whole picture of disease is only permanent *apprehensive depression*, with the same accompaniments as we see in mental agitation in the sane—i.e., loss of sleep and appetite, and failure of the general nutrition. The resemblance to anxiety in the sane person is all the greater because the depression has followed a painful external cause. But we can easily see that the severity, and more especially the duration, of the emotional depression have gone beyond the limits of what is normal. The patient herself sees clearly enough that her apprehension is not justified by her real position in life, and that there is absolutely no reason why she should wish to die.[21]

This patient was experiencing her one and only episode of depressive symptoms; there was "no insane history." In addition to manifesting depressed mood, the patient was suicidal and had insomnia, loss of appetite, and lack of energy ("failure of the general nutrition") and so would qualify for a *DSM* diagnosis of MDD. Although the depressive symptoms began soon after her husband's death, the immediate trigger seems to have been not that but the subsequent need to sell their home and attendant fears of poverty; as we saw in chapter 2, the financial and social consequences of loss can influence the severity of a normal reaction. Once again, the symptoms—including even suicidality, which can occur in nondisordered people who are highly distraught—consist of "the same accompaniments as we see in mental agitation in the sane." Indeed, "the resemblance to anxiety in the sane person is all the greater because the depression has followed a painful external cause."

How, then, did Kraepelin know that this woman was disordered? Although there was a trigger, the reaction, which had lasted about 2 years and included serious suicide attempts, went beyond any possible proportional relationship to the trigger: "the severity, and more especially the duration, of the emotional depression have gone beyond the limits of what is normal." In effect, this meant that the feelings were without cause. This was apparent even to the patient herself: "On quiet consideration, she saw that her fears were groundless. . . . The patient herself sees clearly enough that her apprehension is not justified by her real position in life, and that there is absolutely no reason why she should wish to die." Indeed, the patient had every reason to live, including four healthy children. The case illustrates that when the severity and duration of symptoms are disproportionate to the trigger, they are in effect symptoms "without cause" because the context interacting with normal human nature does not fully explain them. As Kraepelin elsewhere emphasized, "The dejection which in normal life accompanies sad experiences gradually wanes, but in disease even a cheerful environment fails to mitigate sadness, indeed, it may even intensify it."[22]

In sum, Kraepelin maintained the traditional distinction between depressive conditions that were "with" or "without cause." Not symptoms in themselves, but symptoms that became detached from their contexts and took on a life of their own, indicated disorder. Kraepelin offered symptoms as evidence to infer a diagnosis but, in contrast to the *DSM*, he never attempted to define disorders solely in terms of necessary and sufficient symptoms. He clearly recognized normal depressive episodes "with cause" that were proportionate to their triggers and that subsided after the stressor subsided, and he actively grappled with how to distinguish normal sadness from disorder given their possible symptomatic similarity.

Adolf Meyer on Normal and Disordered Reaction Types

Adolf Meyer (1866–1950), a Swiss-born psychiatrist who held the Chair in Psychiatry at Johns Hopkins University, is generally considered the leading American psychiatrist in the first half of the twentieth century. Both the Kraepelinian physiological and Freudian psychological traditions influenced Meyer, and he was known early on for bringing Kraepelinian ideas to American psychiatry, but he was not a full-fledged partisan of either school. By the 1920s, he developed his own distinctive approach that focused more on life course, personality, and patients' capacity for responding to adaptive challenges and less on the particular diseases they might have. Indeed, he reconceptualized psychiatric disorders as impairments in the ability to respond to such everyday problems. Meyer's approach heavily influenced the descriptions of disorders in the first two editions of the *DSM* that preceded the pivotal third edition.

Like psychoanalysts, Meyer emphasized a contextual approach to depression. He thought that the symptoms, causes, and prognoses of depressive illnesses were far too heterogeneous to be encompassed within a single disease condition. Instead, he developed a "biopsychosocial" approach, which stressed how each individual's unique predispositions, environmental circumstances, and specific experiences over the life course produced their conditions. For Meyer, psychiatric disorders, including depression, were maladaptive reactions that arose on the basis of constitutional and psychological predispositions, individual upbringing, and social conditions, as well as from the interaction of individual organisms and their environments. In a definition that accorded with the "without cause" tradition, Meyer defined simple melancholia as "an excessive and altogether unjustified depression" and simple depression as "more or less, excesses of normal depression."[23]

In response to Kraepelin's focus on classification as involving inference to underlying physical pathologies analogous to diagnosis of physical diseases, Meyer included a constitutional (biological) component to stress reactions. Conceiving of mental pathologies as malfunctions in the individual's overall capacity to react adaptively to stressful situations, he developed a general framework for thinking about all disorders that was summarized in the schema, "situation, reaction, and final adjustment."[24] Meyer argued that "the conditions we meet in psychopathology are more or less abnormal reaction types."[25] In talking of reactions and adjustments, Meyer did not include normal sadness in response to loss in his conception of pathology. Rather, conceiving of episodes of disorder as malfunctioning responses to events, he was essentially urging psychiatrists to understand disordered individuals as reacting dysfunctionally to their environmental contexts.

In principle, Meyer and his followers held to a clear, coherent, and traditional distinction between normal reactions that were proportionate and disordered reactions that were excessive and disproportionate. They also clearly discerned that the distinction between normal and disordered depression lies not in symptoms but in the relation to events. Wendell Muncie's Meyerian textbook, *Psychobiology and Psychiatry* (1939), with a foreword by Meyer, defined depressive disorder as a reaction that is differentiated from the universal experience of normal sadness via its disproportionality:

> Depression is a sweeping reaction in which a dominant and fixed mood of sadness or its equivalent appears as the central issue determining a syndrome. . . . The mood may be rather diffuse as sadness, blueness, melancholy, or more topically pointed as worry, or fearful or anxious depression. The reaction presents general slowing and reduction of useful activity, loss of initiative . . . slowness in thinking . . . ideas of unworthiness, and self-depreciation, etc. Pathological depression is to be differentiated from normal depression by its greater fixity, depth, and by the disproportion to the causative factors. Depression is the major reaction most easily appreciated since depression of normal proportions is a universal experience.[26]

Note that Muncie implicitly assumed that the symptoms of normal depression, although proportionate to causes, were similar to those of some pathological depressions. Indeed, he waited until after his symptom description was complete to add criteria for distinguishing the two kinds of depression via the familiar, classic criteria: greater duration ("fixity"), unusual severity of symptoms ("depth"), and disproportion to the cause.

Both Meyer and psychoanalysts focused their concern more on understanding personalities and life circumstances than on distinguishing distinct disease conditions. Their greatest classificatory impact was on the diagnostic manuals that preceded the *DSM-III*, the *DSM-I* and *DSM-II*, which adopted Meyer's "reaction" vocabulary and psychoanalytic ideas about anxiety and defense in some of their definitions, including the definition of depressive disorder.

Initial Psychiatric Classifications

Psychiatric nomenclature in the United States during the first half of the twentieth century did not reflect an intense interest in classification. Instead, the administrative need to keep track of statistics regarding disorders in groups such as hospitalized patients drove the development of diagnostic manuals.[27] Diagnoses focused on the conditions of people found within institutional contexts, the predominant form of treatment of mental disorder at the time, and reflected the fact that most psychiatrists practiced in mental hospitals. Thus diagnostic systems tended to gloss over the less severe neurotic conditions that analysts typically saw in outpatient settings. For example, the first standardized classification system in the United States, the *Statistical Manual for the Use of Hospitals for Mental Diseases*, issued in 1918, divided mental disorders into 22 principal groups, only one of which represented all psychoneuroses.[28]

The *Statistical Manual* contains two categories that covered depressive conditions. First, one of the 2 groups was for non-neurotic disorders of psychogenic origin without clearly defined hereditary or constitutional causes. Manic-depressive psychoses fell into this category (in sharp distinction to Kraepelin's biological view and more akin to psychodynamic approaches). Second, under the general group of *psychoneurosis,* was the category of depression under the label *reactive depression,* in a Meyerian spirit. Its definition of reactive depression is:

> Here are to be classified those cases which show depression in reaction to obvious external causes which might naturally produce sadness, such as bereavement, sickness and financial and other worries. The reaction, of a more marked degree and of longer duration than normal sadness, may be looked upon as pathological. The deep depression, with motor and mental retardation, shown in the manic-depressive depression is not present, but these reactions may be more closely related in fact to the manic-depressive reactions than to the psychoneuroses.[29]

This definition recognized that depressive disorder is to be distinguished from sadness that arises proportionally "with cause" from external circumstances, which is produced "naturally" (i.e., in accord with human nature) and thus is normal and not pathological. The definition also followed tradition in recognizing that a broad range of negative circumstances can trigger normal sadness, offering a clearly nonexhaustive list of examples, including grief, medical illness, and financial reversals, in contrast to recent definitions that no longer recognize the range of potential triggers of intense normal sadness.

The *Statistical Manual*'s distinction between normal and pathological depression, not so different from that of Hippocrates, offered no symptomatic distinction but required pathological depressions to be more severe and of longer duration ("of a more marked degree and of longer duration than normal sadness"). They were not of the depth and severity of manic-depressive illness, yet they were still disorders. An examination of symptoms alone, therefore, could not determine pathology, which was recognized to exist only when symptoms were of disproportionate intensity to their context. The *Manual*, in a tip of the hat to Kraepelin, speculated that pathological depressive reactions may share an underlying etiological factor with manic-depressive depressions, thus explaining their unwarranted intensity and disproportion. Indeed, this definition mirrored the same three kinds of conditions—depressions with cause, without cause, and of disproportionate severity and duration to a provoking cause—that Robert Burton delineated in *Anatomy of Melancholy*; like Burton's definition, it recognized that only the latter two conditions indicated mental disorder.

The *Statistical Manual* guided psychiatric classification from its 1st edition in 1918 through its 10th edition in 1942. By the early 1950s, the center of gravity in American psychiatry had shifted from state hospitals, which focused on psychotic cases, to psychodynamic outpatient therapy of less severe pathology. The classifications of psychotic disorders that dominated the *Statistical Manual* were thus no longer relevant to the vast majority of patients. In 1952, the American Psychiatric Association newly codified mental disorders and produced the first edition of a new manual, the *Diagnostic and Statistical Manual of Mental Disorders* (*DSM-I*),[30] that better reflected the nature of the psychiatric profession's changing patient population.

A combination of psychodynamic and Meyerian approaches dominated the characterization of depression in the *DSM-I*, which generally downplayed biological aspects of disorders and focused on unconscious psychological mechanisms.[31] It contained one category of psychotic affective reactions that, in turn, were divided into manic-depressive reactions and psychotic-depressive reactions. Both of these conditions showed severe symptoms that involved "manifest evidence of gross misinterpretation of reality, including, at times, delusions and hallucinations."[32] The former also featured severe mood swings that were subject to remission and recurrence, whereas the latter did not encompass mood swings but frequently featured environmental precipitating factors.

The manual characterized psychoneurotic depressive disorders, like all psychoneuroses, as stemming from unconscious attempts to deal with anxiety, a basically psychoanalytic perspective. Again in a Meyerian fashion, as a variation of the earlier *Statistical Manual*'s "reactive depressions," *DSM-I* labeled these conditions *Depressive reactions*, which it defined as follows:

> The anxiety in this reaction is allayed, and hence partially relieved, by depression and self-depreciation. The reaction is precipitated by a current situation, frequently by some loss sustained by the patient, and is often associated with a feeling of guilt for past failures or deeds. The degree of the reaction in such cases is dependent upon the intensity of the patient's ambivalent feeling toward his loss (love, possession) as well as upon the realistic circumstances of the loss.
>
> The term is synonymous with "reactive depression" and is to be differentiated from the corresponding psychotic reaction. In this differentiation, points to be considered are (1) life history of patient, with special reference to mood swings (suggestive of psychotic reaction), to the personality structure (neurotic or cyclothymic) and to precipitating environmental factors and (2) absence of malignant symptoms (hypochondriacal preoccupation, agitation, delusions, particularly somatic, hallucinations, severe guilt feelings, intractable insomnia, suicidal ruminations, severe psychomotor retardation, profound retardation of thought, stupor).[33]

This definition of depressive reactions relied heavily on psychodynamic speculations about etiology to define depressive neuroses. The *DSM-I* not only conceived of depressive conditions as ways that people attempt to defend against underlying states of anxiety but also infused the definition of depression with dynamic assumptions that guilt and feelings of ambivalence were central components of the condition. Aside from such etiological defining criteria, much of the definition was taken up with distinguishing psychoneurotic-depressive disorders from psychotic-depressive disorders.

The *DSM-I*'s definition of depressive reaction might appear to be a historical anomaly in that it did not say a word about the distinction between disordered psychoneurotic-depressive reactions and normal reactions to circumstances. This lapse was more apparent than real, however, because the distinction was implicit, based in the *DSM-I*'s underlying psychodynamic etiological assumptions. Spelling out the distinction between normal and disordered depressive responses was superfluous precisely because the *DSM-I* relied on a theory of etiology to identify disorders and to distinguish them, by implication, from normal conditions in which the etiology is absent. The definition, in effect, specified the dysfunctions of psychological mechanisms that caused the intensity of the sadness, including unwarranted guilt and self-deprecation, intense ambivalence about the lost object, and the use of defense mechanisms (including depressive feelings) to avoid the natural anxieties that arise from loss situations. These processes combined to lead to a depressive response that was not merely sadness that was proportional to any actual loss itself (although the "current situation" and the "realistic circumstances of the loss" influenced the response's intensity) but that was, rather, an inflated, disproportionate "degree of reaction" due to the action of these internal psychological dysfunctions. Note that the examples of the triggers of loss responses that might be normal—or, if there were ambivalence about the loss, disordered—are loss of love and of possessions, not bereavement.

The *DSM-I* was the official manual of the APA between 1952 and 1968. Its successor, the *DSM-II*, provides a much more succinct definition of "depressive neurosis," as follows:

> This disorder is manifested by an excessive reaction of depression due to an internal conflict or to an identifiable event such as the loss of a love object or cherished possession. It is to be distinguished from Involutional melancholia and Manic-depressive illness. Reactive depressions or depressive reactions are to be classified here.[34]

The *DSM-II* implicitly recognized the distinction between depressions that were proportionate responses to loss and those that were "excessive" and thus disproportionate. The definition assumed that psychiatrists knew what symptoms constituted depression and attempted neither to specify them nor to suggest that one could use symptoms to distinguish disorder from nondisorder. Again, the definition relied on etiology, in the form of internal conflict, to suggest internal dysfunction, but the definition also recognized that losses may trigger a disproportionate, disordered reaction even in the absence of internal conflict. The definition also noted normal triggers beyond the loss of a loved one, such as loss of a cherished possession. To some extent, the *DSM-II* definition was a return to the classic tradition of simply specifying disordered depression as a disproportionate, "excessive" response.

In sum, 2,500 years of psychiatry held that normal human nature included a propensity to potentially intense sadness after certain kinds of losses. Disorder can be judged to exist, it was widely agreed, only when explanations in terms of triggering events fail to establish a normal cause for the intensity or duration of symptoms. The major influences on psychiatric classification in the first half of the twentieth century—Freud, Kraepelin, and Meyer and the early diagnostic manuals, such as *DSM-I* and *II*, that they influenced—disagreed on many things, but all explicitly or implicitly embraced this understanding of depressive disorder.

The Breakdown of the "With" and "Without" Cause Tradition

The Post-Kraepelinians

During the half-century between about 1920 and 1970, the dominance of the psychodynamic views of Freud and the context-based views of Meyer ensured the general neglect of Kraepelin's system of categorization, which assumed underlying physical etiologies. However, Kraepelin's approach inspired some researchers, especially in the United Kingdom, to pursue an extensive agenda of research into classification of types of depression.

Numerous empirical studies examined symptom patterns in an attempt to discover whether depression consisted of one or more distinct disorders. The work of the psychiatrist Aubrey Lewis was especially influential. In 1934 Lewis published a study of 61 patients treated at the Maudsley Hospital in London.[35] He argued that the distinction between endogenous and reactive depressions was untenable because most supposedly endogenous depressions had external precipitating factors; also, a lifetime of dispositions to depression preceded most reactive depressions. Lewis's research seemed to confirm Kraepelin's claim that almost all depression is one disorder, varying along a continuum of severity from mild to severe but not differing by endogenous or reactive causes. A few researchers, confirming Lewis's contentions, found that depressive symptoms were continuous, and they could not discern patterns that were sufficiently robust to suggest differing underlying etiologies. This group, like Kraepelin, concluded that a rigid division between endogenous and reactive or neurotic and psychotic depressions was unjustified.[36]

Most researchers, however, rejected the notion that all forms of depression fell on a single continuum. Instead, they found that *endogenous* or *psychotic* depression appeared to be a distinct type. The symptoms of psychotic depressions, which often featured hallucinations and delusions, did not correlate with the symptoms of other types of depressions and showed distinct responses to treatment;[37] psychotic depressions seemed more responsive to both electroconvulsive treatment and the antidepressant drug imipramine and less responsive to placebo treatments than other depressed states.[38] Efforts to distinguish psychotic depressions by their lack of environmental precipitants, however, were usually not successful.[39] Instead, stressful life events usually preceded the emergence of all sorts of depressions. Given the paucity of nontriggered depressions that were truly "without cause," the term *endogenous* gradually came to refer to a phenomenological pattern of symptoms, not to a particular cause of symptoms. *Psychotic* or *severe* more accurately characterized the nature of this condition.

Although researchers in this period generally came to agree that psychotic (or endogenous) depressions constituted one distinct type of depression, they could not agree on the nature of nonpsychotic depressions. Gradually, the use of *neurotic* prevailed over *reactive* because precipitating events in the environment provoked the great majority of all types of depression. Some concluded that depression was binary, featuring a neurotic type, as well as a psychotic one.[40] Others felt that three or more distinct types of neurotic depressions existed, although they differed on both the number and the nature of these states.[41] In contrast to the relatively homogenous symptoms found in psychotic depressions, neurotic symptoms were heterogeneous and diffuse across studies.[42] Depending on the study, neurotic depression featured some combination of symptoms that reflected helplessness, low self-esteem, dysphoria, demoralization, anger, hostility, irritation, and disappointment reactions that resisted precise diagnostic schemes.

For our purposes of understanding the roots of current diagnosis, the detailed content and substantive results of this post-Kraepelinian research program are not as significant as its methodology. Although no consensus emerged about the nature of depression from empirical research regarding symptom patterns between 1920 and 1970, the studies did help pave the way for the subsequent revolution in psychiatric diagnoses because of the general approach they took to identifying depressive disorder. These researchers claimed to emulate Kraepelin, but their approach in fact sharply diverged from his. Empirical studies during this period relied on measuring only symptom presentations at a single point in time. Researchers largely set aside issues of course, duration, and, especially, the situational context of symptoms. In contrast, as we saw, Kraepelin rejected using symptoms in themselves to distinguish varying types of depression and emphasized instead the need to examine the course and prognosis of conditions as well as the importance of distinguishing between normal and disordered sadness on the basis of context.

The symptom-based emphasis reflected the way researchers had exploited newly developed statistical methods, especially factor analysis, to analyze whether depression was a single illness or had multiple types.[43] Factor analysis attempts to distinguish various symptom clusters by examining the extent to which individual symptoms tend to occur together with other symptoms. There is no inherent, in-principle conflict between such statistical methods and the consideration of the proportionality of symptoms or the reasonableness of emotional reactions as part of what is statistically analyzed. In actual practice, however, the complexity that such judgments introduced led researchers to deviate from the clinical tradition and rely on symptom patterns alone, without regard to either their context or course, to distinguish different types of depression. Based on the fact that the clinical populations they studied were often hospitalized and in any event generally clearly disordered and had already been diagnosed, researchers who relied on statistical techniques to isolate symptom patterns simply assumed, quite reasonably, that all the symptoms they entered into their models were manifestations of disorder in the sampled populations. But, as we shall see, the kinds of clinical criteria that eventually emerged from these symptom-based analyses came to be applied far beyond the clearly disordered populations from which they were derived to progressively broader groups in which the same symptoms might not mean the same thing.

Lewis's finding that most depressions followed some kind of triggering event made the decision to focus on symptoms easier, because it suggested that perhaps context in the form of "with cause" versus "without cause" was not so important after all.[44] However, Lewis's research never explored the notion of the disproportionality of a response to the nature of the reported trigger, which was at the heart of the classic tradition. Moreover, Lewis's study was of an inpatient, clearly disordered, sample, so it could not reveal differences between the disordered and the nondisordered.

The replacement of the "with cause" or "without cause" distinction by categories based on types of symptoms had especially dire consequences for misdiagnosis of normal individuals because of a major change in the nature of those treated for depression that was occurring at this time. Whereas Lewis's inpatient sample reflected the standard clinical population of depressive patients early in the twentieth century, gradually over the course of the century outpatient psychiatric clinics became the most common settings for treatment for depression. Outpatients, however, presented a far wider range of problems, including substantial numbers of normal sadness states, than the more homogeneous groups of severely disordered inpatients that Kraepelin and Lewis studied.[45] "Psychiatrists today," summarized psychiatrist Hagop Akiskal shortly before the publication of the *DSM-III* in 1980, "are faced with a large number of individuals who are seeking help for poorly defined states of psychic malaise and dysphoria that seem to defy further characterization. . . . Hence the growing vagueness of neurotic depression is paralleled by its increasing clinical visibility."[46] Extending symptom-based diagnostic methods from inpatient settings to far more heterogeneous outpatient clinics, without the simple contextual distinctions used in the past to distinguish the normal from the disordered, created the potential for unprecedented numbers of false-positive diagnoses of depressive disorder.

By the 1970s, a "hodgepodge of competing and overlapping systems" that contrasted psychotic and neurotic, endogenous and reactive, bipolar and unipolar, and many other types characterized the literature on depression.[47] Aside from a consensus that psychotic (or endogenous) depressions were distinct from neurotic states, there was virtually no agreement on the nature of nonpsychotic depressions. Researchers did not agree on whether nonpsychotic depressions were continuous or discontinuous with psychotic forms, on the one hand, or with normality, on the other. They disputed how many forms neurotic conditions took and even whether they had any distinct forms at all. Nor was it known whether some milder forms of depression were early indicators of eventual psychotic forms. In addition, little consensus existed about the particular symptoms that were essential to definitions of nonpsychotic forms of depression. Summarizing the situation in the United States and Great Britain in the mid- to late 1970s, physicians Christopher Callahan and German Berrios noted that "psychiatric diagnostic categories are at best subjective and probably irrelevant."[48] In 1980, responding to this period of confused debate characterized by the highly unsettled state of empirical findings and lack of definitive theory about the nature of non-psychotic depression, psychiatry would nonetheless adopt a definitive set of symptomatic criteria for depression that have remained stable until the present.

Paving the Road to the DSM-III: The Feighner Criteria

The proximate origins of the *DSM-III* criteria lie in the work of a group of research psychiatrists at Washington University in St. Louis who felt that as long as the system of classification remained without precise definitions, there was no hope for psychiatry to become a scientific discipline. Led by two prominent psychiatrists—Eli Robins and Samuel Guze—the group was inspired by the neo-Kraepelinian research tradition of analyzing symptoms statistically, and they wanted to remedy the confusing and divergent definitions of disorders by different researchers. The St. Louis group emphasized the scientific importance of having agreed-on criteria that primarily used symptomatic presentations as the basis for research studies and diagnostic decisions.

In 1972, based on discussions among the faculty regarding how to improve the diagnostic criteria that might be used in their research, a resident at Washington University, John Feighner, codified and published diagnostic criteria for 15 mental disorders, including primary and secondary affective disorders, in what came to be called the *Feighner criteria*.[49] The Feighner criteria were not explicitly formulated for everyday clinical use. Rather, they were an attempt to relieve researchers of the multiplicity of different imprecise definitions then in use and thus to make possible more cumulative, comparable, and reproducible research. The stated goal was a "common ground for different research groups. . . . The use of formal diagnostic criteria by a number of groups . . . will result in a resolution of the problem of whether patients described by different groups are comparable. This first and crucial taxonomic step should expedite psychiatric investigation."[50]

The Feighner criteria divided primary affective disorders into two categories, depression and mania; we consider only the "depression" category. Diagnosis of depression required satisfaction of three criteria. First, the patient must have dysphoric mood marked by symptoms such as being depressed, sad, despondent, or hopeless. Second, at least five additional symptoms must be present (i.e., a total of six for definitive diagnosis; four additional symptoms, or a total of five for probable diagnosis) from among a list including loss of appetite, sleep difficulty, loss of energy, agitation, loss of interest in usual activities, guilt feelings, slow thinking, and recurrent suicidal thoughts. Finally, the condition must have lasted at least 1 month and not be due to another preexisting mental disorder.

Of people who met these symptomatic criteria, only those who had life-threatening or incapacitating medical illnesses were excluded from the diagnosis of primary depressive disorder. One might have thought that this exclusion was based on the fact that being intensely sad is often a normal response to such illnesses. However, it turns out that these patients' symptoms simply warranted a different diagnosis: that of secondary affective disorder. This category encompassed all conditions that met the same symptomatic criteria as primary disorders but that occurred with a preexisting nonaffective psychiatric illness or a life-threatening or incapacitating medical illness. Thus there were, in fact, no exclusions from disorder whatever for those who satisfied symptomatic criteria.

The Feighner criteria for affective disorders differed in significant ways from the criteria in prior empirical research on depression and, in some ways, were in tension with that research. First, all depressive conditions that did not have manic features and that were not preceded by other psychiatric or medical conditions were grouped into a single category. This system conformed to Kraepelin's theory that depression was a unitary disorder but ignored the vast majority of empirical studies that suggested possible distinctions in depressive symptomatic profiles between psychotic unipolar (i.e., not involving mania) depressions and neurotic depressions. However, we have seen that the research was not conclusive and that no consensus existed about possible distinctions between types of depressive disorder.

Where the Feighner criteria most unjustifiably deviated from considered psychiatric judgment was in making no room at all for depressive reactions of more than 1 month in duration that stemmed from normal loss responses, even including bereavement. The criteria did not allow for the possibility that some depressive symptoms were proportionate to their provoking causes even if they lasted a month, whereas others stemmed from dysfunctions. This set a crucial precedent for subsequent criteria sets that built on the Feighner work.

Why the Feighner group ignored the obvious problem of normal sadness in their criteria remains unclear. One possibility is that, to ensure that researchers would widely use the criteria, they fervently strove to avoid any inference about causation in their definitions; they might have concluded that the distinction between normality and disorder implied a particular etiological approach to classification.[51] Another is that they developed the criteria with research samples whose members clearly had some disorder and assumed the criteria would generally be used with similar samples. Or perhaps they simply were following the research tradition that immediately preceded them, which relied on statistical analysis of symptoms without regard to context.

A further possibility is that the Feighner group implicitly recognized the disordered—nondisordered-sadness distinction but assumed that intense sadness of more than 1 month's duration is "prolonged" in Hippocrates' sense and, if it involves the specified number of symptoms, is inherently disproportionate to any possible stressor and thus almost certainly disordered. If so, previous clinical observers did not accept this assumption, and it seems to conflict with the trajectory of normal response to major losses documented in chapter 2; even the *DSM-III* was to allow 2 months of normal symptomatic response to loss of a loved one. In any event, we will see that the *DSM-III* lowered this duration threshold to the much less plausible criterion of 2 weeks. In sum, unlike Kraepelin, Feighner and colleagues provide no background understanding of how to distinguish disorder from nondisorder, nor do they state the need to evaluate whether those satisfying depressive symptom criteria are indeed disordered.

How did the Feighner group develop their influential criteria for depression? One of the ironies of psychiatric history is that the later justification for using the Feighner criteria's symptom-based diagnostic categories as the model for the *DSM-III* was their claimed grounding in empirical research rather than in theoretical speculation.[52] Yet, judging by the citations the article provides, the criteria for depressive disorder, at least, had little empirical support in the prior literature. The article references only four published articles as sources for the depression criteria. (A fifth reference cites an unpublished paper by Robins and Guze from a workshop at the National Institute of Mental Health. In addition, the work gives six citations to publications on mania, which we do not consider here.)

One referenced article asserts that there is no evidence that the particular condition of involutional (i.e., postmenopausal) depressive syndrome is symptomatically distinguishable from other depressive disorders (a question on which Kraepelin had vacillated), and it concludes with a challenge to the general adequacy of symptomatic criteria: "Attempting to group psychiatric patients into clinical entities by symptom pictures has been frustrating as it has never been clear where the dividing lines belong. This is a serious problem in psychiatry."[53] Two other references, coming out of a single research project, indicated that there was some tentative evidence for an endogenous factor that represented the core of depressive symptoms but that the symptoms of reactive depression were most likely to be "phenomenological manifestations of psychiatric disorders other than depression which 'contaminate' the depression syndrome."[54] The findings from these studies, if anything, actually contradicted the Feighner criteria's lumping of endogenous and reactive conditions. The final reference explicitly rejected the use of purely symptom-based definitions of depression that do not embody considerations about the causes of symptoms and their normal versus pathological status:

> In classifying depressive states the first distinction to be made is between normal and pathological reactions. Mourning and grief reactions in general are normal reactions to the loss of a love object—this may be another person, money, the depressed individual's prestige, his cherished hopes, his health—and it is not always possible to distinguish such normal grief reactions from pathological depression on phenomenological grounds alone. A depression is judged to be pathological if there is insufficient specific cause for it in the patient's immediate past, if it lasts too long, or if its symptoms are too severe.[55]

None of the citations that the Feighner article references for depression supports the assumption that purely symptom-based criteria can define depressive disorders. These sources neither justify nor even address the validity of the specific definition of affective disorders in the criteria.

Soon after the publication of the Feighner criteria, the Washington University psychiatrists Robert Woodruff, Donald Goodwin, and Samuel Guze expanded their discussion of their new diagnostic criteria and their general approach to diagnosis in the first symptom-based psychiatric textbook, *Psychiatric Diagnosis.*[56] The chapter on diagnosis of affective disorders emphasized the importance of observing and measuring symptoms without any etiological inferences because of the poor state of knowledge about the causes of depression. This principle perhaps partly explains why the Feighner criteria did not allow even bereavement to be excluded from a diagnosis of depressive disorder.

In a section on differential diagnosis in the affective disorders, the text notes the following regarding bereavement (there is no discussion of other stressors):

> Making the distinction between grief and primary affective disorder can be difficult. However, grief usually does not last as long as an episode of primary affective disorder. . . . The majority of bereaved persons experience fewer symptoms than do patients with primary affective disorder. Furthermore, some symptoms common in primary affective disorder are relatively rare among persons experiencing bereavement, notably fear of losing one's mind and thoughts of self-harm.[57]

Supporting their points about the differences between bereavement and depressive disorder, Woodruff and colleagues cite several articles by psychiatrist Paula Clayton and her colleagues that document the type and duration of depressive symptoms occurring in bereavement.[58] In fact, Clayton found that after 1 month, which was the Feighner duration threshold for diagnosis of a disorder, about 40% of bereaved individuals display full *DSM*-level symptoms. Yet there is little plausibility and no scientific evidence that such a large percentage of the bereaved become disordered. Given the enormous number of individuals who experience bereavement over time, the notion that a "majority" do not experience as many symptoms as the Feighner criteria require of the disordered at the 1-month mark, and the notion that "usually" bereavement at that intense level does not last as long as the Feighner's 1-month requirement, there is no greatly reassuring evidence of its validity. Indeed, it seems to leave the door open to large numbers of false positive diagnoses of the normally bereaved, an issue that goes unaddressed.

The authors' apparent assumption that a 1-month duration and five-symptom threshold for "probable" disorder (six for "definite" diagnosis) was sufficient to discriminate disorder from normal bereavement is unwarranted on the basis of the very studies that they themselves cite. In any event, the text offers no substantive new empirical support for the proposed criteria

for depressive disorder, leaving the validity of the new criteria as empirically challengeable as before. This text, now in its fifth edition, was highly influential in shaping the subsequent *DSM-III*.[59]

Meanwhile, the Feighner criteria clearly served a need in the research community; by 1989, the article in which they appeared was the single most cited article in the history of psychiatry.[60] Their widely influential definition of depressive disorder set the stage for psychiatry's use of purely symptom-based diagnoses, despite the fact that by nature this approach was incapable of distinguishing intense normal from disordered responses.

The Research Diagnostic Criteria

Robert Spitzer was the major translator of the Feighner research criteria into what were to become the clinical diagnostic criteria of the *DSM-III*. The Research Diagnostic Criteria (RDC), which Spitzer created in collaboration with Eli Robins of the Washington University group and published in 1978, was the bridge between these two landmark achievements.[61] In conjunction with the RDC, Spitzer also developed one of the first structured interviews to measure depression, the Schedule for Affective Disorders and Schizophrenia (SADS), an early step toward the development of structured questionnaires that would later be used in epidemiologic studies that applied the new diagnostic approach beyond the clinic to community samples (see chapter 6).[62]

At the behest of the National Institute of Mental Health (NIMH), Spitzer and his colleagues developed the RDC to overcome concerns about the low reliability of psychiatric diagnoses and to create a more sophisticated typology of depression diagnoses. Like the Feighner criteria, the RDC were explicitly aimed at facilitating research, but their clinical application was not hard to see. Building on the Feighner symptom-based approach, they expanded the 15 diagnoses of the Feighner criteria to 25 major types and many more subtypes of disorder.[63]

The symptom criteria for Major Depressive Disorder in the RDC required an episode lasting at least 2 weeks, the presence of a prominent and persistent dysphoric mood or pervasive loss of interest or pleasure, five out of eight additional symptoms (four for a probable diagnosis), help seeking or impaired functioning because of the disorder, and the absence of features that suggest schizophrenia. The major changes in the RDC from the Feighner criteria were stipulations that pervasive loss of interest or pleasure could be substituted for dysphoric mood as a necessary condition (reflecting a growing view that loss of capacity for pleasure is central to depression); that symptoms need only be present for 2 weeks instead of 1 month (an unexplained substantial reduction in required duration that potentially allowed for many more false positive diagnoses of normal individuals but was to find its way into the *DSM-III*); and that the patient had to have either sought help from someone or have impaired social functioning (essentially an early form of the later clinical significance criterion). A number of exclusion criteria that eliminated those with schizophrenia from a depression diagnosis were also added, as were 11 subtypes of MDD. (The nonmutually exclusive subtypes of MDD, the original motivation for NIMH's interest, were primary, secondary, recurrent unipolar, psychotic, incapacitating, endogenous, agitated, retarded, situational, simple, and predominant mood.) Despite the lowering of both the duration and symptom thresholds from the Feighner criteria to levels that would later be incorporated into the *DSM-III*, the RDC's criteria for MDD contained no exclusions for bereavement or any other normal reaction, although they did require researchers to ascertain during their interviews with patients whether bereavement was present.[64]

For reasons we consider in the next section, a major concern in constructing the RDC was reliability of diagnosis, that is, whether different diagnosticians would come to the same diagnosis based on the same information. Studies using the RDC indicated great overall success in achieving reliability. For Major Depressive Illness, the initial reports indicated the remarkable reliability of .97.[65] Other reports indicated reliabilities of about .90.[66] Many considered the apparent improvement of reliability to be a great advance, as the remarks of the noted diagnostician Alvin Feinstein indicate:

> The production of operational identifications has been a pioneering, unique advance in nosology. . . . In the field of diagnostic nosology, the establishment of operational criteria represents a breakthrough that is as obvious, necessary, fundamental, and important as the corresponding breakthrough in obstetrics and surgery when Semmelweis, Oliver Wendell Holmes, and, later on, Lord Lister, demanded that obstetricians and surgeons wash their hands before operating on the human body.[67]

We will see that Feinstein's enthusiasm for Spitzer's accomplishments reflects what was to become Spitzer's greatest achievement, his shepherding of the creation of an entirely new psychiatric clinical diagnostic classification system using the same principles as the RDC to ensure reliability. However, we sound a preliminary caution in anticipation of the discussion of the *DSM-III*: It is true that when symptoms alone are the basis for diagnoses, people can be trained to apply the criteria according to rules and thus to agree, and the reliability of diagnoses may well increase. But are the agreed judgments correct in identifying disorders (i.e., valid)? These studies did not assess the validity of the diagnosis in predicting course, response to therapies, or etiology of depressive conditions. Moreover, the RDC and the Feighner criteria did not involve any systematic attempt to distinguish normal intense sadness from depressive disorder, casting further doubt on the validity of these approaches. Introducing judgments about normal versus disordered reactions to circumstances into diagnostic criteria is challenging to do and would likely lessen reliability, but even so it might substantially enhance validity. To this day, we shall see, psychiatry has not adequately addressed this challenge.

The DSM-III as a Response to the Challenges Confronting Psychiatry

The publication of the *DSM-III* in 1980 is justifiably viewed as a watershed in the history of psychiatric diagnosis.[68] Yet the revision of the *DSM-II* was not seen beforehand as particularly important, and there was no political jockeying from advocates of different theoretical perspectives to be in control of the process. Spitzer's work on the committee charged with revising the *DSM-II*, his prominent role in brokering the removal of homosexuality from that manual, and his development of the RDC criteria led to his appointment as chair of the *DSM-III* task force. Spitzer used the opportunity to create a new kind of diagnostic system that reflected previous decades of thought about how to make psychiatry more scientific.[69]

The *DSM-III* revolution directly incorporated many of the features of the Feighner criteria and RDC into the official psychiatric nosology and specifically embraced symptom-based diagnostic criteria. Spitzer himself recognized that the translation of research criteria into a manual for clinical use required that the diagnostic criteria must reflect "clinical wisdom" as well as evidence from research.[70] His role required not only the skills of a knowledgeable researcher but also those of a master politician attempting to mollify and to find compromise among various clinical constituencies that felt that the new symptom-based system threatened their traditional diagnostic practices.

But what motivated Spitzer to borrow so heavily from the RDC-style symptom-based definitional approach to diagnosis in revising the *DSM?* And why did clinicians, who are concerned with treating individuals and have little interest in reliable classification systems for research, accept the symptom-based classification system that had emerged from the Feighner criteria and RDC?

It turns out that the new system addressed several major problems that clinicians, as well as researchers, faced at the time. By the 1970s, psychoanalytic influence had waned. The psychiatric profession was divided into numerous theoretical schools, and different clinicians shared few assumptions about the fundamental nature, causes, and treatments of mental disorders. The new diagnostic manual, therefore, had to be serviceable for clinicians of many varying perspectives. The lists of explicit symptoms in the *DSM-III* not only improved reliability but also were *theory neutral* in the sense that they did not presuppose any particular theory of the cause of psychopathology, psychoanalytic or otherwise. The new criteria were *descriptive* rather than *etiological* and purged references to postulated psychodynamic causes of a disorder (e.g., internal conflict, defense against anxiety). Defining disorders on the basis of symptoms, regardless of etiology, turned out to be a useful tool in gaining the acceptance of clinicians of varying allegiances who could at least feel that all factions were on a level playing field in using the theory-neutral definitions.

Moreover, psychiatric diagnoses were under attack from a variety of sources. Behaviorists claimed that all behavior, including psychopathology, is the result of normal learning processes and thus that no mental disorders in the medical sense really exist.[71] The "antipsychiatry" movement, inspired by writers such as psychiatrist Thomas Szasz and sociologist Thomas Scheff, portrayed psychiatric diagnosis as a matter of using medical terminology to apply social control to undesirable but not truly medically disordered behavior.[72]

In addition, by 1980 private and public third parties were financing most medical treatment.[73] The murky unconscious entities of the DSM-II and the erosion of psychiatry's medical legitimacy did not provide a solid basis for insurance reimbursement. Although no evidence indicates that insurers influenced the development of the symptom-based disorders of the manual, the new diagnoses provided a better fit with the goal of third parties to reimburse the treatment of only specific diseases. On reflection, clinicians may not have agreed with some features in the new manual, such as the abandonment of contextual criteria, but they realized that the new system had many benefits for them.

Most pressing of all was an erosion of the credibility of psychiatry due to attacks on the meaningfulness of diagnosis. Although he had psychoanalytic training, Spitzer, like the St. Louis group, saw unverified theory and resistance to empirical testing as the major obstacles to psychiatry's attaining scientific status.[74] The central element in Spitzer's vision of psychiatry, pursued in his prodigious research efforts in the 1960s and 1970s and culminating in the DSM-III in 1980, was the development of a *reliable* system of classification in which different diagnosticians would generally arrive at the same diagnosis based on the same clinical information.[75]

Because the DSM-II did not provide specific symptoms that determined psychiatric diagnoses, psychiatrists were forced to use their own clinical judgments in assessing how well each patient fit a particular diagnosis. This led to great disparities in the application of diagnostic labels. For example, the well-known U.S.-U.K. Diagnostic Project, the results of which were published in 1972, studied the ways that psychiatrists in these two countries diagnosed mental disorders. The study demonstrated an alarming lack of agreement between American and British psychiatrists and among psychiatrists within each group. For example, more than five times as many British as American psychiatrists made diagnoses of depressive disorders.[76]

In addition to the U.S.-U.K. study, a great number of studies generally showed remarkable lack of diagnostic agreement in cases in which psychiatrists received the same information (e.g., a videotaped clinical interview).[77] These studies challenged the reliability not only of distinguishing closely related diagnostic categories, such as one affective disorder from another, but also of distinguishing between larger categories, such as affective versus anxiety disorders, and between overall types of disorder, such as psychosis versus neurosis or even psychosis versus normality.

Perhaps the most dramatic and influential such study, now seen as a landmark in the critique of psychiatric diagnosis, directly challenged the ability of psychiatrists to distinguish normality from psychosis. In 1973, psychologist David Rosenhan published a study in the prestigious journal *Science* in which eight normal individuals presented themselves at hospitals and reported only auditory hallucinatory symptoms (they claimed to hear a voice saying things like "thud," "dull," and "empty"), otherwise acting and speaking normally. All of these pseudo-patients were admitted and classified as psychotic (almost all as schizophrenic), and they remained so classified for various periods of time, even though they immediately reverted to normal behavior. Hospital residents, however, did identify several pseudo-patients as likely normals.

To get the flavor of the views prominent at the time, consider a few of sentences in the introduction to Rosenhan's article:

Normality and abnormality, sanity and insanity, and the diagnoses that flow from them may be less substantive than many believe them to be. . . . Based in part on theoretical and anthropological considerations, but also on philosophical, legal, and therapeutic ones, the view has grown that psychological categorization of mental illness is useless at best and downright harmful, misleading, and pejorative at worst. Psychiatric diagnoses, in this view, are in the minds of observers and are not valid summaries of characteristics displayed by the observed.[78]

Based on his results, Rosenhan concluded: "It is clear that we cannot distinguish the sane from the insane in psychiatric hospitals."

The threat of such gross invalidity and, by implication, unreliability (for surely Rosenhan's participants would, under other circumstances, have been judged normal) was not only an acute embarrassment to clinical expertise but also a challenge to the scientific status of psychiatry. Spitzer himself wrote a scathing critique of the methodological flaws in Rosenhan's study.[79] However, such a critique could show only that Rosenhan had not proved his claim that psychiatric diagnosis is by its nature flawed; it could not demonstrate that psychiatric diagnosis, in fact, had an adequately reliable diagnostic system. Much of Spitzer's subsequent effort was to be devoted to the project of creating and nurturing such a system.

Although acknowledging that a reliable system is not necessarily valid, Spitzer emphasized that validity requires reliability. A valid diagnostic system would categorize different syndromes accurately and thereby ought to predict course and response to treatment.[80] But if different diagnosticians could not even agree on the diagnosis, then clearly many of their diagnoses must be inaccurate, and there must be low overall diagnostic validity. Moreover, without reliability of diagnoses across settings, cumulative research could not proceed effectively. Therefore, the primary goal of the psychiatric profession had to be the development of a clear system of diagnostic rules that specified inclusion and exclusion criteria for each diagnosis and promoted a high degree of inter-judge agreement. Even if lacking in validity, such a reliable system could provide a scientifically adequate starting place from which researchers could bootstrap themselves to a more valid system.

However, as many concerned critics pointed out, just creating a reliable system that has clear rules that everybody can follow does not ensure even an approximation of validity; unless the rules are accurate, the reliability might just represent everybody together getting the same wrong answer![81] For example, if symptoms of intense sadness are used to indicate depressive disorder, such symptoms might be identified reliably, but the vast majority of conditions so recognized might not, in fact, be disorders. The field trials conducted before the publication of the *DSM-III*, in which hundreds of psychiatrists had tested the empirical adequacy of the diagnoses, did not compare the effectiveness of symptom-based criteria sets with other alternative ways of conceptualizing depression.[82] They tested only whether different psychiatrists could use the criteria in the same way but did not establish whether they were valid indicators of disorder. As one of Spitzer's collaborators notes: "pathologic conditions (were) redefined *before* empiric investigation (was) conducted."[83] And it is far from certain that such a system, if seriously invalid to begin with, would automatically evolve into a valid system. The implication is that considerations of validity cannot be entirely placed on the back burner while issues of reliability are resolved; both must be pursued together, and the two must inform each other in order to approach more reliable judgments that are also valid.

Between psychiatry's theoretical fragmentation, its diagnostic unreliability, and the antipsychiatry critique, not only psychiatry's claim to scientific status but even its legitimacy as a medical field seemed in jeopardy. The specific criteria of the *DSM-III* appeared to meet these challenges and place the field on a more sound scientific footing. In one fell swoop, Spitzer's incorporation of symptom-based operational definitions of disorders into the *DSM* managed to confront a range of challenges to psychiatry and to facilitate an about-face in psychiatry's status and fortunes, especially coinciding as it did with the advent of new medications that were also bolstering the status of the psychiatric profession.

But even a justified revolution has some unwarranted casualties. Having considered the nature and reasons for the *DSM-III* revolution in general, we now turn to the *DSM-III* criteria for depressive disorder.

The *DSM-III*'s Approach to Depressive Disorder

The *DSM-III* criteria for depression almost completely mirrored the approaches of the Feighner and RDC criteria (the next chapter discusses in detail the similar

DSM-IV criteria). They used symptoms to specify depressive disorder and abandoned or demoted etiological concepts, as well as traditional distinctions such as neurotic versus psychotic and endogenous versus reactive as a basis for different categories of diagnosis. Like the Feighner criteria and RDC, as well as earlier *DSMs*, the *DSM-III* rejected Kraepelin's unification of manic-depressive insanity and depression, instead distinguishing unipolar depressive disorder, or "major depression," from "bipolar" disorders. Although this remains an active area of controversy, family studies, clinical observations, and distinct patterns of medication responses had all served to thoroughly undermine Kraepelin's grand unification of affective disorders long before the *DSM-III.* Moreover, although MDD covered psychotic depression, it was understood that such conditions comprised only a small minority of those falling under the criteria; "simple depression" had come to be the predominant form of depression of concern in the manual.

Likewise, the *DSM-III* abandoned the *DSM-II* distinction between "excessive" versus proportionate reactions to an "identifiable event such as the loss of a love object or cherished possession." This is surprising given that many other categories of disorder in the *DSM-III,* such as some anxiety disorders, use qualifiers such as "excessive" or "unreasonable" to separate disorders from normal responses. Yet the *DSM-III* distinguishes depressive disorders solely on the basis of symptoms regardless of their relationship to circumstances, with the single exception of the bereavement exclusion.

The logic behind the bereavement exclusion, which represents a major improvement over the Feighner criteria and RDC, is that states of grief that otherwise meet symptomatic criteria are not disorders because they represent normal and transient responses to loss. The exclusion seems to have resulted from the work of Paula Clayton, a prominent member of the Washington University group and of the *DSM-III* Task Force on Affective Disorders. Her work had shown that depressive-like symptoms commonly arose during periods of bereavement but that they usually remitted after a fairly short time.[84] As we noted earlier, Woodruff, Goodwin, and Guze mentioned Clayton's work but did not incorporate it into their diagnostic criteria for depression. The *DSM-III* did incorporate Clayton's findings in developing the bereavement exclusion, but did not apply the exclusion to the reactions to any other types of loss that may have the same features as bereavement, such as reactions to marital dissolution, ill health, or financial reversal. So far as we can ascertain, reactions to other stressors simply never came up for discussion by the *DSM-III* affective disorders work group as a possible basis for exclusions.[85] The lack of such exclusions seems to have been a by-product of deriving the *DSM-III* criteria from the exclusionless Feighner and RDC criteria and the symptom-oriented diagnostic spirit of the *DSM-III* effort.

Various reasons have been cited to justify the *DSM*'s failure to allow exclusions from major depression for normal situations other than bereavement. For one thing, such exclusions could pose a serious challenge to reliability; other stressors often lack the relatively clear-cut nature of bereavement, and it would be more difficult to measure their magnitude and to judge their proportionality to the resulting response. However, as we have noted, it makes no sense for reliability to trump validity in constructing diagnostic criteria. In any event, the framers of the *DSM-III*, in creating criteria for "complicated" bereavement, discussed in the next chapter, showed that it is possible to reflect such subtle distinctions within a given stressor type. Similar efforts could have been made to provide guidelines for when reactions to other major stressors represent normal versus disordered reactions.

The question of whether sadness is a proportionate response to real loss is sometimes argued to be an etiological issue that has no place in a theory-neutral manual.[86] But this objection is based on confusion about the nature and point of theory neutrality. The distinction between normal, proportional responses to events and disorders in which sadness derives from an internal dysfunction is not really a theory-laden distinction in the sense relevant to the *DSM-III's* need for theory neutrality. Different theories offer different accounts—whether biological, psychodynamic, behavioral, cognitive, or social—of the nature and etiology of the dysfunction that underlies depressive disorder, and a theory-neutral manual must not accept one theory over another as part of the definition of the disorder. It can, however, acknowledge that all etiological theories share the notion of normal, proportional responses versus dysfunction-based responses. After all, medical thinkers from Aristotle to Kraepelin understood this notion in more or less the same way, and it identifies the common target that rival theories attempt to explain. This distinction is not an etiological hypothesis of the kind that a theory-neutral manual needs to exclude.

Another objection to considering the broader contexts of depressive responses in the *DSM-III* might have stemmed from the impression that psychotropic medication worked on all unipolar depressions, irrespective of the relation to triggering events, so that the "with cause" versus "without cause" distinction was irrelevant to treatment decisions, at least among hospitalized depressives.[87] However, even if medication sometimes works with normal reactions, the normality-versus-disorder distinction can have important prognostic implications for how aggressively to treat a condition and for deciding what kinds of treatments or changes in circumstances might help. Analogously, the fact that, say, Ritalin works on normal and disordered individuals alike to make them more focused, or that growth hormone makes both normal and disordered short children taller, does not imply that diagnosis can justifiably ignore the distinction between normality and disorder.

Finally, the *DSM-III's* ignoring of normal states of intense sadness might have reflected a fear of misdiagnosing the truly disordered as normal, especially given that depressed patients are subject to suicide risk. Yet no effort was made to balance the risks of false negatives with the costs of false positives that arise from labeling normal people as disordered, a cost that is clearer today with the growing apprehension about the possible negative side effects of antidepressive medication and of other treatments for normal sadness, including potential increased suicide risk in some populations.[88] Major psychiatric theoreticians prior to the *DSM-III* felt that it was important to identify normal cases of sadness and to distinguish them from depressive disorders, for good reason. Rather than entirely and unnecessarily ignoring a distinction, it is more prudent to simply use it when helpful but exercise caution so as to err on the side of safety in applying the distinction.

Conclusion

The *DSM-III*'s largely decontextualized, symptom-based criteria stemmed from efforts to enhance reliability, to develop a common language for psychiatrists with a variety of theoretical persuasions, and to bolster the scientific credentials of the profession. But in the urgent quest for reliability, the criteria for the most part inadvertently rejected the previous 2,500 years of clinical diagnostic tradition that explored the context and meaning of symptoms in deciding whether someone is suffering from intense normal sadness or a depressive disorder. The unwitting result of this effort, especially as psychiatry turned from the serious conditions of inpatients to the far more heterogeneous conditions of outpatients and community members, was to be a massive pathologization of normal sadness that, ironically, can be argued to have made depressive diagnosis less rather than more scientifically valid.

5

Depression in the *DSM-IV*

We claimed in chapter 1 that a flawed definition may be facilitating the recent surge in reported depressive disorder and may even lie at its very heart. To justify our claim, we now turn to a detailed examination of the *DSM* criteria for depressive and related disorders. Although the history of depression presented in the preceding chapter logically takes us up to the *DSM-III*, in order to ensure that our discussion applies to current diagnostic practices, we address the criteria presented in the latest edition—the fourth, text-revised edition *DSM-IV-TR* (2000). This does not represent much of a conceptual leap because the current criteria are almost identical to those in the *DSM-III*.

DSM-IV Affective Disorders

We start by placing the *DSM* criteria for Major Depressive Disorder (MDD) in the context of the *DSM*'s approach to affective disorders, also known as mood disorders, the larger category under which depressive disorders fall. The following distinctions are useful to keep in mind:

Unipolar Versus Bipolar Mood Disorders

MDD is "unipolar" depression, which means that the individual has only depressive symptoms rather than oscillating back and forth between depressive and manic symptoms such as elevated mood and grandiosity. Mood disorders that include manic episodes are known as *Bipolar Disorders* (formerly *manic-depressive disorders*), which are relatively rare compared with the claimed rates of unipolar depressive disorder. Bipolar I Disorder is often quite severe; milder forms include Bipolar II Disorder and Cyclothymic Personality Disorder. None of these forms of bipolar disorder is the focus here.

Major Depressive Disorder Versus Dysthymia

MDD generally occurs over time in a series of quasi-discrete symptomatically intense episodes separated by intervals without symptoms or with fewer symptoms. Another, less common form of depressive disorder is Dysthymia, which occurs more or less continuously for long periods of time at a less intense level and which is discussed later in this chapter.

Major Depressive Disorder Versus Major Depressive Episode

The *DSM* defines various subtypes of MDD (e.g., single episode, recurrent) based on the pattern of occurrences of what it calls Major Depressive Episodes (MDE) plus some additional criteria. In fact, it is in the criteria for MDE that most of the diagnostic "action" occurs; the criteria for MDD itself are brief and not very informative:

Criteria for Major Depressive Disorder

A. Presence of a Major Depressive Episode.
B. The Major Depressive Episode is not better accounted for by Schizo-affective Disorder and is not superimposed on Schizophrenia, Schizo-phreniform Disorder, Delusional Disorder, or Psychotic Disorder Not Otherwise Specified.
C. There has never been a Manic Episode, a Mixed Episode, or a Hypo-manic Episode.[1]

In other words, the criteria for MDD simply require that the patient experience at least one Major Depressive Episode, and that the episode is not part of some other psychotic disorder (note that psychotic symptoms can be part of the depression as long as they cannot be better explained as indicating some other psychotic disorder) and is not part of another kind of mood disorder containing manic elements. However, almost all depressive episodes are indicative of MDD and are not part of some other disorder. Thus, in the vast majority of cases, the criteria for MDD essentially come down to the criteria for MDE. We thus examine the much more informative definition of MDE at some length.

DSM-IV *Criteria for Major Depressive Episode*

A. Five (or more) of the following symptoms have been present during the same 2-week period and represent a change from previous functioning; at least one of the symptoms is either (1) depressed mood or (2) loss of interest or pleasure.

1. Depressed mood most of the day, nearly every day, as indicated by either subjective report (e.g., feels sad or empty) or observation made by others (e.g. appears tearful). Note: In children and adolescents, can be irritable mood.
2. Markedly diminished interest or pleasure in all, or almost all, activities most of the day, nearly every day (as indicated by either subjective account or observation made by others).
3. Significant weight loss when not dieting or weight gain (e.g., a change of more than 5% of body weight in a month), or decrease or increase in appetite nearly every day. Note: In children, consider failure to make expected weight gain.
4. Insomnia or hypersomnia nearly every day.
5. Psychomotor agitation or retardation nearly every day (observable by others, not merely subjective feelings of restlessness or being slowed down).
6. Fatigue or loss of energy nearly every day.
7. Feelings of worthlessness or excessive or inappropriate guilt (which may be delusional) nearly every day (not merely self-reproach or guilt about being sick).
8. Diminished ability to think or concentrate, or indecisiveness, nearly every day (either by subjective account or as observed by others).
9. Recurrent thoughts of death (not just fear of dying), recurrent suicidal ideation without a specific plan, or a suicide attempt or a specific plan for committing suicide.

B. The symptoms do not meet criteria for a Mixed Episode.
C. The symptoms cause clinically significant distress or impairment in social, occupational, or other important areas of functioning.
D. The symptoms are not due to the direct physiological effects of a substance (e.g., a drug of abuse, a medication) or a general medical condition (e.g., hypothyroidism).
E. The symptoms are not better accounted for by Bereavement, i.e., after the loss of a loved one, the symptoms persist for longer than 2 months or are characterized by marked functional impairment, morbid preoccupation with worthlessness, suicidal ideation, psychotic symptoms, or psychomotor retardation.[2]

Anyone reporting at least five of the nine symptoms in criterion A, including at least one of depressed mood or loss of interest or pleasure, for a 2-week period is considered to have Major Depressive Episode and thus, generally, MDD. Note that even for those satisfying the symptom criteria, there are the four exclusions in Criteria B through E, eliminating the following from diagnosis: (1) conditions that also include manic symptoms, which are classified under bipolar disorders; (2) conditions that do not cause clinically significant role impairment or distress; (3) conditions that are the direct result of a general medical condition or use of either an illegal substance or prescribed medication; these are diagnosed as Mood Disorder Due to General Medical Condition or Substance-Induced Mood Disorder; or (4) conditions that stem from bereavement, unless the grief has lasted longer than 2 months or involves certain particularly severe symptoms; this is considered a case of "complicated bereavement."

How the *DSM* Criteria for Major Depression Address the Distinction Between Disorder and Normal Sadness

Symptom and Duration Criteria

The *DSM-IV* tries to exclude normal depressive conditions from diagnosis as disorders via the various features of its symptom criteria: (1) its five-symptom threshold for the diagnosis sets a higher threshold than many normal periods of sadness would meet; (2) the specific nature of some of the individual symptoms might inherently suggest pathology, as in feelings of worthlessness, psychomotor retardation, or recurrent thoughts of death; (3) the required duration of 2 weeks, during which five symptoms must cluster together, eliminates shorter periods or sporadic individual symptoms experienced discontinuously over time; and (4) the required severity, intensity, and frequency of the symptoms during at least the 2-week minimal duration—for example, that they must occur "nearly every day" during a 2-week period, be "marked" or "significant," or feature other benchmarks such as a percentage weight loss—also eliminates many milder forms of normal sadness.

There is no question that these features of the symptom criteria do eliminate many episodes of normal sadness from being mistakenly classified as disorders. However, such strategies for distinguishing disordered from normal responses have two disadvantages. First, increases in the symptomatic threshold for diagnosis in order to eliminate false positives can often inadvertently increase false negatives, by which genuine disorders go unrecognized. The disordered status of a condition is not a matter of the number of symptoms because mild disorders with a limited number of symptoms can exist.

Second, although the occurrence of a greater number of symptoms is generally more harmful, it is not always the case that more symptoms, more severe symptoms, or more prolonged symptoms imply dysfunction and disorder. As chapter 2 documented, unusually harsh environmental stressors often produce many intense symptoms in otherwise normal individuals, and the depressive symptoms that occur during normal periods of sadness are generally similar to the depressive symptoms listed in the *DSM* criteria that occur during depressive disorders. Moreover, some people are temperamentally more sensitive and have more severe normal responses to stress than others.

Thus setting high symptom thresholds in terms of number, intensity, or continuity over a 2-week period does not effectively address the dysfunction problem—that is, the problem of distinguishing whether the symptoms are part of a normal sadness reaction or are the result of a dysfunction of sadness-generating mechanisms. Intense normal sadness in response to a variety of major losses can easily include the five symptoms the *DSM* requires, such as low mood, lack of pleasure in usual activities, sleeplessness, lack of appetite, and difficulty concentrating on usual tasks. Nor is the required severity of the *DSM* symptoms, specified in some cases by qualifiers such as "recurrent," "marked," or "diminished," generally of such a distinctive level that it would characterize disordered rather than intense normal sadness responses. Likewise, the 2-week duration does not adequately distinguish potentially normal-range intense reactions to serious losses, such as the end of a marriage or a potentially terminal medical diagnosis, from depressive disorders. Normal reactions to major losses can easily last more than 2 weeks. Certainly, the severity of the symptoms themselves, having five of them, and experiencing them almost every day during a 2-week period does offer a stark contrast to usual functioning and thus may seem on first glance to impart validity. But when the contrast is between depressive disorder and periods of intense normal sadness in response to major losses, normal sadness can easily meet these requirements.

Moreover, many of the symptoms, such as difficulty sleeping and fatigue, have very high base rates in the general population in response to a variety of stresses and are not at all distinctive of depression, normal or disordered, or even of disorder in general. Thus individuals without a depressive disorder might accidentally reach the threshold due to the presence of unrelated symptoms during a period of normal low mood.

It is true that some symptoms, such as complete immobilization, a morbid and unjustified preoccupation with one's worthlessness, hallucinations, and delusions, do not significantly overlap with normal functioning. These symptoms might generally indicate dysfunctions rather than designed sadness, especially if persistent. However, the diagnosis of MDD does not require the presence of such especially severe symptoms.

Exclusion for Bereavement

One way in which the *DSM* attempts to make up for any weaknesses in the symptom criteria's ability to distinguish disorder from nondisorder is through the exclusion clauses. This is the main purpose of the bereavement exclusion. However, like every other mental or physical function, grief can "go wrong" and become disordered. For this reason, the bereavement exclusion has its own exclusion-to-the-exclusion that allows depressive symptoms associated with grief sometimes to be classified as true disorders after all. This occurs when grief responses persist for longer than 2 months, cause marked functional impairment, or include especially severe symptoms, such as morbid preoccupation with worthless-ness, suicidal ideation, psychomotor retardation, or psychotic symptoms.[3] (It is also worth noting that during bereavement transient hallucinations of a lost loved one's presence are not uncommon, and they are not generally considered pathological.)

One might dispute the 2-month limit on normal bereavement, and one might argue that normal bereavement may sometimes include one of the "com-plicated" symptoms that the *DSM* says are sufficient for disorder. However, by far the major flaw in this exclusion criterion is its failure to take into account normal sadness responses to any losses other than the death of a loved one. It would have been easy to generalize the bereavement exclusion clause (and its accompanying exclusion-to-the-exclusion criteria) to cover all severe losses, but this opportunity was foregone, for reasons explored earlier. Consequently, this constructive attempt to validly delineate the normally sad from the disordered is too limited to adequately address the glaring weaknesses in the symptomatic criteria.

Exclusion for General Medical and Substance-Use-Induced Depressions

The exclusion from MDD diagnosis of depressive conditions that directly result from the physiological effects of medical conditions or substance use simply shifts such cases into alternative disorder categories of Mood Disorder Due to General Medical Condition or Substance-Induced Mood Disorder. These catego-ries, although not our focus here, are subject to their own potential confusions. For example, such disorders are sometimes confused with normal sadness re-sponses to having a medical condition or with sadness in response to the prob-lems that result from using or being addicted to a substance. This is an instance of the complex challenges practitioners face in separating symptoms that indi-cate depression from similar symptoms that are not disordered or that are the result of different disorders.

The Clinical-Significance Requirement

Perhaps the most important attempt in the *DSM's* exclusion clauses to distinguish disordered from normal sadness responses is the "clinical significance" criterion, which requires that "the symptoms cause clinically significant distress or impair-ment in social, occupational, or other important areas of functioning." This clause implicitly acknowledges that even nonbereaved cases that satisfy the duration and symptom criteria might still not involve disorder. However, the clause does not ad-dress the basic validity problems of the MDD criteria. It was meant to ensure that the negative consequences of a condition exceed a threshold of significance if the condition is to be clinically relevant and thus potentially classifiable as a disorder, and it does this successfully. But it does not recognize some crucial distinctions. First, periods of sadness in general, whether normal or disordered, inherently entail negative emotions that involve distress. Indeed, it is hard to imagine having five of the specified symptoms without experiencing distress.

Second, intense normal loss responses almost always involve impairment and diminished interest and ability in various areas of functioning; the very prototype of these responses involves social withdrawal and wanting to be left alone (e.g., one does not feel like seeing friends or going to work). Indeed, intense normal loss responses may be designed to cause distress and social withdrawal to enable one to avoid threats and reconsider one's life and goal structure (see chapter 2).[4] Thus the clinical-significance exclusion might eliminate from the disorder category a few conditions whose feeble symptoms occasion no harm. But it is likely to be used quite rarely because the listed symptoms themselves already involve obvious forms of distress and impairment, rendering the requirement of distress or impairment virtually redundant.[5]

The clinical-significance criterion fails to resolve the problem of distinguishing normal from disordered conditions that satisfy *DSM* criteria because, like the symptom and duration criteria, it potentially applies to both kinds of conditions and fails to address the question of dysfunction. Nor is the addition of the qualifier "clinically significant" helpful in making the distinction clearer because the qualifier is left undefined. Thus the phrase can mean only "significant enough to indicate a clinical—that is, disordered—condition," making the criterion circular with respect to distinguishing normal from disordered conditions.

Implications of the DSM's Own Definition of Mental Disorder

Interestingly, our claim that there is a flaw in the *DSM*'s definition of Major Depressive Disorder with respect to distinguishing disordered from normal sadness appears to be implicit in the text of the *DSM* itself. The *DSM*'s preface contains a brief general definition of mental disorder that is supposed to be used to determine which conditions are allowed into the manual in the first place. The *DSM-IV*'s definition of mental disorder reads as follows:

> In *DSM-IV*, each of the mental disorders is conceptualized as a clinically significant behavioral or psychological syndrome or pattern that occurs in an individual and that typically is associated with present distress (e.g., a painful symptom) or disability (i.e., impairment in one or more important areas of functioning) or with a significantly increased risk of suffering death, pain, disability, or an important loss of freedom. In addition, this syndrome or pattern must not be merely an expectable and culturally sanctioned response to a particular event, for example, the death of a loved one. Whatever its original cause, it must currently be considered a

manifestation of *a behavioral, psychological, or biological dysfunction in the individual.* Neither deviant behavior (e.g., political, religious, or sexual) nor conflicts that are primarily between the individual and society are mental disorders unless the deviance or conflict is a symptom of a dysfunction in the individual, as described above.[6]

This definition commendably distinguishes disordered from nondisordered conditions in terms of the presence of internal dysfunction, albeit in a cursory way, without attempting to explain the concept of dysfunction. Given that this is a general definition of the concept of disorder that should apply to each of the manual's categories, it follows that the sets of diagnostic criteria for particular disorders presumably should meet the general rule that only dysfunction-caused symptoms should count as disorders. However, neither the *DSM-III* nor later editions of the manual ever made a systematic attempt to rectify the diagnostic criteria with the general definition of mental disorders. This is unfortunate because it appears that in many instances the definition is more valid than the specific diagnostic criteria sets are.

The definition of mental disorder, which relies on the distinction between symptoms that emerge because of a dysfunction in the individual rather than because of socially expectable or undesirable conditions, is quite similar in some important respects to the "harmful dysfunction" account of disorder that forms the background for our discussion.[7] In particular, the *DSM* definition seems to indicate that even conditions that manifest certain symptoms may not be disorders, because the presence of a disorder depends on whether the symptoms result from a dysfunction. The definition also usefully asserts that a condition cannot be considered a disorder sheerly on the basis of its personal or social undesirability, even if there is distress or impairment or other harmful symptoms. Rather, the condition is a disorder only if a *dysfunction in the person* causes the symptoms. But, according to this definition, it would seem that a person reacting to external stressful events in the way we naturally react, namely, with certain emotional and other reactions of the kind the *DSM*'s symptom list for depressive disorder partly describes, does not have a dysfunction and thus does not have a disorder. Consequently, the *DSM*'s own definition of disorder, combined with the most plausible account of "dysfunction" as failure of natural function, implies that the criteria for MDD are invalid because they misclassify intense but naturally selected loss responses as disorders.

The Precedent of Conduct Disorder

It may seem impossible that the expert diagnosticians who formulated the diagnostic criteria in the *DSM* could arrive at criteria that are not only invalid but also inconsistent with *DSM*'s own stated definition of disorder. However, clinical diagnosis is a quite different task from conceptual analysis of the defining criteria that separate disorder from normality. The two require different skills (just as, for example, recognizing chairs when you see them is very different from formulating a principled definition of the concept "chair" that picks out all and only chairs), and it is thus possible for such errors to enter into the manual. Consider an acknowledged precedent: the *DSM-IV* text itself states that the criteria for an important disorder of childhood and adolescence, Conduct Disorder (i.e., a disorder of antisocial behavior, diagnosed by three or more out of a list of behaviors such as theft, running away, etc.), are invalid and encompass some conditions that should not be diagnosed as disorders despite their satisfying the diagnostic criteria. The problem, the *DSM-IV* informs us, is that the symptomatic antisocial behaviors used to diagnose Conduct Disorder may occur in some conditions that are not due to a psychological dysfunction but only to a normal reaction to difficult environmental circumstances.

Here is what the *DSM-IV* has to say about its own Conduct Disorder criteria:

> Concerns have been raised that the Conduct Disorder diagnosis may at times be misapplied to individuals in settings where patterns of undesirable behavior are sometimes viewed as protective (e.g., threatening, impoverished, high-crime). Consistent with the *DSM-IV* definition of mental disorder, the Conduct Disorder diagnosis should be applied only when the behavior in question is symptomatic of an underlying dysfunction within the individual and not simply a reaction to the immediate social context. Moreover, immigrant youth from war-ravaged countries who have a history of aggressive behaviors that may have been necessary for their survival in that context would not necessarily warrant a diagnosis of Conduct Disorder. It may be helpful for the clinician to consider the social and economic context in which the undesirable behaviors have occurred.[8]

This passage says that the *DSM* criteria for Conduct Disorder are not valid when applied to symptoms that could occur as a normal response to circumstances, as, for example, when psychiatrically normal youths join gangs for self-protection in a threatening neighborhood and engage in antisocial behavior as part of required gang activities. Thus the Conduct Disorder criteria do not always pick out dysfunctions. We are making exactly the same point about the criteria for MDD. The symptomatic criteria do sometimes pick out dysfunctions and thus disorders, but they also pick out a potentially large range of normal responses to problematic environments. As in Conduct Disorder, the problem is not particularly hard to see once one considers obvious examples. Yet it is a profound problem that throws into doubt the meaning of much recent research on depression, as we show in later chapters.

In addition, the criteria for Conduct Disorder contain the same kind of "clinical significance" requirement that appears in the MDD criteria. But the textual comment just quoted implies that the Conduct Disorder criteria are incapable of adequately distinguishing normal from disordered conditions even with the addition of the clinical-significance clause. This clause certainly addresses whether there is sufficient harm for a disorder diagnosis, but it does not address whether a dysfunction causes the harm. In the case of Conduct Disorder, even though the clinical-significance criterion eliminates conditions with symptoms too mild to constitute a disorder, the *DSM-IV* recognizes that a separate question remains about whether or not there is a dysfunction causing the symptoms and thus about whether the symptoms represent a disorder or a normal reaction to circumstances. Precisely the same issue remains in the case of MDD despite the inclusion of the clinical-significance criterion.

How the *DSM* Attempts to Address Contextual Triggers of Sadness

Even if the MDD criteria taken in isolation have the problems we have identified, some would answer our criticisms by suggesting that the *DSM* must be looked at as a whole. They could say that our objections to the criteria are dealt with via other complementary categories or other features of the manual that somehow address the issue of normal loss responses. So, in this part, we consider various other categories and features that the *DSM* uses to handle depressive symptoms. We argue that, far from compensating for the weaknesses in the MDD criteria, these complementary categories and features either do not address the problem at all or in some cases actually make things considerably worse by further broadening the scope of normal sadness responses that can be labeled as pathological.

Textual Mention of Normal Sadness

Textual commentary that accompanies the criteria for MDD and the other Mood Disorders does indeed mention the challenge of distinguishing normal sadness from depressive disorder. However, the way it addresses the issue simply reinforces the problems noted earlier. Under a section on "differential diagnosis," after a lengthy discussion that suggests how depressive disorder can be discriminated from various other mental disorders and from bereavement (here, the text simply repeats the requirements stated in the MDD criteria's bereavement exclusion clause), the *DSM-IV-TR* says the following:

> Finally, periods of sadness are inherent aspects of the human experience. These periods should not be diagnosed as a Major Depressive Episode unless criteria are met for severity (i.e., five out of nine symptoms), duration (i.e., most of the day, nearly every day for at least 2 weeks), and clinically significant distress or impairment.[9]

This passage just reiterates the diagnostic criteria for MDD and reasserts that they are sufficient for disorder. The clear implication is that normal periods of sadness never satisfy the criteria. But, as demonstrated earlier in this book, this is not so. Part of the range of normal variation in sadness, especially in response to severe losses and threats, can easily meet *DSM* criteria. Thus, in stark contrast to the textual comment that accompanies the criteria for Conduct Disorder, the MDD comment seems a half-hearted gesture toward acknowledging the problem of distinguishing depressive disorder from normal sadness; however, it only repeats the original error in the criteria.

Multiaxial System

A second way in which the *DSM* tries to address the issue of development of symptoms in response to stressors is via its multiaxial system of diagnosis. This system rates patients on five distinct dimensions that go beyond the diagnostic criteria. Diagnoses of MDD (and all other mental disorders) are recorded on Axis I, personality disorders on Axis II, general medical conditions on Axis III, psychosocial and environmental problems on Axis IV, and global assessment of functioning on Axis V. The various axes are intended to give the clinician a more comprehensive picture of the context of the patient's problem than the diagnostic criteria alone provide. In particular, Axis IV involves reporting psychosocial and environmental problems that affect the diagnosis, treatment, and prognosis of mental disorders and would include stressors that trigger a loss response.

The problem is that the Axis IV grouping of psychosocial stressors simply places them on a completely separate dimension from the diagnoses of disorders. Symptoms that meet criteria for MDD would have *already* been defined as disordered before Axis IV would come into play. This added information, valuable as it may be, does not in any way address the normal-versus-disordered relation between existing stressors and symptomatic responses, and so it fails to address the problem of whether the condition is a psychological dysfunction or a nondisordered response to a stressor. This axis provides a way for clinicians to take stressors into account in case descriptions, not a means of separating disordered from nondisordered conditions that meet symptomatic criteria.

V Codes for Nondisordered Conditions

Third, the *DSM* contains a short section called "Additional Conditions That May Be a Focus of Clinical Attention," which includes nondisordered conditions for which patients often consult professionals. These categories are often called "V codes" after the letter that precedes their numerical diagnostic codes in the *DSM-III.* Among the V codes is Bereavement, under which it is noted that "As part of their reaction to the loss, some grieving individuals present with symptoms characteristic of a Major Depressive Episode. . . . The diagnosis of Major

Depressive Episode is generally not given unless the symptoms are still present 2 months after the loss."[10] The category of Bereavement thus explicitly recognizes that a condition can satisfy the full set of symptomatic criteria for a Major Depressive Episode and yet not be a mental disorder. But this category is limited to grief after loss of a loved one, and consequently, insofar as recognition of nondisordered conditions goes, it just repeats what the bereavement exclusion clause in the MDD criteria already contains.

Among the other V codes are separate categories for academic, occupational, identity, spiritual, acculturation, and phase-of-life problems. The V codes do not provide any symptom criteria for such nondisordered problems; in each case, they state only that a condition can be classified under the category if it is "not due to a mental disorder." Thus the *DSM-IV* does recognize that many problems in living are not mental disorders. However, it gives no criteria for distinguishing symptoms of mental disorders from those that are nondisordered problems in living. In particular, it makes no provision for overriding the criteria for MDD to classify a condition that satisfies those criteria as a normal response. When the *DSM* states that to qualify as a V code the condition must be "not due to a mental disorder," it in effect means that the condition cannot satisfy *DSM* criteria for a mental disorder, including MDD. Consequently, conditions that meet symptomatic criteria for MDD must be given a specific diagnosis as a disorder and not a V code. Only residual conditions that do not satisfy disorder criteria may be placed under a V code. Therefore, the V codes do not address the problem of normal loss responses that satisfy the *DSM* criteria for MDD. In fact, the V-codes section is exactly where many potential diagnoses of MDD likely belong.

Adjustment Disorder

The main way the *DSM-IV* addresses the issue of sadness responses to stressors is via the diagnostic category of Adjustment Disorder With Depressed Mood. This category in effect attempts to define what the *DSM-I* and *DSM-II* used to call "reactive" depressions that occur in response to circumstances. The challenge in formulating such a definition is that most normal sadness is also "reactive" to circumstances, so the criteria must somehow distinguish disordered from normal reactions. The criteria for Adjustment Disorder With Depressed Mood, however, fail to surmount this challenge and thus inadvertently manage to pathologize (i.e., incorrectly treat as disorder) a vast range of additional normal loss responses beyond those that would fall under the criteria for MDD.

Intended to distinguish pathological overreactions to stress from normal reactions, the overall category of Adjustment Disorder encompasses a set of subcategories, each of which involves a specific kind of symptomatic reaction to a stressor, including depressed mood, anxiety, antisocial conduct, mixed symptoms, and a catchall "unspecified" category for physical complaints, social withdrawal, work inhibitions, and other problematic reactions to stress. Adjustment disorder is a residual "category that should not be used if the disturbance meets the criteria for another specific Axis I disorder," such as MDD.[11]

To qualify specifically as Adjustment Disorder "With Depressed Mood," the condition must meet the general criteria for Adjustment Disorder (discussed next) and, in addition, fulfill the following symptomatic criterion: "This subtype should be used when the predominant manifestations are symptoms such as depressed mood, tearfulness, or feelings of hopelessness."[12] The requirement that any of these symptoms be present is so weak that virtually any normal sadness response would satisfy it. Indeed, in principle, the vague depressive symptom criterion allows diagnosis with just one common sadness-response symptom, such as depressed mood or crying.

However, diagnosis also requires satisfying the general Adjustment Disorder criteria, and the validity of Adjustment Disorder With Depressed Mood thus hangs on these general criteria, which are as follows:

A. The development of emotional or behavioral symptoms in response to an identifiable stressor(s) occurring within 3 months of the onset of the stressor(s).
B. These symptoms or behaviors are clinically significant as evidenced by either of the following:
  1. Marked distress that is in excess of what would be expected from exposure to the stressor
  2. Significant impairment in social or occupational (academic) functioning
C. The stress-related disturbance does not meet the criteria for another specific Axis I or II disorder.
D. The symptoms do not represent Bereavement.
E. Once the stressor (or its consequences) has terminated, the symptoms do not persist for more than an additional 6 months.[13]

Adjustment Disorder, unlike MDD, is specifically limited to conditions that are reactions to triggering events. Clause C formalizes the "residual" character of the diagnosis and implies that Adjustment Disorder With Depressed Mood can be diagnosed only if the individual does not satisfy criteria for MDD. As in the criteria for MDD, the only exemption from disorder status is bereavement; reactions to any other losses that satisfy the criteria are considered disordered.

It is certainly true that the process of adjusting to stressors, or "coping," can go awry and become pathological. The critical issue is whether the criteria for Adjustment Disorder succeed in their intended purpose of distinguishing such disordered reactions from normal-range but intense coping responses that can accompany stressful events.

The criteria require that the symptom(s) must occur within 3 months of the stressor and must end within 6 months of the termination of the stressor. These timing criteria are designed to ensure that the symptoms are indeed a reaction to a stressor and not independent of it. The problem is that the vast majority of normal loss responses are characterized by a close temporal relationship to the stressor that triggers them; they tend to start soon after the occurrence of the stressor and to subside soon after the stressor abates. Thus the timing requirements potentially encompass the vast majority of episodes of normal sadness and do not distinguish disordered from nondisordered reactions to loss. The requirement that the reaction cease within 6 months of termination of the stressor (or its consequences) is of particular concern because one of the best indicators that a reaction might be considered pathological is that it does *not* gradually subside after the stressor ceases but takes on a life of its own independent of events.

The temporal requirements aside, the distinction that the *DSM* Adjustment Disorder criteria make between normal and disordered coping comes down entirely to whether the condition satisfies at least one of the two specified "clinical significance" criteria under criterion B. To be classified as a disorder, the reaction must include either "marked distress that is in excess of what would be expected from exposure to the stressor" or "significant impairment in social or occupational (academic) functioning."

Regarding the "excess distress" criterion, even normal reactions to stressors are inherently prone to be distressing, and when the stressor is a marked one, normal responses are (by the principle of proportionality) prone to be, or at least capable of being, marked. So this criterion's ability to distinguish normal from disordered reactions comes down to its requirement that the distress in disordered conditions is "in excess of what would be expected" for that stressor. The problem is how to construe this criterion. It cannot be understood as requiring that the symptoms are "in excess of what is expectable in a normal reaction," because that raises the question of how these criteria are supposed to distinguish normality from disorder. One obvious alternative is to construe "in excess of what is expectable" as a statistical requirement. However, the statistical interpretation would allow the top half or third (say) of the distribution of normal responders to be classified as disordered. But having greater than the typical or expected level of reaction does not necessarily imply that one's reaction is due to a disorder. For example: (1) the individual's meaning system and values may make a stressor much more problematic or threatening than it is for most people; (2) the individual may exist within a problematic environment in which the stressor is more serious or more enduring than usual; (3) the individual may come from a more expressive cultural background or family than other individuals do; or (4) the individual may temperamentally respond more intensely than most people do to life events.

A more charitable interpretation is that, by an "expectable" response, the *DSM* means whatever is a "proportionate" response when all the factors, including the nature and context of the stressor itself, as well as the subjective and cultural meanings of the stressor, are taken into account. We argued earlier that rough proportionality is one of the earmarks of a nondisordered loss response.

If the first component of criterion B is interpreted as specifying that a reaction "in excess" is outside the range of proportional responses, then, taken by itself, it is potentially a valid indicator of dysfunction and does correctly place some disorders into the Adjustment Disorder category and avoid obvious false positives.

But then there is the problem of criterion B's second component, impairment in social or occupational functioning. This, by itself, is offered as a sufficient alternative for classifying a condition as disordered. Unfortunately, it fails to exclude great numbers of normal loss response conditions. Whenever major stressors occur, it is likely that people will suffer impairment in their social, occupational, or academic functioning. Just the time and concentration it takes to deal with the stressor, the emotional feelings that make it difficult to focus on routine tasks, and the real-life changes that people must make can easily lead them to resist usual tasks and roles. Moreover, the issues and challenges that major stressors trigger may make some role functioning seem temporarily insignificant by comparison, causing a loss of motivation and interest. Virtually any low mood might have such consequences. Thus, even if the "marked distress" criterion is charitably interpreted, the flaws in the alternative impairment criterion ensure that a vast number of normal loss responses can be diagnosed as Adjustment Disorders.

We conclude that the criteria for Adjustment Disorder and for its subtype Adjustment Disorder With Depressed Mood potentially classify as disordered an enormous number of normal responses that are triggered by stressors and that subside after the stressor ends, just as such responses are designed to do. And they do so on the basis of as little as one symptom that reduces role functioning. Indeed, any normal loss response of any consequence that does not fall under the *DSM* criteria for MDD is almost sure to fall under the criteria for Adjustment Disorder With Depressed Mood.

The flaws in the Adjustment Disorder category are so apparent that researchers and epidemiologists have largely ignored it. They have clearly "voted with their feet" that Adjustment Disorder is not of interest, judging from the very low numbers of research studies on it and the lack of growth in those numbers, which stand in stark contrast to the growth of research on other *DSM* categories in general and on MDD in particular. In 1980, 80 medical articles contained "adjustment disorder" in their titles, a number that actually declined to 55 articles in 2005.[14] By the latter year, nearly 158 articles appeared with "depression" in their titles for each article about adjustment disorder. In short, MDD, not Adjustment Disorder With Depressed Mood, has become the operative category for the field when it comes to studying depressive states. This neglect of Adjustment Disorder by researchers appears to be justified. The diagnosis suffers from such glaring problems in distinguishing normal from disordered conditions that it has collapsed as a serious target of research under the weight of its own invalidities. However, within the clinical realm, the diagnosis of Adjustment Disorder may nonetheless sometimes still be useful as a way of providing a potentially reimbursable label for reactions to stressful circumstances that may or may not be genuine disorders but that often deserve and need clinical attention.

Other Depression-Related Categories and Features of the *DSM-IV*

Subthreshold Diagnoses I: Minor Depression

Conditions that fail to meet the full symptomatic or duration criteria for MDD but that include some symptoms mentioned in the criteria are called "subthreshold" conditions. The *DSM-IV* placed a new category, Minor Depressive Disorder, which would subsume such conditions in an appendix on "Criteria Sets and Axes Provided for Further Study." It would require only two, instead of five, symptoms from the nine criteria for MDD, as long as one symptom is either depressed mood or diminished interest or pleasure. In other respects, such as the duration requirement and various exclusions, it is essentially the same as Major Depressive Disorder.[15]

As we shall see in the next chapter, various arguments in the recent literature propose that subthreshold conditions should be defined as genuine disorders. None of these recommendations seriously addresses the problem that allowing subthreshold conditions opens the floodgates to diagnosing as disorders normal sadness responses that are not even particularly intense or enduring. Indeed, such a category could encompass virtually all significant loss responses or periods of sadness. Thus far, however, the *DSM* has not adopted minor depression as an official category.

Subthreshold Diagnoses II: Mood Disorder Not Otherwise Specified

Nevertheless, the *DSM* does already specify that mental health professionals at their discretion can classify as depressive disorders subthreshold conditions that do not meet the *DSM* criteria for MDD. This is due to the fact that, as it does for many other kinds of categories, the manual includes an additional "wastebasket" category of Mood Disorder Not Otherwise Specified (NOS). One of the main purposes of this category is to diagnose "disorders with mood symptoms that do not meet the criteria for any specific mood disorder."[16]

The manual's introduction includes a section titled "Use of Not Otherwise Specified Categories" that identifies the situations in which an NOS diagnosis may be appropriate. The first applies to conditions for which there is

> Enough information available to indicate the class of disorder that is present, but further specification is not possible, either because there is not sufficient information to make a more specific diagnosis or because the clinical features of the disorder do not meet the criteria for any of the specific categories in that class.[17]

The intention here was no doubt the legitimate one of giving clinicians the flexibility to diagnose occasionally clear disorders that do not quite meet the official threshold for a more specifically named condition in a class. But applying the NOS category to depressive disorder, with no precautions about distinguishing it from normal reactions, could allow clinicians to diagnose as disorders many normal responses that are not intense enough to meet the five-symptom, 2-week threshold.

The second situation the manual specifies as one in which the NOS category can be used is when "the presentation conforms to a symptom pattern that has not been included in the *DSM* classification but that causes clinically significant distress or impairment."[18] This is equally problematic because both normal and disordered sadness can easily possess significant distress and role impairment. So, when it comes to loss responses, the Mood Disorder NOS category in effect gives clinicians carte blanche to classify normal reactions as disorders.

Dysthymic Disorder

A second category of depressive disorders in the *DSM-IV* is Dysthymic Disorder. Conceived in part as a concession to psychodynamic clinicians, this disorder was substituted for the traditional category of neurotic depression (and actually appeared under the title "Dysthymic Disorder (or Depressive Neurosis)" in the *DSM-III*).[19] Its criteria are quite different, however, from those for traditional neurotic depressions, which included excessive but often time-limited reactions to specific stressors. Diagnosis of Dysthymic Disorder requires a disturbance of mood and only two additional symptoms, but it also requires that the symptoms must have lasted for at least 2 years (1 year for children and adolescents) and during that time must have been present for most of the day on most days. Like MDD, Dysthymic Disorder is diagnosed solely on the basis of symptoms, without reference to such factors as chronic stressors (e.g., the gradual decline and death of an ill child) that might distinguish normal from disordered states of chronic depressive symptoms. Nor do the symptomatic criteria allow a distinction between depressive disorder and normal-range melancholic personality or temperament, the latter identified since the time of Aristotle. These problems present major challenges for the validity of the Dysthymic Disorder category itself, and certainly its inclusion as a category of milder but chronic depressive conditions does nothing to fix the problems that stem from the lack of adequate distinction between normality and disorder in the MDD criteria.

Melancholic Major Depressive Disorder

For some persons who meet the MDD criteria, the *DSM* specifies a "With Melancholic Features" subcategory. This classifies an individual who either has lost pleasure in all or almost all activities or who does not react to usually pleasurable stimuli and who displays three additional symptoms from a list that includes a distinct quality of the depressed mood in contrast to usual sadness, greater severity in the morning, early-morning awakening, marked psychomotor retardation, weight loss, and excessive guilt.

The subcategory of melancholia was intended to correspond to traditional cases of *endogenous depression*, which were considered to be particularly clear instances of depressive disorder.[20] However, the *DSM* does not actually use the term *endogenous* because, by tradition, that term connotes certain types of "vegetative" or seemingly physiologically based symptoms and a lack of any external triggering circumstances, all of which do indeed suggest disorder but involve an etiological assumption. Instead, the *DSM* uses symptoms alone to diagnose the melancholic subcategory. Consequently, many conditions that the *DSM*'s symptomatic criteria classify as melancholic do have associated precipitating stresses and would not traditionally be considered "endogenous."

It is possible that, due to their special symptomatic requirements, *DSM* melancholic depressions may, on average, be actual disorders more often than other types of depression. But melancholic depressions make up only a small fraction of *DSM* Major Depressive Disorders. Thus the distinction between melancholic and other depressive conditions cannot yield any solution to the validity problems of the overall MDD criteria.[21]

Would it have helped to resolve the problem of distinguishing normal from disordered sadness if the *DSM* had formulated the criteria for melancholic depression to reflect the traditional notion of "endogenous" in contrast to "reactive" depressions? As we argued in chapter 1, the endogenous-reactive distinction does not adequately distinguish disorder from nondisorder because, although endogenous depressions are generally disorders, so are many reactive depressions by virtue of a disproportionate symptomatic response to the magnitude of the triggering loss. The *DSM* justly abandoned this distinction but, unfortunately, did not find an adequate replacement for it.

Conclusion

The symptom-based diagnoses in the *DSM-III* and *DSM-IV* in many ways improved previous efforts to classify depression. They overcame the cursory and ambiguous definitions of depression found in previous manuals. Explicit criterion sets enhanced communication among researchers and clinicians about the meaning of depression. Researchers could create more homogeneous populations of participants, and clinical diagnoses had greater chances of referring to the same types of conditions.

These undoubted advances, however, also had costs. The main cost was that the symptom-based diagnoses did not validly distinguish depressions that indicate the presence of disorder from expectable reactions to situational contexts. The many features of the *DSM* that deal with responses to stressors fail to resolve this problem. The manual's own definition of mental disorders, combined with the empirical data cited in chapter 2, suggests that its criteria for depressive disorder are not valid. The multiaxial system does not help because it uses the relevant axis of psychosocial stressors only to supplement, not to modify, a diagnosis of disorder. The category of Adjustment Disorder merely compounds the problem because it pathologizes even those normal reactions that display fewer than the usual symptoms and that go away when the stressor ceases. Nor does the inclusion of V codes overcome the fundamental problem that all conditions that meet diagnostic criteria must be diagnosed as disorders. It would have been easy enough for the definition of MDD to have included a more extensive set of exclusion criteria comparable to the exclusion for bereavement, but this was not attempted. The result is a major invalidity that leads to the pathologization of intense normal sadness.

Kraepelin conceptually embraced the "with cause" versus "without cause" distinction, although it was not an important practical consideration in classifying his inpatient populations. By the time the *DSM-III* was published in 1980, outpatient therapy was much more common, and, consequently, the range of the problems people brought to psychiatrists had enormously expanded. Just when it would have been most useful to further develop the "with cause" versus "without cause" distinction so as to avoid false positive diagnoses, the *DSM-III* abandoned the distinction and thus inadvertently reclassified as mental disorders many conditions that were problems of living. The resulting problems went unremedied in subsequent editions of the manual. But the problem of pathologizing normal sadness does not end there. The next step in transforming normal unhappiness into mental disorder came when the symptom-based logic behind the *DSM-III* and *DSM-IV* went beyond the clinic and formed the basis for studies of depression among untreated individuals in the community.

6

Importing Pathology Into the Community

The transformation of intense normal sadness into depressive disorder occurred in several stages. The development of influential symptom-based research criteria for affective disorders in the Feighner criteria and RDC provided an initial step. Such criteria lacked the contextual assessment that had traditionally protected diagnosis from misclassifying intense sadness as disorder and thus created the potential for false positives. Research on depression was, however, primarily concerned with hospitalized patients and quite severely afflicted community members who were clearly disordered. Within this context, the symptom-based criteria worked well to distinguish affective disorders from other serious disorders, and the potential for false positives was not immediately realized. The second step occurred when the *DSM-III* applied the symptom-based logic to clinical practice in general, including burgeoning outpatient practices and community clinics in which therapists might see all forms of mental distress. Applying decontextualized criteria to this heterogeneous group of outpatients made it more likely that these diagnoses would be applied to those suffering from normal sadness.

However, several factors work to minimize the overapplication of the *DSM*'s criteria to normal sadness in outpatient clinical settings. Patients tend to self-select, so although many individuals do seek help for normal sadness, more often they seek treatment only after they attribute their symptoms to internal problems and not to stressful situations.[1] Moreover, clinicians themselves, in spite of enticements by insurance reimbursement to see depressive disorder wherever possible, can still use their commonsense judgments to correct for flaws in the *DSM* criteria and to recognize when a patient is not disordered but perhaps just in need of reassurance and support to alleviate painful but normal and likely transient feelings.

It is not, then, in the clinical context that the confusion between what is normal and abnormal is most in danger of occurring. Instead, the most radical transformation of ordinary sadness into pathology happened when the *DSM*'s criteria, developed primarily for treated cases, were lifted out of the clinical context with its special constraints and applied to studies of depression in the community among people who had not sought professional help for their conditions.

The field of psychiatric epidemiology viewed the symptom-based logic of the *DSM* criteria as an opportunity to achieve its long-pursued goal of assessing prevalence of mental illness in the general population through the use of relatively simple, lay-administered checklist questionnaires. Such checklists eliminated the need for mental health professionals to diagnose large populations and made the cost and logistics of such studies much more achievable. By using the *DSM* criteria, epidemiological instruments were supposed to uncover the same disordered conditions in the community that were presumed to exist among treated patients. But, as we shall see, in the change of context from the clinic to the community, the false-positives problem latent in the *DSM* criteria emerged with a vengeance; in fact, the new epidemiological instruments equally identified both pathological depression and widespread intense normal sadness that exists in community members, and thus they grossly overestimated the number of depressive disorders in untreated populations.

Community Studies Prior to *DSM-III*

To understand the enormous impact of *DSM* depression criteria on epidemiological studies of how many people in the community have depressive disorders, it is useful to step back and consider the history of psychiatric epidemiology. At a certain historical moment, the goals of epidemiology and those of the *DSM* converged, and the *DSM* criteria offered epidemiologists both improved criteria and a seeming solution to problems that confronted their field.

In the early days of psychiatric epidemiology during the first half of the twentieth century, estimates of rates of mental disorder were based on surveys of various treatment settings and relied on the diagnoses contained in medical charts.[2] However, it soon became apparent that surveys of treated patients provided a poor indicator of the degree of mental disorder in a community. Not everyone who has a disorder seeks treatment—for reasons having to do with stigma, cost, or the failure to recognize that the problem is a disorder—and many who might seek treatment do not have professional services readily available. Moreover, many of those who do seek treatment for various problems are not disordered. Thus, in order to guide mental health policy and estimate the need for services, as well as to gain a better understanding of the etiology and prevalence of mental illness, epidemiological studies attempted to surmount these problems by directly surveying the community at large.

Community studies try to determine the amount of mental illness among people who are not in clinical treatment but whose conditions are presumed to be diagnosable in a way comparable to the conditions of people who are being treated. To accomplish this aim, researchers must develop measures that can assess psychiatric symptoms among individuals who often neither consider themselves to be mentally ill nor seek mental health treatment and so have never been professionally diagnosed. Because some disorders affect a small number of people, surveys must study quite large numbers to obtain accurate estimates of the amount of specific kinds of mental disorder in a population. Since the beginning of psychiatric epidemiology, formulating valid indicators of disorder to use in such surveys has represented a major challenge to the ingenuity of researchers.[3]

The major impetus for attempts to measure the amount of depression and other common mental disorders in community populations lay in the experiences of World War II military psychiatrists who had treated and studied what they labeled *combat neuroses,* a combination of depressive, anxious, and psychophysiological symptoms that resulted from battlefield experiences. Similar war neuroses had been familiar to psychiatrists from earlier wars—for example, Freud occasionally used them as a model for his thinking about trauma—but they did not take on central theoretical importance in the psychiatric profession until World War II.

In that war, very high proportions of previously normal soldiers who were exposed to highly stressful combat conditions were found to develop psychological problems. Overall, nearly 1 million American soldiers suffered neuropsychiatric breakdowns: in combat divisions, admission rates to hospitals for psychiatric conditions numbered 250 per 1,000 soldiers.[4] Moreover, up to 70% of soldiers exposed to long stretches of combat suffered mental breakdowns. One report in 1946 estimated that the average soldier would have a psychiatric breakdown after 88 days of continuous combat. Not considering any other sources of casualties, the report also estimated that 95% of soldiers would break down after 260 combat days. "Practically all men in rifle battalions who were not otherwise disabled," the report added, "ultimately became psychiatric casualties."[5]

Furthermore, no preexisting psychological characteristics predicted which soldiers would break down and which would not.[6] Instead, it was the intensity and duration of combat experiences that led to the development of combat neuroses. When faced with sufficient stressors from the environment, all individuals could become seriously disturbed. "It would seem," military psychiatrists Grinker and Spiegel asserted in 1945, "to be a more rational question to ask why the soldier does *not* succumb to anxiety, rather than why he does."[7] Their wartime experiences turned the attention of psychiatrists away from the qualities of individuals toward the qualities of stressful environments.

The typical response to psychiatric casualties during World War II was to provide these soldiers with hot food, rest and sleep, showers, and reassurance. Such responses, "which basically consisted of resting the soldier and indicating to him that he would soon rejoin his unit," did not require extensive psychiatric training.[8] The most careful postwar study indicated that over half of psychiatric casualties returned to duty with virtually no treatment and that over two-thirds of those given rest and sedation returned to their units within 48 hours after treatment.[9]

Surely, many of these individuals whose conditions endured had developed mental disorders. One might ponder, however, whether the majority who recovered quickly and spontaneously without any real treatment had extreme normal stress responses in reaction to truly abnormal circumstances.[10] But what is important historically for the development of psychiatric epidemiology is that psychiatrists came to view all such psychological consequences of combat as mental disorders.[11]

After the war, socially oriented psychiatrists saw combat stress disorders as a useful model for the mental disorders of civilian life and equated the extraordinary stressors of war with the ordinary stressors of postwar life.[12] The theme that "every person has his breaking point" was transferred from soldiers to ordinary citizens. The combat neuroses thus provided a new paradigm for the mental health field for the next several decades that remains influential to the present.[13] Failing to recognize that most soldiers who suffered breakdowns recovered with minimal or no treatment, postwar psychiatrists came to emphasize the point that any stressful experience among normal people could precipitate serious, enduring breakdowns if not subject to early intervention. They turned their attention to creating theories and measures to study numerous environmental stressors in everyday life that they presumed would lead to psychiatric disorders.[14]

This erosion of the distinction between normal distress and disorder was furthered by another basic theme of researchers from the 1940s through the 1970s that derived from the psychodynamic tenets of Freud and Meyer: mental health and illness were not categorically distinct but lay on a continuum of symptom severity, from mild to severe.[15] Only rare individuals who were entirely symptom free were considered to be entirely mentally healthy.[16] All other points of the continuum were viewed as disordered or, at least, as less than fully healthy. An important aspect of the continuum concept was that if placed under stress persons who had symptoms at the mild end were at risk of developing more severe conditions in the absence of professional intervention. A consequent article of faith among community-oriented psychiatrists at the time was that early treatment of mild disorders in community settings could prevent the development of more serious conditions.[17] It became a major goal of psychiatry to develop instruments that could identify individuals most at risk for becoming mentally ill and to treat them before their conditions became more severe. The continuum notion, coupled with the assumption that sociocultural stresses caused mental disorder in the normal and caused the mildly symptomatic to become severely disordered, meant that virtually the entire population could be conceived as ill to some degree and at risk for becoming more seriously mentally ill.

Thus the evolving philosophy of community psychiatry made it imperative to study factors that determine the risk of presumed pathology among untreated populations. In the 1950s and 1960s, teams of dynamically oriented psychiatrists and social scientists jointly focused on studying how sociocultural factors caused many distressing conditions in the general population. To study the symptoms of modern urban populations, the psychiatrist Thomas A. C. Rennie and sociologists Leo Srole and Thomas Langner developed the Midtown Manhattan project, which surveyed more than 1,600 residents of Manhattan.[18] A second major project, the Stirling County study, was another collaboration between psychiatrists and social scientists that correlated types of stressors with the distribution of psychological symptoms among the population of a rural area of the Canadian province of Nova Scotia.[19]

The two major purposes of these initial postwar community studies were, first, to ascertain the magnitude of mental health problems in the population and, second, to test the hypothesis that sociocultural factors caused mental disorders.[20] Before they could answer these questions, these studies had to address the problem of how to define a psychiatric case among untreated individuals. The official psychiatric manual at the time, the *DSM-I*, did not provide any explicit criteria to measure specific types of mental illness. Clinicians used general and vague standards that were heavily dependent on their idiosyncratic judgments. Community studies could not rely on these judgments because they would produce far too much variance in outcome from interviewer to interviewer when used to establish rates of mental illness in untreated populations. Such studies also faced a significant practical problem: relying on mental health professionals to conduct large numbers of interviews was far too expensive to be an efficient option in community studies. For both practical and substantive reasons, these studies had to develop standardized measures that lay interviewers could administer.

Decontextualized, symptom-based measures of mental illness have tremendous practical appeal for surveys of mental illness. They provide standardized outcomes that do not vary from interviewer to interviewer. Because they do not require (or even permit) probes about the personal meaning of responses, interviewers do not need any clinical training or experience. This considerably lowers the cost of administering surveys, an especially important consideration in large epidemiological research. Studies developed questions that lay interviewers could ask in standardized formats, which could then be used to categorize respondents as disordered or not. The decision of these studies to use decontextualized measures of symptoms stemmed from considerations of practicality and cost, not from tests showing that these methods were accurate.[21]

The definition of depression in the *DSM-I* posed an additional obstacle for these community studies that strove to determine the influence of sociocultural factors on rates of distress. The *DSM-I* defined neurotic depression as "psychoneurotic depressive reaction," stating that "this reaction is precipitated by a current situation, frequently by some loss sustained by the patient. . . ."[22] When situational causes *by definition* precipitate nonpsychotic depressions, it is impossible to separate the influence of social from other, intraindividual, causes because the former must be implicated in all cases.[23]

Epidemiological studies tried to solve this problem in the *DSM-I* by first removing etiology from the definition of depression and then assuming that *all* symptoms were pathological. Situational factors were not taken into account in the definition of what counted as a disorder in the first place but, instead, were viewed as one type of cause of the symptoms. This decision meant that symptoms that were reactive to losses and other contextual factors, as well as those that were not, all counted as disordered. This solution allowed epidemiologists to achieve their goal of showing the relative influence of social and nonsocial factors in causing symptoms. At the same time, it created the problem of making disordered and nondisordered symptoms indistinguishable. Isolating symptoms from their context and assuming that they indicated disorders abandoned the historical recognition that only "excessive" or "disproportionate" symptoms were signs of disorders. The result was that sadness, by definition, could not be a normal response to a stressful situation but must indicate a disordered condition.

Thus the problem of decontextualization and consequent muddying of the distinction between depressive disorder and normal sadness that was to occur later in the clinical arena with the advent of the *DSM-III* actually occurred for independent reasons within the discipline of psychiatric epidemiology even before the *DSM-III*. Indeed, the problem was worse in these community studies because they did not account for the degree of severity, duration, and other requirements—that is, the extended criteria sets—that the *DSM-III* took pains to identify. Instead, individual symptoms themselves were taken as sufficient indicators of disorder, a situation that soon led to what were widely acknowledged to be absurd estimates of levels of pathology.

The earliest community studies did not measure specific types of mental illness (such measures were not yet available) but instead developed broad, continuous, and nonspecific measures of psychological distress interpreted to indicate levels of disorder.[24] They used scales containing general symptoms of depression, anxiety, and psychophysiological problems to develop global measures that they arrayed on a continuum from mild to severe.[25] Many of these items, such as "trouble getting to sleep," "in low or very low spirits," "can't get going," or "wonder if anything is worthwhile," can often be signs of normal distress. Because these studies defined all symptoms, including everyday unhappiness, as signs of pathology, they unsurprisingly found massive rates of disorder. In the Midtown Manhattan study, only 18.5% of respondents were "well," that is, reported no symptoms.[26] In contrast, 23.4% of respondents were "impaired," an additional 21.8% displayed "moderate" symptom formation, and the remaining 36.3% were "mildly" impaired. The Stirling County Study reported even higher rates, asserting that 57% of the sample was likely to be comparable to psychiatric cases.[27] Both the Midtown Manhattan and Stirling County studies found strong correlations between low socioeconomic status and poor social conditions and high rates of presumed mental illness.

These studies justified their findings of such high rates of disorder by the fact that control groups of treated psychiatric patients also reported large numbers of similar symptoms, presumably providing criterion validation for the symptom measures. Yet had these studies used as their control groups untreated community members who were not disordered but who had suffered recent life events such as bereavement, romantic breakups, or unemployment, they would also have found highly elevated rates of symptoms. They could have easily concluded that they measured ordinary unhappiness rather than mental disorder.

The high rates of putative disorders in community studies in the 1950s and 1960s generated considerable skepticism at the time. "If all persons who cough," noted the renowned epidemiologist Rema Lapouse, "are counted as cases of tuberculosis, both incidence and prevalence rates will skyrocket. Fortunately, the laboratory provides a safeguard against that kind of diagnostic extravagance. Psychiatric diagnosis as yet has no such safeguards."[28] Even Stanley Michael, a psychiatrist associated with the Midtown study, questioned its results:

> The uncovering of mental and emotional symptoms in four-fifths of the sample representing an urban population suggests that either a degree of psychopathology is the norm in the statistical sense of the population average or that mental mechanisms which by psychodynamic derivation can be considered pathological may be a mode of normal adjustment.[29]

The assumption that normal people would be symptom-free regardless of their life circumstances indicated a thoroughgoing confusion about normality and disorder. The fatal error of community studies was to define all symptoms as pathological without considering the context in which they arose and persisted.

Despite the problems inherent in the use of decontextualized symptom measures, subsequent community studies quickly adopted them and treated mental disorder as a continuum from less to more severe conditions. They regarded all points along the continuum as indicating pathology. Critiques of these studies, instead of trying to distinguish symptoms that indicated a disorder from those that were appropriate responses to stressors, focused on the nonspecific nature of the symptom scales. They claimed that the scales were so broad and unspecific that it was not clear how they were related to specific psychiatric conditions.[30] It was this particular flaw—the vagueness of the symptom measures with regard to actual diagnoses—that set the stage for a shift to *DSM*-style criteria sets for specific disorders.

Diagnoses Enter Community Studies

Using continuous distributions of highly generalized symptoms was incommen-
surate with the radically new paradigm of criteria sets for specific categories of
mental disorder that the *DSM-III* implemented in 1980. But earlier community
studies already shared the new manual's underlying assumptions that decontextualized symptoms must be the basis for diagnosis. The congruence of the
symptom-based approach epidemiologists used and the *DSM-III*'s symptom-
based measures perhaps accounts for the fact that epidemiologists quickly
adopted *DSM* criteria in the new wave of community studies that emerged in the
1980s.[31] The comparatively seamless transition from the dynamically oriented
yet symptom-based community studies in the 1950s and 1960s to the symptom-
based community studies of the 1980s was likely due to the fact that, unlike
their psychodynamic counterparts in the clinical community, community psychiatrists had already adopted a model that equated decontextualized symptoms
with the presence of some degree of pathology. In contrast, the *DSM-III* emerged
only after a protracted battle between the neo-Kraepelinians, who purged etiological assumptions from the manual, and the dynamic psychiatrists, who resisted their efforts.[32]

Because the *DSM-III* required that conditions satisfy an extended criteria
set before being classified as a specific disorder, psychiatric epidemiologists
expected *DSM* diagnoses to provide not only category-specific diagnoses but
also more realistic estimates of the amount of mental disorder in the community. For example, the five symptoms necessary for diagnoses of Major
Depressive Disorder seemingly set far more stringent standards than the one
symptom that characterized a "mild" condition in the Midtown Manhattan
study. Indeed, because the *DSM* criteria were generally accepted as authoritative and reasonably valid, psychiatric epidemiologists could base their questionnaires on these criteria without having to do elaborate validity studies of
their own and without much independent assessment of whether the criteria
in fact yielded valid results in the community context, with its great differences
from clinical contexts.

The categorical system of the *DSM-III* was thus the basis of all large American
community studies of psychiatric disorders that have been implemented since the
late 1970s. Simultaneously with the development of the *DSM-III*, the National
Institute of Mental Health decided to launch the first study that would measure
the prevalence of particular types of mental disorder in the community.[33] Researchers from Washington University—the same institution that produced the
Feighner criteria that underlay the *DSM-III*—constructed the Diagnostic Interview Schedule (DIS) that the new epidemiological studies used. This instrument
measured specific diagnostic conditions in community populations that were
supposed to be comparable to the major clinical entities found in the *DSM-III*,
including Major Depression and Dysthymia.

Because *DSM-III* diagnoses were based entirely on symptoms, epidemiologists could, with little change, simply translate criteria developed for diagnosis of clinical patient populations into questions for surveys of the general population, using a symptom checklist approach similar to that of earlier studies but with more complex algorithms for making a diagnosis. Their core assumption was that a structured diagnostic interview would allow researchers "to obtain psychiatric diagnoses comparable to those a psychiatrist would obtain."[34] The results would presumably provide good estimates of how much untreated mental disorder existed. These estimates, in turn, would provide policy makers with knowledge of how much unmet need existed for psychiatric services.

The DIS, founded on the same symptom-based logic of the *DSM-III*, uses closed-format questions that trained lay interviewers can administer to gather information about symptoms. Identical questions are asked in precisely the same way: "The interviewer reads specific questions and follows positive responses with additional prescribed questions. Each step in the sequence of identifying a psychiatric symptom is fully specified and does not depend upon the judgment of the interviewers."[35] This standardization is necessary because even minor variations in question wording, interviewer probes, or instructions can lead to major differences in results.

The DIS was the basis of the first national study of the prevalence of specific mental illnesses in the community—the Epidemiologic Catchment Area (ECA) study launched in the early 1980s.[36] The ECA surveyed more than 18,000 adults in the community and 2,500 persons in institutions in five sites (New Haven, Durham, Baltimore, St. Louis, and Los Angeles). It used estimates of the amount of disorder in these five sampled sites plus sophisticated statistical analyses to generate national estimates of prevalence. The second major community study of the prevalence of specific psychiatric disorders was the National Comorbidity Survey (NCS), which the NIMH fielded in 1991 with a 10-year follow-up begun in 2001.[37] The NCS, a sample of about 8,100 persons meant to represent the population of the United States, used the Composite International Diagnostic Interview (CIDI), an instrument similar to the DIS. Its age range of 15–54 years was somewhat different from the 18–65 age range that the ECA sampled.

The NCS illustrates how these *DSM*-based community surveys measure depression. It uses two steps to obtain diagnoses of depression based on *DSM-III-R* criteria.[38] In the first, respondents must affirm at least one stem question that appears at the beginning of the interview. These questions ask: "In your lifetime, have you ever had 2 weeks or more when nearly every day you felt sad, blue, or depressed?" "Have you ever had 2 weeks or more when nearly every day you felt down in the dumps, low, or gloomy?" "Has there ever been 2 weeks or more when you lost interest in most things like work, hobbies, or things you usually liked to do?" and "Have you ever had 2 weeks or more during which you felt sad, blue, depressed or where you lost all interest and pleasure in things that you usually cared about or enjoyed?" Given the broad nature of these questions and the fact that they have no exclusion criteria for the circumstances in which they arose, it is not surprising that 56% of the population reported at least one "yes" response to them.[39] Later, in the second step of the interview, this group is asked questions about symptoms of appetite and sleep disturbances, fatigue, and feelings of sadness, worthlessness, hopelessness, and the like, which are comparable to the symptoms in the *DSM* criteria for Major Depression. A computer program then determines whether respondents meet the criteria for a diagnosis of depression.

The NCS estimates that about 5% of participants had a current (30-day) episode of Major Depression, that about 10% had experienced this disorder in the previous year, that about 17% had had an episode over their lifetimes, and that about 24% reported enough symptoms for a lifetime diagnosis of either Major Depression or Dysthymia.[40] Likewise, a study in New Haven that was a precursor to the ECA found lifetime rates of 20% for Major Depression.[41] Rates from the ECA were lower, with 6.5% of respondents reporting Major Depression over the preceding year and about 11%, either Major Depression or Dysthymia over their lifetimes.[42] The findings from the ECA and the NCS are the basis for the estimates regarding the prevalence of mental disorder that the scientific, policy, and popular literatures now widely cite.

The Myth of the Equivalence of Community and Clinical Diagnoses

Are the many cases of putative Major Depression that post-*DSM-III* community studies uncover equivalent to treated clinical cases? If so, do they present an accurate picture of the total amount of mental disorder, as epidemiologists assume? Even some of those who design and execute such studies have started to worry that the reported symptoms may often represent transient normal responses to stress.[43] Such concerns are well justified because current epidemiological instruments inherit and greatly magnify the problems in distinguishing disorder from nondisorder that afflict the *DSM* criteria on which they are based and because diagnoses arrived at in such studies have none of the mitigating circumstances that exist in clinical diagnosis to reduce the practical effects of such invalidity.

As mentioned before, people who seek help from clinicians are by definition self-selected, and they use all sorts of contextual information to decide for themselves whether their conditions exceed ordinary and temporary responses to stressors. Sociologist David Karp, for example, found that depressed people seek help from psychiatrists only after they attribute their symptoms to internal psychological problems and not to stressful situations:

> Once it becomes undeniable that something is really wrong, that one's difficulties are too extreme to be pushed aside as either temporary or reasonable,

efforts begin in earnest to solve the problem. Now choices to relieve pain are made with a conscious and urgent deliberation. The shift in thinking often occurs when the presumed cause of pain is removed, but the difficulty persists. Tenure is received, you finally get out of an oppressive home environment, a destructive relationship is finally ended, and so on, but the depression persists. Such events destroy theories about the immediate situational sources of depression and force the unwelcome interpretation that the problem might be permanent and have an internal locus. One has to consider that it might be a problem of the self rather than the situation.[44]

Patients who enter treatment thus have already decided that their problems go beyond normal reactions to social stressors.

In addition to patient self-selection, in clinical practice contextual probes are usual, and all of the *DSM* manuals assume, with varying levels of explicitness, that clinicians will use their commonsense judgments in applying diagnostic criteria. Clinicians can, for example, reassure highly distressed people whose marriages are unraveling that their problems are mainly situational rather than internal. In treatment settings, the symptom-based logic of diagnoses need not be rotely applied.

In contrast, symptom-based diagnoses in community studies consider all persons who report enough symptoms as having the mental disorder of depression and thus cannot separate intense expectable responses from disorders. The context in which the symptoms developed (aside from bereavement), their duration (beyond a 2-week period), or their remission after a stressor has ended are irrelevant to a decision about whether or not a disorder exists. The computer scoring of the participant's symptoms of depression in survey research lacks any discretionary checks over whether symptoms indicate a mental disorder. Interviewers can neither exercise clinical judgment nor use flexible probes about responses. Indeed, they are forbidden to make any judgments about the validity of respondent answers. Even if the respondent seems to have misunderstood the question, the interviewer is instructed to repeat the question verbatim.[45]

The rigid standardization of structured interviews has the advantage of improving the consistency of symptom assessment across interviewers and research sites and the consequent reliability of diagnostic decisions.[46] However, the standardized questions and scoring procedures in community studies preclude the possibility of using discretion and thus treat all symptoms, regardless of their context, as signs of pathology. The sorts of experiences that produce normal sadness responses—breakups of romantic relationships and marriages, job losses, severe physical illness, disappointed career goals, and the like—are rampant in community populations. Many, perhaps most, community members have experienced major losses at some point in their lives that produce nondisordered episodes of sadness, some severe enough to qualify for a diagnosis of Major Depression and therefore to contribute to the seemingly high rate of depressive disorders in community populations.[47]

In short, the inflexibility of symptom ascertainment and criteria application greatly increases the chances of false-positive diagnoses. Not surprisingly, agreement between clinical diagnoses and diagnoses of depression that use standardized measures is generally weak.[48] Standardization may produce more reporting of depressive symptoms, but many of them may be normal sadness responses. A respondent might recall symptoms such as depressed mood, insomnia, loss of appetite, or diminished pleasure in usual activities that lasted for longer than 2 weeks after the breakup of a romantic relationship, the diagnosis of a serious illness in an intimate, or the unexpected loss of a job. Although these symptoms might have dissipated as soon as a new relationship developed, the intimate recovered, or another job was found, this individual would join the many millions of people who suffer from the presumed disorder of depression each year. Because the kinds of symptoms that presumably indicate depressive disorders are often common products of ordinary stressors, the number of people who do not have mental disorders but who are diagnosed as depressed must be assumed to be quite high until proven otherwise and might even exceed the number of people who are accurately classified as depressed.[49]

Diagnostically oriented community studies did not demonstrably uncover high rates of depressive disorders so much as plausibly demonstrate that the natural results of stressful social experiences could be distressing enough to meet symptom criteria for a disorder. Yet, without adequate consideration of the nature of the reported conditions, the high untreated rates of depression are used to argue that depression is a public health problem of epidemic proportions, that relatively few people who are depressed seek appropriate treatment, that untreated depression creates vast economic costs, that the amount of mental health services is inadequate, and that many people ought to take prescription medications to overcome their depression.[50]

Back to the 1960s: Eliminating *DSM* Symptom Thresholds in Community Studies

Whatever its shortcomings, the *DSM* does make a good-faith effort to construct diagnostic criteria that indicate disorders as distinct from transient unhappiness, using a symptom threshold as its major tool. Indeed, the *DSM* criteria are genuinely more stringent than the earlier epidemiological single-symptom approach. The groundwork, however, is currently being laid for an erosion of even this progress and for a much more radical expansion of the symptom-based approach to diagnosing depressive disorder in the community. The argument for this new approach—which is not really so new at all but is, in fact, a throwback to the single-symptom measures of the 1950s—is unfolding currently in research journals, in psychiatric conferences, and in programs that screen for the presence of depressive disorders. It is, above all, based on epidemiological findings that start from symptom-based criteria and that argue for including as disorders conditions with even fewer symptoms than the number required by *DSM* criteria for MDD. This approach would largely abandon the constraints of the *DSM's* symptom thresholds and would classify below-threshold conditions as disorders.

The community studies of psychiatric conditions in the 1950s and 1960s had framed mental illness as a continuum from mild to severe depending on the number of reported symptoms rather than as a set of discrete disorders that were categorically distinct from ordinary distress. In contrast, the major community studies since the 1980s have reported their results as categories that corresponded to *DSM* definitions. Cases of Major Depression required five or more symptoms, which meant that persons with fewer than five symptoms were not considered disordered. Epidemiologists expected that this change would eliminate the obvious inflation of disorder estimates that the continuum approach produced.

However, the symptom threshold that is at the heart of the *DSM's* approach to depression diagnosis is now itself seen as a problem. Even the most avid proponents of the *DSM's* categorical diagnosis of MDD recognize that the particular number of symptoms required for distinguishing disorders from nondisorders is somewhat arbitrary and largely a matter of diagnostic convention.[51] In clinical practice, specifying an objective cutoff point is convenient in order to generate diagnoses, decide on treatments, and receive reimbursements. But there is no compelling scientific reason for why that point for MDD is set at five rather than, for example, at four or six symptoms. Indeed, even the *DSM* implicitly recognizes that conditions with fewer than the required five may be depressive disorders and allows them to be diagnosed under the "Affective Disorders Not Otherwise Specified" category.[52]

The arbitrariness of a symptom cutoff for diagnosis of depressive disorder is less problematic in clinical settings than in community studies, because clinicians can use their judgment as to the pathological or nonpathological nature of a case, and, at least prior to recent use of aggressive screening and case-finding methods, people with mild cases with very few symptoms were unlikely to enter professional treatment in the first place. Most (though by no means all) treated patients with depression have tended to show long-standing symptoms, chronic courses, and frequent relapses and thus have been less likely to be false-positive cases—people who meet diagnostic criteria but who do not have mental disorders.[53]

In contrast, symptoms among untreated community members lie on a continuous distribution that ranges from mild to severe and from few to many, with the number who report a small number of symptoms far exceeding those who report many symptoms.[54] For example, 8.7% of ECA respondents reported one depressive symptom over the previous month compared with the 2.3% of respondents who met the full criteria for major depression.[55] Likewise, although the average duration of symptoms among treated outpatients is between 6 and 9 months, diagnostic standards in community studies require only a 2-week duration.[56]

The continuous distribution of symptoms in the general population, along with the fact that the preponderance of conditions fall toward the mild end, poses a challenge for the categorical classification of depression for two reasons. First, the smoothness of the curve of symptom distribution itself, with no particular discontinuity, makes it difficult to justify a categorical symptom cutoff because the symptoms themselves do not naturally suggest the break between categories. Second, and central to recent analyses, the harm associated with different levels of symptoms, such as degree of social, occupational, and health disabilities, also appears to increase smoothly and proportionately as symptom number rises.[57] When there is no clear demarcation point in the distribution of impairments at different symptom levels, it seems hard to justify a categorical concept based on the number of symptoms. Milder cases, it is argued, just represent milder disorders, not normality.[58] The use of impairment as a validating criterion inevitably leads to pressures to measure depression as a continuous rather than a categorical disorder.

Consequently, a flood of studies since the mid-1990s have argued for expanding the notion of depressive disorder by lowering the symptom threshold for diagnosis. In essence, these new studies have reinvented the notion from the community research in the 1950s that depression is a symptomatic continuum from few symptoms (well below the current five-symptom threshold) to many. The proximate origin of this movement lies in studies that showed that people in primary medical care who have depressive symptoms, but not depressive disorders, have much functional impairment.[59] Indeed, the degree of disability associated with depressive symptoms without disorder exceeded that of eight common, chronic medical conditions such as hypertension or diabetes. The *DSM* criteria for Major Depression, however, excluded this large and seemingly very impaired group of people from the ranks of persons who were considered to have disorders. Such findings generated suspicion that the arbitrary boundaries of categorical criteria could raise the number of false negatives: people who have disorders but who are not counted as disordered because they report fewer than five symptoms.[60]

Thus a fear that the categorical criteria of epidemiological studies actually underestimate the number of depressive disorders underlies the considerable body of depression research that has now accumulated. The first theme of this new research is that depressive disorders vary along a continuum that ranges from minor to major. "To accept depression as disease," psychiatrist Peter Kramer concludes, "is to see pathology or risk in minor versions."[61] *Minor* or *subthreshold* depression includes persons who report between two and four symptoms of depression but who do not meet the full criteria for MDD or Dysthymia.[62] Other studies extend the category of minor depression even further, counting persons with one or more symptoms of depression, including mood disturbance, as impaired.[63] At the extreme, reporting a single depressive symptom of any type qualifies one as having a disorder.[64] The basic argument is that fewer symptoms represent milder versions of depressive disorder along a diagnostic continuum that contains no sharp boundary between disorder and nondisorder. Applying Kraepelin's argument for his inpatient samples to untreated community samples, some researchers assert that "depressive symptoms at the major, mild, Dysthymic and subthreshold levels are all part of the long term clinical structure of major depression."[65] Any sign of sadness is an aspect of a unitary depressive disorder.[66]

As a second theme, the new research emphasizes that all points along the continuum are *disorders* because they are associated with increasingly higher rates of disability. The justification for lower cutting points for depressive disorder stems from the gradations in impairment that follow from increasing numbers of symptoms.[67] Studies indicate that subthreshold conditions are associated with significantly higher levels of household strain, social irritability, and financial difficulties, as well as limitations in physical and job functioning, restricted activity, and poor health status.[68] Likewise, the NCS data show a gradient of increasing impairment among persons with 2–4 symptoms, 5–6 symptoms, and 7–9 symptoms, as indicated by the interference of these symptoms with life activities and by whether or not the patients had seen a physician or some other mental health professional or were taking medication.[69] "The fact that the correlates of mD (minor depression) and MD (Major Depression) are similar," assert one group of researchers, "means that mD cannot be dismissed as simply a normal reaction to environmental stress while MD is seen as something quite different."[70] Impairments such as social and occupational disabilities, physical disorders, and future hospitalizations increase continuously as the number of symptoms increases.[71] Even one symptom of depression, compared with no symptoms, is associated with more adverse outcomes on most measures of disability.[72] Therefore, attention must be paid to the full range of depressive conditions, not just to conditions that meet the *DSM* criteria for MDD.

A third aspect of the new wave of community studies is their focus on mild conditions as risk factors for future disorders of greater severity and their lowering of the threshold of disorder because of these risks. For example, in the ECA, people who reported two or more lifetime symptoms were far more likely to develop Major Depression during the following year than those who reported fewer symptoms.[73] In this study, more than 50% of cases of first-onset Major Depression were associated with prior depressive symptoms. "Our findings," the authors conclude, "tentatively suggest that if depressive symptoms could be identified and treated before major depression first develops, many cases of first-onset major depression could potentially be prevented."[74] The NCS data, as well, indicate that mild cases of disorder at the first period predict more serious cases at the follow-up period.[75] The "development of early interventions to prevent progression along a given severity continuum might reduce the prevalence of serious cases."[76]

Not surprisingly, lowering the criteria for depression greatly increases prevalence rates. In a *1-month* period, nearly a quarter of the population (22.6%) in the ECA study report at least one putative symptom of depression.[77] At some point in their lives, about one in every four people in the ECA who do not meet criteria for MDD or Dysthymia report enough symptoms to qualify for a diagnosis of subsyndromal depression.[78] Likewise, when the disorder of "mild depression" is defined as the display of two to four symptoms, the lifetime prevalence of depression increases dramatically from 15.8% to 25.8%.[79] In some populations, especially among the elderly, rates of minor depression exceed 50%.[80] The high prevalence of mild depression, coupled with the accompanying adverse outcomes, the increased risk for full-fledged mood disorders, and the increased social disability that accompanies it, leads to arguments that this condition is "a truly hidden, unrecognized public health problem that has an enormous 1-year prevalence in the society" that should be a focus of research and preventive efforts.[81]

These major themes of psychiatric epidemiology in the early twenty-first century almost precisely echo those of the initial postwar community studies in the 1950s and 1960s, except that what was then tended to be construed as a disorder caused by environmental stress now tends to be viewed as a disorder caused by biological malfunction. To sum up these common themes: (1) mental disorder is continuous, and all points along this continuum should be viewed as problematic; (2) mild conditions at one time are likely to become major conditions at another; (3) even a single symptom of depression is worrisome because it is associated with future disability and can be a risk factor for major depression; (4) because of its extremely high prevalence, social policies should focus on preventing depression from developing in the general population. Psychiatric epidemiology has come full circle, returning to its concern with even the mildest presumed conditions of depression.

Fallacies Behind the "Minor Depression" Movement

What is right and what is wrong in the proposed expansion of disorder to include "minor depression" that has fewer symptoms than the *DSM* requires? What is right about it is, first, that we do need to be alert to subthreshold conditions in some circumstances in which they can help predict future problems. But the fact that a condition is a risk factor for future problems does not make it a disorder, a point to which we return subsequently.

Second, and most important, the *DSM* cutoff is somewhat arbitrary and is not a magic dividing line between pathology and normality. No doubt some subthreshold conditions deserve to be diagnosed as disorders; also, *DSM* criteria for depressive disorder likely do yield some false negatives, in addition to the false positives we have emphasized. More generally, viewing depression as continuous rather than categorical has a number of theoretical advantages.[82] Many disorders, such as depression, might naturally be based on underlying, continuous dimensional processes rather than on dichotomies, and so continua might be more likely than diagnoses to "carve nature at its joints" and yield fruitful research and theory.

However, the assertion that, because there is a linear relationship between number of symptoms and impairment, each point along the continuum therefore represents a *disorder* is highly problematic. When all symptoms are counted as disordered, ordinary sadness is hopelessly confounded with genuine dysfunction, and prevalence rates reach even more untenable levels than they do now. For example, in the ECA study, the most common symptoms are "trouble falling asleep, staying asleep, or waking up early" (33.7%), being "tired out all the time" (22.8%), and "thought a lot about death" (22.6%).[83] College students during exam periods (particularly those studying existential philosophy), people who must work overtime, those who are worrying about an important upcoming event, or respondents who take a survey around the time of the death of a famous person would all naturally experience some of these symptoms. Symptoms that neither respondents nor clinicians would ever consider as reasons for entering mental health treatment nevertheless can indicate disorder in community surveys. Moreover, the duration criteria require that the symptom last for only a 2-week period, ensuring that many transient and self-correcting symptoms are counted as disordered.

Given the common nature and brief persistence of many putative symptoms of depression, it is difficult to imagine that there are many people who have *not* experienced episodes of mild or subthreshold depression at some point in their lives, although there certainly are some people with temperaments that seem to virtually preclude intense sadness. Indeed, the very high rates of depression found when cutting points are lowered almost certainly *underestimate* the number of people who experience putative symptoms of depression. One reason for undercounts is that respondents do not recall all symptoms that have occurred at some point in their lifetimes. One group of researchers, for example, found that most respondents who reported episodes of lifetime depression at the baseline interview in the ECA failed to report any lifetime episodes at the 12-year follow-up period.[84] The majority of respondents simply forgot previous depressive states. If respondents accurately recalled all episodes of depression, lifetime prevalence rates of depressive disorder would exceed 50% in the ECA data. A second reason for the undercount of symptom prevalence is that respondents disregard the instructions of surveys, apply their own contextual criteria for symptoms, and fail to report symptoms that they attribute to life crises or medical conditions.[85] Epidemiologist Rema Lapouse's critique of the postwar community studies—"If all persons who cough are counted as cases of tuberculosis, both incidence and prevalence rates will skyrocket"—holds as well for contemporary psychiatric epidemiology's continuous concept of depressive disorder in which no provision is made for distinguishing normal sadness from mild disorders.[86]

The major justification for treating all symptoms as disordered is that they are associated with current or future disability. This assumes that any psychological condition that is related to a problematic outcome must be a mental disorder. Yet it is entirely possible, for example, that a temperament prone to somewhat more sadness, and thus to normal-range depressive symptoms in response to life's vicissitudes, may also be somewhat more vulnerable to the development of depressive disorder; but that does not make temperamental variation a disorder. Moreover, this conclusion would be warranted only if symptoms of normal sadness are not impairing. Yet *both* disordered and nondisordered depression can vary continuously on a number of dimensions, including severity, duration, and impairment, and can certainly cause social role disabilities. One need only consider grief as an example, but surely more moderate forms of normal sadness also incline people to withdraw from social interaction, to become less capable of concentrating on routine role performances, and to develop other impairments.[87] Such interference with role functioning and productivity does not make sadness a disorder.

Aside from associated disability and impairment, epidemiological studies justify their decision to treat subthreshold symptoms as disorders with the argument that mild conditions at one point are likely to become more serious conditions that reach the *DSM* threshold for disorder in the future; they argue that the milder condition is therefore part of a larger disease process and that early detection of and intervention with mild conditions can make it possible to stop disorders from developing.[88] Perhaps this is sometimes true. However, a basic problem with this as a general argument about minor depression is that, especially given the potential invalidity of MDD diagnoses themselves, even when a subthreshold condition does precede a full-syndrome condition, it is unclear whether either condition is an actual disorder or not, much less what the relationship of one condition is to the other. For example, a person might feel bad as a troubling situation at work, a marital conflict, or a physical illness in a loved one develops, might report two or three symptoms, and then, when the trouble gels into a loss, might have a more intense response. Both the initial sadness and the later, more intense reaction might be perfectly normal, and yet an epidemiologist might interpret the sequence as one in which a minor depressive disorder led to a major depressive disorder. The fact that a few sadness symptoms are later followed by more intense sadness symptoms tells us little by itself about whether the earlier, milder condition or the later, more severe condition or both or neither are disorders. Valid criteria in either case must go beyond symptoms.

Moreover, subthreshold symptoms do not necessarily predict *DSM* Major Depression diagnosis at a later time; in fact, evidence for the prediction of later major depression is quite weak. Many, or even most, symptoms uncovered in community studies will be transient and limited in duration to the context of the stressful situations that gave rise to them. In the ECA study, one-half of people with mild depression became asymptomatic during the following year.[89] In this study, only 10% of persons with minor depression with mood disturbance and only 2% with minor depression without mood disturbance developed Major Depression in the 1-year follow-up, and because of the ECA's *DSM* symptom-based criteria, we do not know how many of those were truly disordered. Conversely, over one-third of the group with Major Depression became asymptomatic, and nearly 40% fell into the group with minor depression.[90]

These findings indicate that more serious conditions are more likely to become less serious conditions than the converse. Because of the extraordinary instability of "caseness," with people slipping in and out of varying states of severity, there are no reliable ways of identifying which conditions will get worse and which will not. Although persons with mild depression might be more likely than those without symptoms to develop future cases of Major Depression, the vast majority of people with a small number of depressive symptoms will *not* develop Major Depression in the future. Indeed, studies indicate that, in the absence of any intervention, up to two-thirds of depressive symptoms naturally remit.[91] For example, in the ECA study mentioned earlier, 97 of 114 participants diagnosed as depressed in the initial interview recovered during the follow-up period.[92] Symptoms that result from life problems typically go away when these problems are over, even though they might initially meet clinical criteria.

It is difficult to understand the logic of the argument that because some subthreshold conditions might be disorders rather than normal sadness, all should be classified as disorders. The explanation seems to be that the minor-depression movement rejects *DSM* symptom thresholds but tenaciously clings to the *DSM*'s basic assumption that context-free, symptom-based criteria can best diagnose depressive disorder. Consequently, the extension of depressive disorder to subthreshold conditions, which may eliminate some false negatives, comes at the price of a much greater likely expansion in false-positive diagnoses of nondisordered sadness as disorder. Yet those who advocate diagnosing minor depression have notably disregarded the problem of how to avoid misdiagnosis of normal sadness as disorder. Only if a more valid approach to the disorder-nondisorder distinction is first put in place will it be justifiable to encompass low-symptom conditions within the disorder category.

Because of these weaknesses in the current approach to minor depression, the policy implications that stem from the use of the continuous concept of depressive disorder are questionable. The highest priority of good public policy ought to be to provide mental health services to persons who are most in need of them. When the concept of a continuum of mental health problems was applied in the 1960s, the result was the pathologization of a large proportion of the population, the extension of services to many people with problems of living, and a consequent diminution in services provided to the seriously mentally ill.[93] The minor-depression movement could be laying the groundwork for the same mistake again.

Advocates for the mentally ill, the NIMH, and psychiatric researchers have been receptive to findings of high rates of Major Depression in community surveys because they think these findings will help to decrease the stigma associated with labels of mental disorder and to obtain public and legislative support for funding mental health programs.[94] Yet extending definitional thresholds for depressive disorder downward in community studies so that even more people are counted as depressively disordered might, like the already high prevalence rates from *DSM*-based epidemiological studies of Major Depression, have the opposite effect of undermining the political will to deal with the problem due to fears among public and private funders about the huge costs of providing services to such a large population.[95] As psychologist James Coyne emphasizes, "improving the outcomes of known cases of depression should take precedence over increasing the detection of depression," and this is all the more true when what is being detected is likely not depressive disorder at all.[96] We should heed the warning of Rema Lapouse, writing in the original era of the continuous concept:

> Rates which include a large proportion of equivocal or mild cases, or actually nonsick individuals, may even have the deleterious effect of encouraging the deployment of the limited mental health forces for the treatment of those who are least sick and have the best prognosis.[97]

Conclusion

There is nothing wrong per se with the use of symptom continua in research and theory on depression. However, such continua are not in themselves a substitute for the distinction between disorder and nondisorder. The problem of false positives has its root in the failure to connect symptoms and associated disabilities to the context in which they arise, an issue that surfaces at all points on the symptom severity continuum. The problem of false positives becomes progressively worse, however, as fewer and fewer symptoms are used to define disorders. Indeed, if consideration of context is abandoned, all normal sadness responses potentially can be seen as a sign of pathology; the very possibility of normal sadness is lost.

We have thus far considered the unintended consequences when the *DSM*'s decontextualized symptom-based criteria were applied to untreated samples in the community, with the resulting great expansion of the group labeled as having pathological depression. But the consequent inflated epidemiological prevalence estimates have not remained mere scientific abstractions. Instead, they have become the basis for sweeping and intrusive new social policies toward depression, to which we now turn.

7

The Surveillance of Sadness

If you are a typical resident of New York City, the chances are that you'll visit your primary care physician at some point over the next year. If your doctor follows the advice of the New York City Commissioner of Mental Health, he or she will ask you to fill out a questionnaire that asks: "Over the past 2 weeks, how often have you been bothered by any of the following problems?"[1] Each of nine symptoms are rated as 0 (*not at all*), 1 (*several days*), 2 (*more than half the days*), or 3 (*nearly every day*). Here are the nine symptoms:

1. Little interest or pleasure in doing things.
2. Feeling down, depressed, or hopeless.
3. Trouble falling or staying asleep, or sleeping too much.
4. Feeling tired or having too little energy.
5. Poor appetite or overeating.
6. Feeling bad about yourself, or that you are a failure or have let yourself or your family down.
7. Trouble concentrating on things, such as reading the newspaper or watching TV.
8. Moving or speaking so slowly that other people could have noticed; or the opposite, being so fidgety or restless that you have been moving around a lot more than usual.
9. Thoughts that you would be better off dead, or hurting yourself in some way.

The instrument is scored as follows: if five or more of the nine symptoms, including one of the first two, score 2 or 3 (a total score of at least 10), then you would receive a diagnosis of Major Depressive Disorder; you would be diagnosed with minor depressive disorder if at least two questions, including one of the first two, fall in the 2 or 3 range (a total score of at least 4). For example, if you felt down and tired most days for the past 2 weeks (i.e., for 8 days or more), you would qualify for a diagnosis of minor depressive disorder; if on most days for the past 2 weeks you felt down and tired and bad about yourself and also had trouble falling asleep and trouble concentrating on things, you would qualify for Major Depressive Disorder.

The city claims that individuals whose scores are high enough to indicate likely disorder will be referred for a clinical assessment. However, because these symptoms are so common, it is hard to see how enough resources would be available to assess the potentially enormous number of referrals. Moreover, most people who report having the specified symptoms likely are experiencing them because of some immediate loss or problem that is preoccupying them and causing them to be sad, distracted, and so on. Yet physicians could be easily tempted to prescribe medication even to those with minor depression, a diagnosis that a substantial proportion of primary care patients would warrant. Thus the tentative labeling of the individual as depressed without taking into account that individual's circumstances can set in motion a clinical response that is based on inadequate substantive information.

New York City's program is part of a national movement toward screening adults and children for depression that a Presidential Commission report supports.[2] In this chapter we explore the depression-screening movement and some of the problems that result because of its use of decontextualized, symptom-based criteria for identifying depressed individuals.

The Depression-Screening Movement

Epidemiologists, as we saw in chapter 6, failed to adequately distinguish normal sadness from depressive disorder in community studies. As a result, they presented mental health policy makers with surprisingly high estimates of the number of people who have untreated depressive disorders. Fearing that there was an enormous unmet need for mental health services among people who might not even recognize that they were suffering from a disorder, these policy makers in turn placed a high priority on finding ways to identify people with untreated disorders in the community and to bring them into treatment. And it was decided that if people would not come in for diagnosis, then diagnosis must go to the people. The result has been a set of screening programs that, in principle, aim to diagnostically evaluate every single person in America for the presence of depressive disorder.

Several assumptions underlie the attempt to identify and treat previously unrecognized cases of depression. One is that, unless brought into treatment, people who meet symptomatic criteria in community studies may develop chronic, recurrent, and deteriorating conditions.[3] Another is that individuals with unrecognized cases of depressive disorder are suffering needlessly and can benefit from available medications and therapies.[4] A concern that untreated depressive disorders could have very negative outcomes such as suicide also drives the urgency for treatment. Moreover, untreated depression has significant hidden economic costs: patients with undiagnosed depression overutilize the health care system, have many unnecessary medical evaluations, and drive up the costs of medical services.[5]

The major question facing initiatives that deal with unmet need for treatment is how best to identify and make contact with untreated cases of depression. Efforts that target entire populations, such as public service announcements, educational campaigns, and direct-to-consumer advertisements, are one way to reach such cases. Pharmaceutical companies and other concerned organizations were quick to take this approach and to plant in the public's mind a quite broad notion, based on common *DSM* symptoms, of the possibility that, even unbeknownst to oneself, one might have a depressive disorder and ought to consult one's physician. Such appeals encourage people to monitor themselves and their families and associates for signs of sadness and to interpret these common signs according to the worrisome meanings derived from expansive definitions of depressive disorder. No doubt such initiatives do encourage some individuals with depressive disorder to beneficially enter treatment. They likely have contributed to increased rates of treated depression and prescriptions for antidepressant medication over the past two decades.[6] However, in the end, such efforts are of limited effectiveness because they depend on individuals themselves to recognize that they might be depressed enough to warrant medical treatment.

The screening movement, therefore, has focused on extending medical authority beyond the usual response to spontaneous help seeking. This is a critical goal of the movement because current diagnostic criteria do not correspond to what most laypeople believe is disorder.[7] Thus many people whom the *DSM* would classify as disordered do not themselves believe that they have signs of mental disorder, do not raise such questions with their physicians, do not seek help, and thus do not present themselves as targets of treatment. Because of this, assessment must go out into the community, somehow be externally imposed, and proceed on the patient's behalf.

We turn now to how this new surveillance via screening is conducted and how specific screening programs help to redefine the experience of intense sadness as disorder for the lay population. Before proceeding to examine how such screening works, we need to mention one important caveat regarding the limits of our argument. Our analysis specifically concerns the redefinition of the experience of normal sadness as a disorder that results from using current *DSM* criteria, including subthreshold criteria, in community screening programs. Our analysis could easily be mistaken for a critique of depression screening in and of itself. However, the desirability of screening is a separate issue that depends on whether screening, either in its current form or in some future form, can be shown to yield benefits in preventing or alleviating suffering that demonstrably outweighs its costs. At present, such empirical support does not exist; there is simply no evidence that mass screening for depression is effective in achieving any major mental health goal. This chapter thus addresses not the pros and cons of screening per se but the problem of the pathologization of normal sadness that results from screening solely with symptom-based criteria.

Prescreening and Diagnostic Screening for Depressive Disorder

The goal of depression screening is to reveal those persons in the community who either do not recognize that they have depressive disorders or for some other reason have not acted to get help for their disorders. Having mental health professionals clinically diagnose each and every person in the community would be far too expensive and time-consuming to be practical. Thus briefer tests, or screening instruments, must be used to decide whether someone has a higher than usual probability of having a disorder, and only those people who test positive are then fully diagnosed.

Screening is an ambiguous term that can refer to two distinct processes (although we will see later that these two processes often collapse into one). First, it can mean giving community members a test that is sufficient by itself to provide a likely diagnosis of a target disorder. For example, various businesses have health-screening days when employees can get their blood pressure checked and their blood cholesterol level measured, with tests that diagnose high blood pressure and hypercholesteremia more or less accurately. Similarly, tuberculosis screening can involve teams of physicians who, equipped with mobile X-ray machines and other necessary equipment, go into the community to provide underserved populations with medical tests that establish a likely diagnosis of tuberculosis if it is present. We refer to such screening as *diagnostic screening*. One important feature of diagnostic screens is that a positive result is taken to indicate pathology and thus is sufficient to justify treatment.

But *screening* also commonly refers to mass testing that provides only some initial indication of whether there might be a problem and thus whether an individual requires a referral to a professional for further diagnosis. Such screening does not provide a likely or presumptive diagnosis by itself and often generates a large number of positive results that are ultimately not confirmed in later diagnostic testing. For example, positive results on patch tests for tuberculosis only provide some indication that a disorder may be present; they are not diagnoses. Further follow-up diagnostic assessments are required to establish the presence of a disease, and many people who show positive on the patch test end up testing negative for tuberculosis. Similarly, mammograms that detect lumps in the breast indicate the need for further evaluation, but a large proportion of detected lumps are benign, so diagnosis must await a further test, such as a biopsy. We refer to such nondiagnostic screening that serves as a stage prior to actual diagnosis as *prescreening*. Only the second-stage evaluation, not the prescreen itself, justifies referral for treatment.

Prescreening instruments can be better or worse at correctly detecting the likely presence of disorder. There is a complex trade-off in the design of pre-screens. On the one hand, it is desirable to eliminate as many normal people as possible from the pool of those who require further diagnostic screening. The costs and sometimes the risks of diagnostic testing are such that one wants to minimize the number of false positives on the prescreen—that is, those who test positive on the prescreen and are sent on for diagnostic screening but are not ultimately found to be disordered. On the other hand, one wants to avoid miss-ing any disordered individuals; ideally, one wants to send all such individuals on for diagnostic screening.

Of these two goals, prescreening instruments for depressive disorder have emphasized the goal of not missing any cases of disorder. Consequently, they have been designed to use the fewest possible screening questions to detect any possibility of depressive disorder. The unintended result, as we will see, is an im-mense number of individuals who test positive on the prescreen and who thus require further diagnostic evaluation but who have no disorder (false positives).

Unlike screening tests for most physical disorders, which provide information that respondents would not otherwise know, typical questions in depression pre-screening instruments ask people variants of the question, "Are you depressed?" For example, in the first major study of screening, the three (of eight) items in a first-stage prescreen that were most highly correlated with receiving a second-stage diagnosis of depression according to *DSM* criteria were: "I felt depressed"; "In the past year, have you had 2 weeks or more during which you felt sad, blue, or depressed . . ."; and "Have you had 2 years or more in your life when you felt depressed or sad most days. . . ."[8] Because almost anyone who has a true de-pressive disorder has symptoms of this type, such questions ensure that truly depressed people will prescreen positively.

The flip side of this inclusiveness is that the great majority of individuals who score positively on the prescreen and who thus must be clinically evalu-ated do not end up receiving a diagnosis of depressive disorder when diagnosti-cally screened. This is to be expected given the ubiquity of sadness. Unlike many screening programs for physical disorders, there is no "gold standard," such as a biological test, that can show when symptoms of sadness indicate depressive disorder and thus can ensure that normal people are not prescreened or ulti-mately diagnosed as disordered.

For example, an early study that used an eight-item prescreen for depressive disorder in primary medical care settings found that a second-stage diagnostic assessment using *DSM* criteria confirmed only 29% of those identified as possi-bly having Major Depression and only 25% of those possibly having Dysthymia as actually having these disorders.[9] In other words, over 70% of the cases that the prescreen indicated as possibly disordered were not ultimately diagnosed with a disorder, despite the fact that potentially overly inclusive *DSM* criteria were used in the second-stage assessment.

Further studies of screening confirm such findings. An overview of screening studies in primary care settings concludes that, under the assumption of a 5% prevalence rate of depression, 31 of every 100 patients will prescreen positively for depression but that second-stage interviews will diagnose only 4 patients in this group with Major Depression.[10] Expectedly, the number of MDD false positives is especially high when prescreening involves a very small number of questions. A recent study that used two prescreening questions about experiencing 2 weeks or more of sadness during the preceding year or of losing interest in things that are normally enjoyed shows in follow-up that about 73–82% of those who prescreen positively do not have MDD.[11] The fact that so many normal individuals may be sent on for a second stage of clinical evaluation is itself a massive intervention that may have unanticipated side effects.

Studies find wide variability in the proportion of patients who prescreen positively for depression, ranging from 15 to 50%. For example, one large study that compared three different screening instruments found that 20, 25, and 36%, respectively, of primary care patients prescreened positively for depressive disorder.[12] Some studies that used just two questions report that nearly half of patients have positive prescreens.[13] The implication for the broader question of misdiagnosis is that the prescreen stage, whatever it accomplishes, does not eliminate anyone who might constitute a *DSM* false positive.

Prescreening is of interest within our broader argument for three reasons. First, prescreening itself constitutes a minipathologization of normal emotional experiences that can lead to labeling, stigma, or self-doubts and other concerns. Because prescreens are often based on a small number of questions about common symptoms of sadness, they identify virtually all intense sadness as a potential red flag. The effect is to at least raise the question of possible disorder and thus make every individual who experiences normal intense sadness a potential candidate for diagnosis. Even those who screen positively and then do not later qualify for a *DSM* diagnosis may have some concerns about what made professionals suspicious enough about their mental health to warrant a diagnostic interview. The prescreening process itself creates a space of pathological possibilities that did not previously exist. No research is available that assesses the potential negative effects of such interventions.

Second, prescreening in mass venues, such as the primary care and school settings we discuss later, sends on for second-stage *DSM* diagnosis all those in the community with intense sadness responses, whether or not they themselves feel disordered. Consequently, the second-stage diagnostic screening applies the *DSM* diagnostic criteria to virtually every individual in those settings who might qualify for diagnosis. This means that the flaws in the *DSM* criteria can no longer be dismissed as merely theoretical anomalies, challenges to research validity, or loopholes of limited clinical impact that are useful for getting reimbursement for those wanting treatment. Rather, the aggressive use of minimal-symptom prescreening in effect transforms what might have remained a relatively esoteric conceptual confusion into a tool of emotional surveillance and potential misdiagnosis for each and every one of us.

Third, the pressures of time and money have led to what amounts to a bait-and-switch tactic in which instruments initially presented as prescreens are actually used as the full diagnostic screens. Discussions about possible screening programs to be launched in a community initially claim that all those who prescreen positively will be clinically evaluated for disorder and thus not summarily diagnosed. However, once such programs are inaugurated, the trend is for the costly second-stage diagnostic screens to be eliminated or reduced and for the minimal prescreen itself to become the basis for diagnosis and treatment decisions. The following sections illustrate how prescreening and diagnostic screening have been pursued within two community venues, primary medical care and school settings, and how prescreening instruments often become full diagnostic instruments in these settings.

Screening for Depression Among Medical Patients

Depression in Primary Care Settings

Primary medical care settings have been the major locus of screening programs to identify and treat depression. These settings seem ideally suited for such efforts. General physicians are in a particularly strategic position to detect and treat previously unrecognized depressive disorder in large segments of the population because most people make a primary care visit over the course of any given year.[14] Moreover, people with depressive symptoms are especially likely to make such visits: studies show that they are between two to three times as likely as others to visit primary care settings.[15] Thus many experts believe that there are many unidentified primary care patients who do indeed have depressive disorders; various studies claim that from 10 to 35% of primary care patients have these disorders, a rate that jumps to about half among those who visit general physicians most often.[16]

Primary care settings are also a good locus for follow-up interventions after individuals are diagnosed with disorders, because many people with presumptive depressive disorder receive their only treatment in the general medical sector.[17] General physicians are the sole treatment providers for one-quarter to one-half of the people whom community surveys identify as depressively disordered.[18] Primary care settings are seen as especially good places in which to implement preventive efforts for persons with little income and education, for ethnic and racial minorities, and for the elderly, because these groups are relatively unlikely to seek treatment from mental health professionals but are more likely to seek help from their general physicians.

However, despite the large proportion of primary care patients who are presumably depressed and the seemingly ideal nature of the general physician's office for depression intervention, the ability to recognize and treat depression in general medical settings is generally regarded as poor.[19] Studies repeatedly report that general practitioners recognize only from one-third to one-half of their patients who are depressed.[20] One reason for this could stem from patient reluctance to present emotional symptoms and greater willingness to express physical complaints. Another is that physicians' medical training naturally leads them to focus and place higher priority on treating somatic complaints. Their busy office schedules also do not allow them the time to sort out psychological from physiological illnesses, so they naturally concentrate on the physical complaints. Studies further emphasize the inadequate treatment that primary care physicians provide to patients whom they do recognize and diagnose as depressed. Less than half of these patients receive antidepressant medications or other standard types of depression-specific care, and even those who are medicated often receive the wrong types or inadequate doses of medication.[21]

The concern about unmet need for services, combined with the deficiencies of general physicians' responses to depression, has led to many initiatives that try to improve the recognition and treatment of depression in primary care settings.[22] All such diagnostic screening efforts depend on the development and use of instruments that allow physicians to identify cases of depressive disorder in primary care settings that would otherwise remain undetected. Because of the many time pressures in typical office practices, these screening instruments, if they are to be useful, must be short, easy to administer, and take little physician or patient time.[23] Typically, they attempt to perform what essentially amounts to a brief version of a *DSM* diagnosis using a reduced set of self-administered questions about common symptoms of depression that are assumed to be roughly equivalent to the full *DSM* criteria.

Developers of screening initiatives in primary care face two major decisions. First, how broad a population should receive them? That is, should they be applied to as many primary care patients as possible, or only to patients who are viewed as being at special risk for having unrecognized disorders? Second, what level of criteria should yield positive screens at the prescreening and diagnostic stages? The trend has increasingly been both to broaden the population that is subject to screening and to use more liberal criteria for positive screens.

Beginning with the NIMH-sponsored Depression Awareness, Recognition, and Treatment (DART) campaign in 1987, a number of initiatives have tried to focus attention of patients and providers on the underrecognition and undertreatment of depression in primary care settings.[24] The initial efforts were notable for their cautious attitude toward screening, and none recommended widespread screening in primary care.[25] "The conclusion to be drawn," the summary of the first volume devoted to this issue indicates, "is that depression questionnaires should not be routinely administered to ambulatory medical patients. There is merit, however, to such assessment practice in selected circumstances and with well-defined populations."[26]

These early efforts were just as concerned with the problems created when too many people were wrongly diagnosed with depression as they were with accurately identifying people who were actually depressed.[27] To this end, these programs recommended using cutoff points for depression that were higher than those used in community populations.[28] One study concluded:

> In sum, it does not appear, at least from the data produced by this study, that enough of an advantageous balance of sensitivity and positive misclassification rates of these screens can be achieved at this time to enthusiastically recommend them for use in screening for affective disorders in primary care populations.[29]

Screening initiatives during the 1990s, however, ignored these warnings and urged the routine use of screening among as broad a group as possible.[30] The World Health Organization (WHO), for example, urges that every patient who visits primary care be screened for depression.[31] At the same time, the criteria used in these more recent screening efforts have become more liberal. Many initiatives came to use criteria for detecting cases of possible disorder in untreated groups that were well below *DSM* standards, in effect encompassing almost anyone who experienced intense sadness for a couple of weeks. The U.S. Preventive Services Task Force, for example, recommends that physicians ask patients just two questions to prescreen for possible cases of depression: "During the past 2 weeks, have you felt down, depressed, or hopeless?" and "During the past 2 weeks, have you felt little interest or pleasure in doing things?"[32] Likewise, the WHO suggests that all primary care patients should be asked whether they had experienced 2 weeks or more during the preceding year when they felt sad, empty, or depressed or lost interest in things they normally enjoyed and whether these symptoms had occurred for 1 week or longer during the preceding month.[33]

Such minimal prescreens, when positive, are supposed to be followed by a full diagnostic assessment. Diagnostic interviews that use *DSM* criteria to validate positive prescreens typically find that about 10–20% of primary care patients meet full criteria for MDD.[34] The trend toward expanding prescreens to encompass subthreshold diagnoses with only two or more symptoms, however, has greatly increased the number of positive second-stage diagnoses, so that about one-quarter of primary care patients are found to have some sort of depressive disorder. For example, the Michigan Depression Study, which used *DSM-III* criteria, found that 13.5% of family practice patients had MDD and that 23% had some kind of depressive disorder.[35]

As a practical matter, however, using two stages of screening has not proven to be a feasible method of detecting cases of depressive disorder in primary care. In actual medical settings (as opposed to research studies), it is prohibitively expensive to subject the one-quarter to one-third of all patients who screen positively for depression to a second-stage screening instrument. General physicians, who see four or five patients in an hour, do not have time to interpret the results of prescreenings or to conduct full follow-up diagnostic interviews, and most practices do not have specialized mental health personnel available to conduct such interviews.[36] Therefore, the trend has been toward collapsing screening and diagnosis into a single stage using very brief instruments.

Robert Spitzer's PRIME-MD (Primary Care Evaluation of Mental Disorders), one of the first screening instruments designed specifically to be used in primary care settings and still one of the most popular of such instruments, was the initial effort to encompass within one instrument a two-stage process that first performs a prescreen and then, if the prescreen is positive, yields full diagnoses of mental disorders, roughly according to *DSM* criteria.[37] It asks patients to respond to a one-page, self-administered questionnaire that contains 26 yes-or-no questions about common psychiatric symptoms they have experienced over the preceding month. Two of the questions prescreen for the presence of depression. They ask whether patients have often been bothered in the past month by having "little interest or pleasure in doing things" and by "feeling down, depressed, or hopeless." Positive responses to either of these questions trigger a clinician-administered depression module that yields diagnoses of major depression, dysthymia, or subthreshold conditions. Reflecting *DSM* criteria, there is no allowance for the context in which the prescreen symptoms developed, so that their presence in themselves is enough to trigger the use of the diagnostic interview. The clinician instrument takes only about 8 minutes to administer, so it appears to be a very efficient way for busy physicians to screen for possible psychiatric disorders.

The overall PRIME-MD prescreening scale detects symptoms that occur so commonly that 81% of 1,000 primary care patients in the developmental trials screened positively for some disorder; only 19% were not given the second diagnostic stage. In effect, physicians would almost always administer the entire two-stage process. Results at the second stage show that about 25% of primary care patients, ranging from 19 to 35% across different sites, receive diagnoses of Major Depression, Dysthymia, or both.[38]

Even the 8-minute PRIME-MD interview, however, was too lengthy for routine use in regular medical settings, in which entire appointments average just 15 minutes. Spitzer subsequently developed the Patient Health Questionnaire (PHQ), which contains a nine-item depression module based on *DSM* criteria that does not involve a two-stage screening procedure but that directly ascertains self-reported symptoms of MDD and subthreshold depressive conditions.[39] The nine particular symptoms are found in the example at the beginning of this chapter. As noted, the PHQ diagnoses Major Depression when at least five symptoms, including depressed mood or anhedonia, are present and diagnoses "other depression" when only two or more symptoms exist, again as long as one is depressed mood or anhedonia. In validation studies, the PHQ provides somewhat lower estimates of all depressive conditions than the PRIME-MD, averaging 16% across eight sites with a range of from 11 to 28%. The use of such single-stage interviews is now becoming common practice in primary care settings. This compression of the process, which immediately makes a final diagnosis based only on the PHQ, leaves even less opportunity to evaluate the possibility that a nondisordered patient might receive a false-positive diagnosis.

In addition, the transformation of *DSM* criteria into a screening instrument that is as brief and easy to administer and score as possible can unintentionally weaken the criteria. For example, the *DSM* requires that most symptoms occur "nearly every day" within the preceding 2 weeks, whereas the PHQ allows a symptom to support diagnosis if it occurs on "most days." In some instances, the *DSM* includes severity modifiers such as "marked," which the PHQ does not include; and, although the PHQ presents a clinical-significance question analogous to the *DSM*'s clinical-significance criterion, it does not use this question in scoring.

In addition, the PHQ's two-symptom threshold for diagnosis of "other depressive disorder" illustrates the growing acceptance of the use of subthreshold symptomatology as sufficient in and of itself for diagnosis. This trend toward using fewer criteria to identify depressive disorders has remarkable implications when the recommendation to screen all primary care patients is taken into account. In 2001, about 84% of the U.S. population made at least one visit to a doctor's office or an emergency room or had a home visit by a physician.[40] If current policy recommendations to screen all primary care patients at least once a year were actually followed,[41] roughly *60 million people* would screen positively for either MDD or a subthreshold depressive disorder in a single year! Moreover, the more often patients are screened for depression, the higher the probability is that they will receive a false diagnosis of depression based on transient normal symptoms.[42] Indeed, it seems likely that, with repeated screening, a large proportion of the population will be falsely considered to be depressively disordered at one time or another and possibly treated for a disorder that they do not in fact have.

The Problem of False-Positive Diagnoses in Primary Care Screening

There are good reasons to expect that many primary care patients will have symptoms that meet *DSM* criteria for depressive disorder yet that do not truly indicate major or minor depressive disorders. Stressful life events, which can produce high levels of intense normal sadness, precede many entries into primary care. Although rates of help seeking from mental health professionals have grown exponentially in recent decades, many people still regard their primary care physicians as the first line of help when problems of living arise.[43] Severe life events such as bereavement, marital disruption, and job loss are more likely to precede the onset of symptoms among family practice patients than among psychiatric patients, suggesting that cases of normal sadness are found more in medical than in psychiatric settings.[44] And, of course, depressive symptoms often arise as reactions to the stresses of having medical conditions. Because normal sadness often manifests the same symptoms as depressive disorders, including not only symptoms such as feeling depressed and losing interest in doing things but also a variety of somatic complaints such as fatigue and problems with sleeping and appetite, many people who have experienced recent stressful life events will be likely to consult their physicians and may meet *DSM* diagnostic criteria for Major Depression despite not having a disorder. (Note that when the symptoms do result directly from a medical condition or substance, neither MDD nor minor depression should be diagnosed; rather, the appropriate diagnosis is depressive disorder due to a general medical condition or to substance use, a challenging discrimination for the physician to make quite independently of any issues with screening but one that screening for depressive symptoms may bring to the fore.)

The problem is not just the false-positive diagnoses that result from primary care screening for depressive disorder but also the skewing of the resulting decision-making process regarding treatment for those who are thus diagnosed. About 40% of individuals who visit primary care settings are now screened for depression and other behavioral problems.[45] In everyday medical practice, less than a quarter of persons diagnosed with depressive disorders receive referrals to specialty care.[46] Primary care physicians, who are far more comfortable using medication than any other modality to treat depression, themselves treat the great majority of diagnosed patients.[47] The typical result of a depression diagnosis is therefore likely to be a prescription for antidepressant medication. Consequently, individuals treated for depression were 4.5 times more likely to receive a psychotropic medication in 1997 than in 1987.[48] Many of these people who receive medications may not have depressive disorders but may be facing serious life challenges.

It could, of course, be argued that people who report normal sadness, as well as those who suffer from depressive disorders, can benefit from and will not be harmed by treatment. The evidence does indicate that the benefits of treatment exceed those of placebo for persons with serious cases of depression. However, depression among many patients in primary care is in the less severe range, and in this range there is no demonstrated advantage for treatment over placebo.[49] Wayne Katon, an expert on screening for depression in primary care, summarizes:

Research suggests that half the patients initiating antidepressant in primary care have minor depression. In these patients, active treatments have not been shown to be more effective than placebo and disease management programs have not been shown to be more effective than usual care.[50]

Moreover, in recent years, those who have been prescribed medication by general physicians are tending to get less personal contact, with many never seeing their physicians or seeing them only one or a few times.[51] Thus patients suffering from normal sadness who are on medication may fail to get the accompanying counseling and support that their circumstances often warrant. In any event, the decision to take medication is best made with as accurate an understanding of the nature and prognosis of the condition as possible and with all reasonable options for treatment considered. Diagnosis of a depressive disorder tends to quickly foreclose such discussions in the direction of medication as the most appropriate response, when normal sadness may require more flexible responses for optimal treatment.

Even for those primary care patients whose depressive symptoms are severe enough to satisfy full *DSM* criteria, the fact that they are not actively seeking treatment of their depressive conditions is a potentially important consideration. Studies of the effectiveness of therapy generally use persons who voluntarily seek treatment, and patients' attitudes toward treatment can influence treatment effectiveness. In particular, patients with negative attitudes toward antidepressants actually have worse outcomes in intervention programs than those who get no treatment at all, suggesting that effective medication therapies require motivated participants.[52] In actual practice, half of patients have such negative attitudes.[53] If many patients in primary care settings submit to physician-recommended treatment but are not spontaneously motivated to receive treatment for their unrecognized depression, therapy could be ineffective.

It is possible that treating normal sadness as if it were depressive disorder can not only be wasteful but also have costs for patients that must be balanced against any benefits. Screening and identifying otherwise unrecognized cases of depression may undermine normal recovery by intensifying a person's feelings of distress and disrupting normal coping processes and use of informal support networks.[54] Providing results that indicate that people are depressively disordered can alarm and stigmatize them, especially if they themselves do not experience their feelings as disorders. It is thus perhaps not surprising that many people who screen positively resist being treated for depression.[55] Others might start taking medications but then discontinue treatment after a short period of time.[56] Such "noncompliance," although certainly of concern in some cases, in other instances might result from an accurate recognition of conditions that result from ordinary life stressors and a choice to approach the problem in an alternative way.

The primary care depression screening movement is a well-intentioned effort to develop and deploy psychological instruments that enable us to prevent potentially harmful outcomes of unrecognized, untreated depressive disorder in the general population. Despite the limitations and concerns raised here, the enormous efforts invested into the development and dissemination of screening instruments may have an increasing payoff as the instruments are refined. In particular, screening in primary care may well be made more worthwhile in the future if contextual indicators of normal reactions can be built into instruments so as to allow better identification of likely cases of disorder. Aside from context, it may be presumed that if symptoms are chronic, recurrent, or unusually severe, the condition is more likely to stem from a depressive disorder. Focusing resources on preventing recurrence in cases with multiple prior episodes, for example, may be a more efficient policy goal than screening all primary care patients for depression.[57] Pending the development of better screening instruments and considering scarce resources, efforts to improve the treatment of self-presenting cases of depressive disorder should take priority over mass screening programs.[58] Most important, when physicians screen for depression, and contrary to the current advice to attend only to symptom scores, they should be cautioned to attend also to the context of the reported symptoms and urged to use their diagnostic common sense and a policy of "watchful waiting" rather than blindly following DSM criteria-based results and reflexively prescribing medication.

Screening for Adolescent Depression

Schools are a second major target for screening of depressive disorder. Adolescents provide a particularly attractive focus for screening and preventive efforts because they appear to have high rates of depressive disorder, yet at the same time they are rarely treated for their conditions.[59] Suicide among adolescents provides another rationale for depression screening. About 4,000 American children and adolescents commit suicide each year, making it the third leading cause of death among 15- to 24-year-olds and the fourth among 10- to 14-year-olds; over half a million adolescents attempt suicide with sufficient seriousness to require medical attention.[60] Moreover, enormous publicity is accorded to rare but shocking school shootings by adolescents who in some instances have been depressed, imparting an additional urgency to arguments for preventive screening efforts. The belief that, in addition to these immediate problems, untreated adolescent depressive disorder is also likely to persist into adulthood and become chronic motivates screening efforts, as well.[61] Early identification and treatment are claimed to stop the downward spiral of increasingly worsening problems. Finally, all adolescents are mandated to attend school, and everyone is an adolescent at some time, so the schools provide a readily available opportunity to screen a population that over time will include virtually all individuals. Consequently, it is claimed, "prevention of the entire spectrum of depressive problems experienced by adolescents is of paramount importance if the needs of the largest number of adolescents are to be met."[62]

Concern about teenage depression in general and suicide in particular has led to major policy initiatives. The 2003 President's New Freedom Commission Report recommends that every adolescent in the entire country ought to "have the opportunity for early and appropriate mental health screening, assessment, and referral to treatment." Already several state legislatures have adopted measures with the goal that "every child should be screened for mental illness once in their youth in order to identify mental illness and prevent suicide among youth."[63] In 2004 President George W. Bush signed a bill authorizing $82 million to fund such screening programs beginning in sixth grade, with the goal of preventing suicide among young people.[64]

Our concerns about these well-intentioned efforts to help adolescents are similar to those that arise with respect to primary care screening. These efforts tend to ignore the distinction between disorders and conditions that are normal reactions to real losses. They thus focus clinical resources on many who are in transient normal states and they trigger interventions that tend to emphasize medication rather than addressing possible real problems in the adolescent's circumstances that might be causing intense distress. Moreover, the decontextualized instruments used to prescreen youths for depressive disorder or suicidal potential cast such a broad net that they identify much of the adolescent population as potentially at risk and as in need of further evaluation, confusing normal emotions with likely mental disturbance. A second-stage diagnostic screening may eliminate many of these errors but also applies symptom-based *DSM* criteria to adolescents' labile emotions, possibly still yielding substantial false-positive identifications of depressive disorder and suicide risk. Nor thus far is there scientific evidence that provides support for the effectiveness of teen screening.

Pathologizing Adolescent Distress

The primary justification for screening and preventive efforts in schools lies in the high perceived prevalence of depression among adolescents. A review of 52 studies from more than 20 countries indicates that about 20% of adolescents have depressive disorders according to *DSM* criteria.[65] Studies undertaken after 1990 showed even higher mean prevalence rates of 26% for some depressive disorders. Some researchers estimate that up to a third of adolescents will experience episodes of MDD by age 20.[66] Nearly half of one large sample of adolescents report having either a subthreshold or full diagnosis of depression.[67] For most researchers, these data support an obvious conclusion: "It is clear that depression is a major, pervasive, and perhaps increasing problem for youth."[68]

However, as in primary medical care, the nature of the screening and diagnostic instruments used for adolescents ensures that they are far more likely to uncover transitory and self-limiting cases of normal sadness than depressive disorders. These instruments do not inquire about the context in which symptoms develop. Thus, they cannot distinguish disorder from normal distress that arises from common adolescent stressors, such as arguments with parents, perceived betrayals by friends, or not being chosen for a valued activity, club, or athletic team. For example, many adolescents who have recently broken up with a boyfriend or girlfriend surely do not have depressive disorders, but nevertheless they may report enough symptoms in the ensuing period of time that screening and diagnostic instruments count them as depressively disordered.[69] Indeed, the potentially misleading nature of the statistics on adolescent depressive disorder is strikingly illustrated by the fact that the recent breakup of romantic attachments is the *strongest* predictor of depression in a large, national sample.[70]

Unlike typical cases of disorder, symptoms of adolescent depression are extremely unstable. Studies commonly find that most high scorers on self-report measures change their status when retested soon after.[71] Only about a third of adolescents remain depressed after only 1 month.[72] The relative emotional lability of adolescents, which would naturally lead to higher rates of transient negative emotions than in other groups, compounds the problem of using measurements that do not take context into account. The instability of symptoms among adolescents suggests that they are more likely to be transient responses to stressful life circumstances than the results of internal dysfunctions.

Research also fails to support claims that mild symptoms at one point in time are likely to become more severe at later periods. Most adolescents who initially report mild symptoms of depression report a year later that their symptoms are minimal or mild—that is, that their symptoms have decreased or remained the same; conversely, most adolescents who initially report severe symptoms report after a year that their symptoms have decreased rather than remained severe.[73] Nonetheless, a minority of adolescents with mild symptoms does get worse, and a minority with severe symptoms remains severe after a year. We might surmise that this minority of cases tends to include the truly disordered. The focus in screening research should be on developing more fruitful strategies for identifying and targeting this minority for intervention.

Columbia University TeenScreen

One major motivation for widespread screening of adolescents is to prevent suicide, and recently screening instruments have been developed that are specifically designed to detect suicidality and related mental disorder in teens. The President's New Freedom Commission cites the Columbia University Teen Screen program as a model and urges its use in every school in the country. We therefore take a closer look at TeenScreen as an example of the current state of the art in adolescent screening.

The TeenScreen program has developed two scales for use in prescreening adolescents. Both are derived from questions on a child diagnostic survey, the DISC (Diagnostic Interview Schedule for Children), and both require administration of the DISC as a second-stage diagnostic screening for those who test positive on initial evaluation. One, the DISC Predictive Scale (DPS), diagnoses eight mental disorders. With respect to depression diagnosis, it is very similar to the prescreening instruments we considered in the previous section on primary care. It asks very general questions at the beginning of the instrument, such as "In the past six months, were there times when you were very sad?" or "In the past six months, has there been a time when you weren't interested in anything and felt bored or just sat around most of the time?"[74] Any "yes" answer to these questions leads to several further questions about specific symptoms, such as having "a time when nothing was fun for you, even things you used to like" or being "so down that it was hard for you to do your schoolwork" or "grouchy or irritable . . . so that even little things would make you mad."

Although designed as a prescreen instrument, the DPS has come to be seen as a potential stand-alone diagnostic instrument. The executive director of Teen-Screen, Laurie Flynn, in testimony before a congressional committee, stated: "In 2003, we were able to screen approximately 14,200 teens . . . ; among those students, we were able to identify approximately 3,500 youth with mental health problems and link them with treatment."[75] Flynn here equates a positive prescreen with having "mental health problems," yielding about a 25% rate of such problems among a general student population. Yet studies show that the DPS yields four to five false-positive diagnoses for every DISC-confirmed diagnosis. Moreover, the DISC itself is simply an application to children and adolescents of *DSM*-style symptom-based criteria, and we have seen the questionable validity of these "confirming" criteria. If the DPS is widely used as either a prescreening or diagnostic instrument, the result is likely to be a massive pathologization of normal adolescent sadness and distress.

The other major TeenScreen instrument, the Columbia Suicide Screen (CSS), a brief 11-item (or sometimes 8-item; the number varies with the version) prescreening instrument self-administered by students, is designed to prescreen for risk factors that specifically increase suicide risk, including depressive disorder. To avoid making it obvious that the instrument is about suicide, the operative questions are embedded within a broader set of health questions and the instrument itself is labeled a "health survey." The CSS asks whether the individual has ever attempted suicide, has thought about suicide within the past 3 months, has experienced any of a short list of depressive symptoms (e.g., "unhappy or sad," "withdrawn"), anxiety symptoms, or substance use symptoms within the past 3 months, or feels a need to talk to a professional. Any student who answers "yes" to any one of the questions about suicide attempt, suicidal ideation, or need for help or "yes" to three of the questions about symptoms of depression, anxiety, or substance use is "positive" and is referred to a professional for further diagnosis and possible treatment.

How well does the CSS accomplish its goal of identifying those students with significant risk of suicide? If the numbers are any indicator, the answer is "not very well." In a major test of the CSS by its originators, 28% of 9th- to 12th-grade students tested positive on prescreening for risk of suicide, with the rate approaching half of all students (44%) in one school.[76] Seventeen percent of students report either thinking about suicide in the preceding 3 months or attempting suicide sometime in the past. The fact that nearly one in five adolescents reports either suicide attempts or suicidal ideation and that over 10% report thinking about suicide in the previous 3 months alone is either truly alarming or, more likely, indicative that the questions are not assessing what they are trying to assess and instead are tapping thoughts and feelings that many adolescents who are not truly at risk occasionally experience.

A further problem for both the CSS and the confirming DISC is the surprisingly low reliability in the answers to the relevant DISC questions. When the same questions about suicidal potential are asked at 8-day intervals, only about half of students who provide positive answers at one time also score positively just a week later! Given the extraordinarily unstable nature of the responses about suicidal ideation on the TeenScreen instrument, even the designers of TeenScreen admit that: "Poor test-retest reliability could be related to the ephemeral nature of suicidal ideation and depressive feelings among teens."[77] The low reliability means that we cannot be sure how seriously to take either the CSS or the follow-up DISC results. And we have seen that the DISC's *DSM*-style decontextualized criteria, especially when applied to emotionally reactive and labile teens, are of questionable validity in ferreting out the disorders among all those who are transiently distressed for a variety of normal reasons. Even though the DISC does reduce the percentage of positive diagnoses to 4% of the student population, it is impossible to have confidence that they are the right 4% who are really at risk or disordered. One way to check the validity of the DISC is to compare its results with clinicians' diagnoses. Disturbingly, despite the fact that clinician diagnoses themselves are generally based on *DSM* criteria, studies indicate extremely low levels of agreement between DISC and clinician diagnoses, further eroding confidence in the validity of even the two-stage TeenScreen procedure.[78]

TeenScreen researchers, aware of many of these problems, suggest at one point that perhaps even the enormous number of false positives generated by the CSS without DISC verification is not such a bad thing after all: "It is important not to lose sight of the fact that many of these so-called false-positive cases may be experiencing painful depressive symptoms with social and academic impairment and are likely to benefit from treatment."[79] This passage suggests that even if the CSS were used as a stand-alone suicide screen without a second DISC stage, teens who are not disordered may nonetheless benefit from treatment, and the same argument could be applied to DISC false positives. But the treatment of false positives may not be so innocuous.

Recall that the goal of screening programs, now being enacted into law, is to screen "every child in America" for depression and suicide potential.[80] Once TeenScreen identifies cases of putative depression and suicidal tendencies, the most common next step would be to treat with antidepressant medication, and this does seem to be TeenScreen's goal: "For antidepressant medication to be used effectively, cases of depression need to be identified, adding to the importance of screens of the type described here."[81] Although many normal but troubled youths can benefit from talking with a counselor, the possibility of treating nondisordered adolescents in large numbers with antidepressant medication for normal situational reactions that are likely transient and that might be dealt with in other ways raises special issues and concerns. There are real questions as to whether antidepressant medication works effectively in teenagers.[82] Most studies of this issue show no greater benefits of antidepressant medications compared with placebo.[83] Those studies that do find that medication benefits depressed adolescents are limited to voluntary samples with diagnoses of MDD that are stable over time. And even here the differences between treated and placebo groups tend to be minimal.[84] Moreover, as we saw with respect to primary care screening, the screened-positive populations may be different from, and may react to treatment differently than, self-referred clinical populations. Indeed, the U.S. Preventive Services Task Force does not recommend screening children or adolescents for depression or suicide.[85]

Evidence is also beginning to emerge that the risks of drug treatments may be greater for children than for adults.[86] Although clinical trials of medications have not yet reported any actual suicides, they do appear to show higher rates of suicidal ideation and other adverse events among groups taking antidepressant medication compared with placebo.[87] In some cases, such as school shootings, which are sometimes used to justify the need for screening, perpetrators were already using SSRIs that at least a few experts believe might even have contributed to the murderous state of mind of those particular teens.[88] If millions of adolescents were diagnosed as depressed and then medicated, the possibility that a number of teens would newly develop suicidal thoughts would have to be balanced against the number whose suicidal thoughts drugs would effectively control. The alarm generated by these findings has led regulatory agencies in Great Britain to warn physicians not to prescribe most antidepressant medications for persons younger than 18. Likewise, in the United States, the FDA now requires warnings on every bottle of pills about the possible adverse effects of antidepressants on younger persons. This whole area remains highly controversial, but the possibility of vast increases in the number of teens taking such medication due to invalid screening raises these concerns with a vengeance. At the least, the questionable or minimal effectiveness of antidepressant medications for children and adolescents, coupled with the possible effects of these medications on increasing adverse events and the as-yet-unknown effects of imposing long-term medication regimens on large numbers of still-developing teenagers who may not be disordered, are reasons for pursuing cautious rather than sweeping screening programs until more information is available. These considerations also argue for prudence in the treatment recommendations those programs may be used to support.

With regard to our focal issue of the overdiagnosis of depressive disorder, anyone who reports a few depressive symptoms on the CSS, even without suicidal behaviors or thoughts, is sent on for a DISC. In effect, the CSS is a way, motivated by the urgency of the desire to prevent suicide, of screening vast numbers of teens for depressive disorder with the associated false-positive problems we have identified. Yet unlike in epidemiologic research, the result of a TeenScreen "false positive" is not merely theoretical or statistical. The result is the personal identification of a specific young person as having a major mental disorder and perhaps as being in danger of further deterioration or suicide. This in turn can suggest a reconceptualization of the nature of that youth to him- or herself, his or her parents, and school officials; can alert parents, as well as school personnel, to the individual's presumed disorder; and possibly (if treatment is not refused) can lead to treating the individual with medication or psychotherapy that has unknown impact on a normally developing youth.

As the news media's sensational stories remind us, there is a very small but real possibility that undetected mental disorder in one's own children or in their classmates could lead to some horrific outcome such as suicide or homicide. The desire to do something to make our children safer from such threats is understandable. The problem is that the science does not yet exist to allow us to predict and intervene in ways that are known to prevent such tragedies. Moreover, screening programs that are justified by assurances that the results will be carefully evaluated clinically to eliminate false positives tend over time to be reinterpreted as conclusive diagnostic instruments and used as triggers for treatment in their own right.

Yet none of the currently available instruments for screening young people takes the context of distressing feelings into account. Thus none can discriminate normal adolescent emotionality from mental disorder. The result is a potential for a profound intrusion into our children's emotional lives using diagnostic labeling that is of questionable validity.

Conclusion

Routine screening for depression in the general population at locations such as schools and doctors' offices is now viewed as a major policy goal and an almost unqualified good. Given that such initiatives can influence the lives of millions of people, it is important to consider their possible costs and to critically scrutinize their underlying assumptions. Screening programs have repeated the mistake made in epidemiology of failing to seriously reassess validity when transporting the *DSM*'s criteria to the new context of community screening. They monitor the nuances of changing emotional reactions in us and our children in response to life's vicissitudes and label a considerable number of them as pathological without adequate contextual constraints. As these programs become part of our lives, they potentially influence our self-concepts and our judgments of others and offer a new form of social penetration of our private emotions. This form of influence is hard to quantify but real nonetheless. The ultimate effect could be to reconstitute our view of the normality of distressing feelings and to expand psychiatry's power to monitor, classify, and perhaps control our emotions in order to prevent even transient role impairment.

Screening initiatives might be beneficial or they might not be; at present, we just do not know. Remarkably, there currently exists no controlled scientific study that shows that these massive screening and treatment programs improve overall outcomes of depressive disorder or suicide. Nor does evidence exist that the benefits of such programs outweigh the costs of the inappropriate diagnosis and treatment they may initiate. This should especially trigger alarm bells when it comes to teen screening.

If one looks for historical analogies, this new surveillance of sadness is arguably comparable in its magnitude, its penetration of our intimate lives, and its encouragement of both professional and family hypervigilance of ordinary life to the much-discussed surveillance and medical pathologization of childhood masturbation that typified the sexual fears of the Victorian era. Just as that misconceived sexual control distorted children's natural sexual development even as it claimed to prevent or cure disorder, current campaigns to screen for depression, although they sometimes identify true disorder, have the potential to distort reactions to the natural experience of sadness in normal individuals and to disrupt any constructive features of normal sadness.

The challenge in effectively targeting preventive efforts via screening is to create instruments that are sufficiently sensitive to context so that they are able to distinguish the truly disordered from the normally distressed within the population of individuals who do not spontaneously present themselves for treatment. Policy efforts should promote pilot projects to develop scales that will be sensitive to the context and duration of symptoms and that will distinguish depressive disorders from normal sadness, thus better identifying those individuals who truly need professional help.

8

The *DSM* and Biological Research About Depression

Research into the biological causes of depressive disorder, such as its grounding in neurochemicals, receptors, genes, and the structure and function of the brain, holds great promise of contributing to our growing understanding of behavior, as well as of leading to new and more effective treatments. Such studies include, for example, those that use magnetic resonance imaging (MRI) to explore brain activity in depressed patients, examinations of neurotransmitters and their role in depression (bolstered by the success of medications in influencing the level of neurotransmitters), and research on the genetic influences on depressive disorder.

Around the same time as the publication of the *DSM-III* in 1980, biologically grounded models of depression began to dominate psychiatric theory and practice, and the influence of psychosocial models began to wane.[1] Moreover, a number of leading figures in the construction of the *DSM* were also leading biologically oriented psychiatrists. It is thus tempting to see the two as conceptually linked. Yet, as we have seen, the *DSM* definition was not in fact intended to imply any particular cause of depression. Instead, it was designed to be theory-neutral and compatible with social and psychological, as well as biological, causes of symptoms.

Nonetheless, the *DSM* criteria have played a prominent role in research studies on the biology of depression. The presence of agreed-on, theory-neutral criteria that could form a basis for communication among researchers has certainly been beneficial to biological research, as to all psychiatric research. However, on the other side of the ledger, we argue that the conflation of normal sadness and depressive disorder in *DSM* criteria has handicapped biological research and created confusion that can potentially lead researchers to draw misleading conclusions from their data.

The basic problem is simply that biological processes underlie nondisordered, as well as disordered, human traits. No doubt disordered sadness reactions often are due to underlying biological malfunctions. But the same symptoms of sadness are present in both normal and disordered conditions. The biological processes that are specific to disorder must be distinguished from the biological processes that underlie normal sadness. For example, studies show that many normal emotions and attitudes, such as introversion, religiosity, and even political beliefs, have a genetic component.[2] Genetic influences also explain to some extent why people naturally grieve when a beloved intimate dies.[3] The fact that there is a genetic basis for grief does not show that grief is a disorder—rather, bereavement is biologically grounded in normal, not in defective, genetic processes. Thus research that shows a biological or genetic correlate of a sadness condition says nothing in itself about whether or not that condition is a *disorder.*

Similarly, brain scans used in studies that induce states of sadness in normal participants indicate biological changes comparable to those found among persons with depressive disorders.[4] Thus the MRI of a normal individual who has suffered a severe loss resembles the MRI of a depressively disordered individual, most likely because of their similar subjective experiences.[5] The pattern of brain activity associated with symptoms consequently cannot be used as a basis to infer disorder, unless the context of the brain images is taken into account. The same point applies to studies of neurotransmitter levels; changes in neurotransmitter levels may occur during periods of normal intense sadness, as well as of depressive disorder, and some more complex underlying processes that involve neurotransmitters that are not properly responsive to environmental circumstances are liable to be present in disorders. If scientists consider only the correlation between biological markers and *DSM* criteria without taking into account the context in which they occur, they could wrongly conclude that a marker indicates disorder rather some phenomenon common to normal sadness and disorder.

This chapter considers some of the most common ways that biological psychiatry has attempted to show how depression is grounded in abnormalities of brain functioning. These include studies of twins and adoptees, of neurochemical deficiencies, of genetic defects, and of anatomical lesions. We argue that an adequate context-based distinction between normal sadness and depressive disorder would enhance each of these styles of research.

Twin and Adoption Studies

For most of the twentieth century, biological research focused on using twin and adoption studies in attempts to show the genetic basis of depression. The central goal of these studies was to separate the impact of genetic and environmental factors in the illness. Twin studies capitalize on the fact that there are two kinds of twins that have known, but different, degrees of genetic similarity. Dizygotic

(DZ) twins, like regular siblings, share 50% of their genes, whereas monozygotic (MZ) twins are genetically identical. Both types of twins presumably share the same family environment. To the extent that genetic factors influence depression, MZ twins ought to have twice the concordance rate as DZ twins. Conversely, if environmental factors are predominant causes, both types of twins should exhibit comparable levels of depression.

The logic of adoption studies derives from the fact that the parents who transmit genes to their children are not the same parents who raise these children. Therefore, findings that show high rates of depression among children born to depressed mothers but raised by nondepressed adoptive parents would indicate that depression has a genetic component. In contrast, rates of depression among adopted children that more closely resemble those among their adoptive than among their natural parents would indicate that environmental factors have a stronger influence than genetic ones.

The voluminous literature on twin and adoption studies regarding the genetic contribution to depression yields ambiguous findings. Some twin studies show strong genetic but weak environmental influences, others show the reverse, and many show only a slightly higher concordance among MZ than among DZ twins.[6] Likewise, some adoption studies indicate a higher concordance in rates of depression among adopted children and their natural parents than among those children and their adoptive parents,[7] whereas others indicate just the reverse.[8] But overall, it appears reasonable to conclude that the heritability of depressive disorder can lie in the range of about 30–40%.[9]

Even if it were possible to draw definitive conclusions from these studies, we would still not know whether what is genetically or environmentally transmitted is a depressive disorder or normal sadness. No evidence demonstrates that depressive disorders have a higher probability of inheritance than tendencies to become sad. Indeed, it appears that people inherit predispositions to be on the high or low range in the distribution of sadness responses or to have depressive disorder to about the same degree. Twin studies indicate that personality traits related to sadness, such as introversion, have heritabilities of about 40–50%, quite similar to those of depressive disorder.[10] Therefore, showing that some trait has a high probability of being inherited says little about whether that trait is a disorder or a normally distributed personality characteristic. Before researchers can legitimately conclude that their biological findings reflect the genetic basis of conditions that are *disorders,* they must *first* use a definition of depression that adequately separates their research groups into those with depressive disorder and those with normal sadness.

Depression Stems From a Chemical Imbalance

Current biological research has the potential to be more informative than twin and adoption studies about the specific causes of depression because it directly examines genes and brains, rather than inferring genetic contributions from the degree of relatedness among individuals. Nevertheless, it suffers from the same conceptual problems as these studies. One typical kind of study searches for neurochemical levels that are related to depressive disorders.[11] But in order to reach appropriate conclusions, we must understand the context in which various levels of chemicals arise. Showing an association between some brain state and depressive symptoms cannot in itself answer the question of whether the symptoms are normal responses to stressful environments or indicators of a disorder. The findings of current studies of neurochemicals and depression are often uninterpretable because they do not adequately make this distinction.

One of the most popular theories posits that a chemical imbalance in the brain, specifically deficient amounts of the neurochemical serotonin, causes depression. It follows, then, that drug treatments targeting serotonin, the selective serotonin reuptake inhibitors (SSRIs), which presumably correct this chemical imbalance, are the appropriate response to depressive disorders. This theory is relentlessly promoted in many ways: pharmaceutical advertisements emphasize how correctable chemical imbalances cause depressive disorders, public service messages stress that depression stems from flaws in brain chemistry rather than in character, and mental health advocacy groups advance the message that depression is a physical, brain-based illness, just like diabetes or asthma.[12] These ubiquitous messages have led to the widespread impression that research has actually shown that chemical deficiencies are the cause of depressive disorders and that drugs work because they correct these impairments in the neurotransmission system. Therefore, it might seem that one way to separate depressive disorders from normal sadness would be to examine levels of serotonin in the brain.

The chemical deficiency theory of depression originated with psychiatrist Joseph Schildkraut's hypothesis, published in 1965, that low levels of amines were associated with the development of depressive disorders. His paper is still one of the most frequently cited articles in the history of psychiatry.[13] Interestingly, Schildkraut thought that norepinephrine, not serotonin, was the neurochemical implicated in depressive disorder:

> The "catecholamine hypothesis of affective disorders," proposes that some, if not all depressions are associated with an absolute or relative deficiency of catecholamines, particularly norepinephrine at functionally important adrenergic receptor sites in the brain. Elation conversely may be associated with an excess of such amines.[14]

The major source of evidence for the chemical deficiency hypothesis stems from the success of drug treatments, which raise levels of amines, in alleviating depressive symptoms. Schildkraut himself recognized that "even if the drugs are effective in treating the disorders, that does not necessarily imply that their mode of action involves correction of the underlying abnormality."[15] Nevertheless, many subsequent arguments relating to serotonin rely on the premise that if enhancing its transmission improves depression, then a deficiency in the serotonin system may be responsible for the initial emergence of the condition.

Many problems beset such theories. One is that the SSRIs cause immediate changes in levels of serotonin, but the resulting effects on depression typically take several weeks to transpire. The impact of the drugs on depression, therefore, might not result from the change in neurotransmitter levels that they create but instead from a number of other processes associated with the change in amine activity. Another is that some drugs that do not affect either serotonin or norepinephrine, the major amines involved in the catecholamine hypothesis, also can alleviate depression.[16] Indeed, some antidepressant drugs developed after the SSRIs influence dopamine and other amines, but not serotonin. A third difficulty is that the drugs used to treat depression work with at least equal effectiveness on other disorders, including those of anxiety, eating, attention deficit, substance abuse, personality, and a host of other conditions that may or may not be comorbid with depression. This suggests that the drugs are not correcting a specific neurochemical abnormality that underlies depression but are instead acting on very general brain functions that influence many emotional and behavioral systems. No theory explains how such a single abnormality in brain chemistry could be related to such a wide range of resulting problems. In addition, measures typically show that only about 25% of depressed patients actually have low levels of norepinephrine or serotonin.[17] Even if the deficiency hypothesis is proven to be correct, it would explain only a portion of depressed cases, as Schildkraut himself recognized in his original article.[18]

Another fundamental problem is that the hypothesized deficiencies of serotonin or other brain chemicals quite possibly may be the consequences, rather than the causes, of depression. No evidence thus far has demonstrated that chemical imbalances actually precede and cause depressive disorders.[19] Instead, depression itself, as well as the drugs used to treat it, could be responsible for the inferred deficiencies that exist in patients with depression. Because most research participants have long histories of medication treatment, it is impossible to know what their unmedicated brains looked like before they began using antidepressant drugs.

The most serious conceptual problem with the neurochemical deficiency hypothesis, from our perspective, is that no adequate contextually grounded standard exists for normal versus disordered levels of serotonin or other amines. High or low levels of any neurochemical are not abnormal in themselves, but only in relation to a particular set of circumstances and to the way the brain is biologically designed to respond to those kinds of circumstances. The mechanisms that underlie levels of serotonin (and other neurochemicals) likely are biologically designed to be quite responsive to their contexts: the brains of normal people who are experiencing serious losses would expectably show depleted states of serotonin. The normality of amine levels can be established only relative to the environmental context in which they occur.

For example, as the studies considered in chapter 2 show, serotonin levels among primates vary substantially as a function of social situations: gains and losses of social status are associated with rising and falling levels of serotonin, respectively.[20] Thus low levels of serotonin in humans also could reflect the emotions that normally accompany a recent change in social status rather than a depressive disorder. Likewise, baboons living in the wild show highly elevated levels of glucocorticoids (stress hormones) after experiencing bereavement, loss of social rank, or other stressful events.[21] These levels return to normal after the affected animals resume grooming behaviors with members of their social networks. In these cases, extreme levels of neurochemicals do not indicate disorders but show instead the way that normal brains respond to stressful situations.

Conversely, disordered states are associated not with extreme levels of neurochemicals alone but also with extreme levels that are inappropriate responses to environmental contexts. The sorts of changes in the brain that result from depressive disorders are similar to responses to acutely stressful situations.[22] Indeed, an extreme amount of serotonin or other amine in response to a stressor can be adaptive in the situation in which it occurs.[23] The difference between normal and abnormal levels of neurochemicals lies not in the level of the neurotransmitter per se but rather in the fact that the neurotransmitter level has escaped from usual restraints and become more chronic and removed from environmental circumstances.

Statements that depression is a "flaw in chemistry" or a "physical disease" are premature; cognitive, psychodynamic, social, or other factors that enduringly disrupt biologically designed sadness reactions but that may or may not correlate with brain abnormality may well cause at least some depressive disorders. "The truth is," notes psychologist Eliot Valenstein, "that it is really not known how drugs alleviate the symptoms of mental disorders, and it should not be assumed that they do so by correcting an endogenous chemical deficiency."[24] But for future research to have a better chance of confirming or disconfirming that some deficiency in neurotransmitter systems is causally related to cases of depressive disorder, researchers will have to use criteria that can separate cases in which various levels of neurochemicals result from normal brains operating in stressful environments from those in which some abnormality leads to inappropriate brain functioning.

The Genetic Basis of Depression

Studies of the genetics of depression have entered a new era. Major breakthroughs in genetic research during the 1990s have allowed researchers to directly map specific genes and examine their connection to the development of symptoms.[25] Yet, despite these advances, current research on the genetics of depression remains handicapped by its failure to distinguish under which circumstances genetic factors lead to biologically selected responses to loss or to mental disorders. Current *DSM* symptom-based definitions of depression do not adequately distinguish intense normal sadness from disorder, yet much important genetics research relies on population-based samples that are likely to be composed of predominantly normal individuals. Thus researchers are in jeopardy of mistakenly identifying findings about the roots of normal sadness as discoveries about the causes of depressive disorder.

To illustrate how this error might occur, we focus on a single article, "Influence of Life Stress on Depression: Moderation by a Polymorphism in the 5-HTT Gene" by psychologist Avshalom Caspi and colleagues.[26] This article's influence on the general scientific community may be greater than that of any genetic study of any mental illness that has been conducted to date. *Science* magazine named it, along with two other articles on the genetics of mental illness, the second most important scientific breakthrough of 2003 (after only an article about newfound insights into the nature of the cosmos). The National Institute of Mental Health's (NIMH) Web site cites the study as one of the great accomplishments of the agency's focus on the biological basis of mental illness. Thomas Insel, the director of the NIMH, claims that: "What they have done is going to change the paradigm for how we think about genes and psychiatric disorders."[27] Another NIMH psychiatrist calls the study "the biggest fish yet netted for psychiatry."[28] The study's findings were broadly disseminated and featured in both U.S. and worldwide media.[29]

The research stems from a longitudinal study of a cohort of 847 Caucasians in New Zealand born in the early 1970s and followed from birth into young adulthood. The researchers' central concern was to examine the association between stressful life events, depression, and the 5-HTT gene when cohort members were 26 years old. The 5-HTT gene was chosen for study because it controls the way that serotonin, itself the focus of much genetic research on depression, passes messages through brain cells. Previous research suggested that the gene is associated with reactions to stressful stimuli in mice, monkeys, and people undergoing brain imaging, although no prior studies had found a direct link between the gene and depression.

The 5-HTT gene has three genotypes: in the New Zealand sample, 17% of respondents had two copies of the short allele; 31%, two copies of the long allele; and 51%, one short and one long allele. The study measured stress through an additive index of 14 life events, including employment, financial, housing, health, and relationship stressors that participants experienced between ages 21 and 26. It also used the Diagnostic Interview Schedule (DIS), designed to perform *DSM* diagnoses, to determine whether or not participants had experienced an episode of Major Depression over the preceding year. The study also reported on number of depressive symptoms, on suicidal ideation, and on informant reports of depression. Its central hypothesis was that people who have one or two of the short versions of the 5-HTT allele might be especially vulnerable to highly stressful environments, whereas those with genes containing the long version might be more resistant to adverse environmental stressors.

The study found that 17% of this population sample of 26-year-olds reported episodes of depression severe enough to meet MDD criteria over the preceding year. It showed no association between the 5-HTT gene and those who became depressed. There was, in other words, no direct genetic effect on depression: people with two short alleles, two long alleles, or one of each allele had equivalent chances of becoming depressed. The study also found no relationship between the 5-HTT genotype groups and the number of stressful life events that participants experienced, so the genotype should not account for differential exposure to stressors. That is, it was unlikely that possessing a given genotype was the cause of the number of stressful life events that respondents reported.

The study did find a strong positive relationship between experiencing more stressful life events and developing depression. As the number of life stressors increased from zero to four or more, rates of MDD increased from 10% to 13, 15, 20, and 33%, respectively. Put another way, people who experienced four or more stressful life events were about three and a half times more likely to develop depression than those who experienced no stressful events.

The study's major finding, and the one that generated much attention, was a significant gene-by-environment interaction. Among the 15% of the sample who experienced four or more stressful life events after their 21st and before their 26th birthdays, those with one or two copies of the short allele on the 5-HTT gene were significantly more likely to have MDD, as well as self- and informant-reported depressive symptoms, than those with two copies of the long allele. In the group that faced four or more stressful life events, 43% of individuals with two short alleles and 33% with one short allele became depressed compared with 17% of those with two long alleles who did.

In summary, the study did not find a direct effect of the 5-HTT gene on depression. It did find a fairly strong relationship of stressful life events with depression, so that people who experienced more stressful events had a greater chance of becoming depressed. And it found that the 5-HTT gene interacts with the number of life events to predict depression; at high levels of stressful events, possession of the short gene leads to more depression.

The authors viewed their finding as confirmation of the "diathesis-stress theory of depression," which predicts that experiences of higher levels of stress will elevate the vulnerability of depression much more among people who are at high genetic risk than among those at low genetic risk.[30] The short allele on the 5-HTT gene presumably makes people more sensitive to stress, whereas the long allele protects them from the impact of stress. Therefore, the short allele is the stress-sensitive genotype associated with depression.

But this interpretation of the short allele is open to question, at least for the most classic case of depressive disorder, endogenous depression. The study found that about 10% of the 263 people who had experienced no negative life events over the preceding 5 years developed depression. This 10% was the group who most clearly had depressive disorders as opposed to normal intense sadness, yet there was no impact of the 5-HTT genotype on this group's response to stress. If there is a genetic cause of endogenous depression, it does not seem to show up here, so this particular type of depressive disorder appears unrelated to the 5-HTT gene or, at least, to the widespread variants of it that Caspi et al. studied.

There is a much more fundamental problem with Caspi et al.'s interpretation of their findings: it is not clear that the identified gene has much to do with depressive disorder at all. The study used *DSM* criteria for depression, which contain no systematic distinction between normal sadness and depressive disorder. The extraordinarily high rate of depression among the young people in this study—17% of the entire community sample of 26-year-olds met *DSM* criteria for MDD—itself suggests that many of these cases actually reflected normal intense sadness, not depressive disorders. Nor was there some unusual situation that might explain high rates of depressive disorder: the research took place in a modern and prosperous country during a period of tranquility when there were no wars, major economic downturns, or cultural upheavals,[31] and it excluded the Maori, a deprived ethnic minority that would be expected to have high rates of depression. The fundamental question of whether the measure of disorder was valid and thus whether the observed interaction reflected normal variation or disorder remains entirely unaddressed and unanswerable based on the existing data.

Concluding that the short allele is a genotype for depressive disorders is especially premature because of the particular kinds of stressful life events the Caspi et al. study measured. Most of the 14 stressful life events that the study measured were associated with inadequate financial resources, such as problems with debt, not having money for food and household expenses, lacking money for medical expenses, and difficulty paying bills. Consequently, many of these events might be co-occurring results of a single stressor, such as unemployment or long-term poverty. In many cases, reports of four or more stressors would indicate not an additive increase in stressful life events but the experience of a particular kind of financial stressor connected with many of the measures the study uses. The short allele's impact, therefore, might not be associated so much with experiencing *more* stressors as it is with experiencing particular *kinds* of stressors that are linked to financial problems that are especially likely to be related to normal sadness.

Although this study does not report the association of social class with these life events, other studies of similar age groups find strong relationships between low socioeconomic status and the number of major life events that young adults experience.[32] The Caspi et al. study may actually mainly show how people with limited economic resources are exposed to the kinds of stressors—financial debt, social inequality, and poverty—that might naturally lead people to report symptoms of normal sadness. If correct, this interpretation has important implications for prevention or treatment efforts, because over two-thirds of the population has at least one short allele. The Caspi et al. article focuses on the possibility of medication, noting that "more knowledge about the functional properties of the 5-HTT gene may lead to better pharmacological treatments for those already depressed."[33] But if the 5-HTT gene is largely responsible for normal sadness that emerges because of social inequality rather than depressive disorders, preventive efforts, at least, would best address social conditions and not exclusively focus on medicating a presumed internal genetic defect.

In any event, the meaning of the Caspi et al. findings remains ambiguous. Whether the studied genes interact with certain types of stressors or stressors in general rather than revealing the genetic underpinnings of depressive disorder, the findings could be interpreted equally well as revealing normal genetic variations in the tendency for people to become sad when they are under intense stress. The study's data are entirely consistent with the possibility that the short and long alleles represent two roughly equal, fitness-enhancing variations on the pattern of sensitivity in normal loss responses. Subsequent attempts to replicate the study's findings display serious discrepancies both among themselves and in relation to the original study, yielding a confusing rather than scientifically congealing picture.[34] The resulting ambiguities may stem from the fact that all this research failed to separate natural from dysfunctional conditions and thus likely encompassed some heterogeneous mix of normal and disordered sadness with varying genetic determinants. The use of measures that separate normal sadness from disordered depression could help clarify this problematic situation.

Anatomical Brain Abnormalities as the Basis for Depressive Disorder

A final type of biological research looks for anatomical abnormalities in various brain regions, in particular the prefrontal cortex, the hippocampus, and the amygdala, to demonstrate the biological basis of depressive disorders. The prefrontal cortex helps regulate evaluations of rewards and punishments, fear states, and changes in mood, including those that occur when people display normal states of sadness.[35] Therefore, abnormalities in this area should affect processes that are integrally involved in depressive disorders. The hippocampus has a central role in learning and memory, which could help explain the cognitive deficits that often accompany major depression.[36] Finally, the amygdala has an especially important role in processing negative affect, which should obviously have a critical role in sadness and depression.[37]

As early as the nineteenth century, studies of brain anatomy had already indicated the major localized regions associated with different brain functions.[38] More recently, brain images from MRIs that are able to pinpoint the brain circuitry associated with depressive feelings are coming to dominate articles in psychiatric journals. Studies that use MRIs and other imaging techniques can use computer analysis to visualize living brains at the level of subcellular molecules, neurons, and genetic material. An extensive body of research suggests that particular lesions might be the primary sites of aberrant mood regulation among people with depression.[39]

We saw in our examination of the Caspi et al. research that genetics researchers who rely on *DSM* criteria are in jeopardy of interpreting features of normal sadness as characteristics of depressive disorder.[40] There is a second kind of error that can also derive from reliance on the *DSM* criteria for depressive disorder in biological research: if results of research on brain lesions that are confirmed for a clearly disordered clinical population are mistakenly generalized to all those who satisfy the *DSM* criteria and are thus presumptively disordered, then the lesion may be mistakenly attributed to many who are experiencing normal sadness.

We examine a heralded study of brain circuitry by anatomist Grazyna Rajkowska and colleagues, "Morphometric Evidence for Neuronal and Glial Prefrontal Cell Pathology in Major Depression," to illustrate the possibility of this second kind of error. Rajkowska's study was published in 1999 as a special "priority communication" in the journal *Biological Psychiatry*. Peter Kramer, in his book *Against Depression*, cites it as the most important work yet done on depression because it "changed the way doctors view their patients."[41]

Rajkowska et al. compared brain tissue from 12 chronically depressed patients who died suddenly with brain tissue from 12 normal controls who also died suddenly. They found that the depressed group had distinct pathological characteristics associated with brain abnormalities. In particular, these patients had abnormal levels of glial cells, which help mediate between neurons and their environment, in the prefrontal cortex. These deficits can contribute to a variety of pathological changes in this brain region. Elevated levels of glucocorticoids, in turn, can cause damage to the hippocampus, so that patients who are depressed have significantly smaller volume in the hippocampus than control participants.[42]

Other research finds that the reduction of glial cell density and neuronal size is especially acute in patients with MDD compared with patients with bipolar disorder and schizophrenia, as well as with normal control participants, suggesting the specific kind of lesion that might indicate a particular disorder.[43] Moreover, modifications of the brain associated with MDD are present even when the symptoms of the illness no longer are. Studies have observed brain changes in individuals with MDD when the illness is in remission, suggesting that the disorder has caused permanent damage to particular regions of the brain.[44] Some research also shows that participants with depression have enlarged amygdalas, which might be related to hippocampal volume loss.[45] Major Depression, such evidence suggests, is a disruption in a defined circuit in specific regions of the brain.[46]

The evidence that depression is related to a brain lesion, however, has ambiguous implications for the causes of depressive disorders. Many researchers assume that the demonstrated morphological changes are more likely to be the consequences, rather than the causes, of depression, although this issue remains unsettled.[47] As Rajkowska emphasizes, no evidence shows that anatomical abnormalities precede and predispose people to depression; it only suggests that brain damage is associated with depression.[48] In addition, because the patients in such studies are generally being seen by clinicians, it is possible that the abnormal brain reorganization observed among people with depression could be the result of exposure to long-term treatment with antidepressant medications rather than the consequence of depressive disease.[49] We simply do not know what the brains of depressed people looked like before they started extensive regimens of medications.

But, these doubts aside, if the findings that a neuroanatomical substrate is associated with, or causes, depressive disorder are confirmed in the population Rajkowska studied, what would be the range of their applicability? Kramer's discussion of Rajkowska's work simply assumes that because Rajkowska studied MDD patients, the results likely have wide applicability to virtually all patients who fall under the diagnosis of MDD, even subthreshold conditions. This interpretation supports Kramer's view of the deeply pathological nature of all depressive states. Depression at every point in the spectrum, according to Kramer, is "debilitating, progressive and relentless in its downhill course" across the entire range of presentations.[50] All criteria, including the number of symptoms, their severity, and their duration, fall on continua that are assumed to indicate some degree of pathology at each level.[51] Moreover, while many minor states are dangerous on their own, whereas others are likely to degenerate into major states, every point on the continuum represents a state of high risk of developing the kinds of lesions that the Rajkowska study demonstrated in extremely severe cases. "To accept depression as disease," asserts Kramer, "is to see pathology or risk in minor versions."[52]

In assessing such claims, it is important to consider the nature of those individuals in the Rajkowska sample whose brains showed pathology. These were patients in long-term treatment for chronic conditions. Despite treatment, 7 of the 12 who were depressed died as a result of suicide. Three of the five individuals who were not suicides were taking antipsychotic medications at the time of their deaths. Only two members of the depressed sample were neither suicides nor presumably suffering from psychosis. The group was thus almost entirely composed of extremely severe cases of what were very likely true depressive disorders.

So how far can the results of these studies be generalized? Given the heterogeneous mix of not only mild and severe cases but also normal and disordered sadness that currently falls under the MDD diagnostic criteria, it is unlikely that the Rajkowska results apply to the entire category of MDD cases, not to mention subthreshold conditions. There is no evidence that the demonstrated brain abnormalities affect more than a small minority of those who satisfy the *DSM* criteria and who are the most clearly disordered. No one has ever shown, for example, that most people who experience symptoms of depression that satisfy these criteria have lost glial cells; one would expect this theory to fail to generalize to those who meet *DSM* criteria but are in fact experiencing intense normal sadness.[53] Nor, regarding Kramer's remark about risk, has any study ever shown that people with normal states of sadness are more likely than others to develop later anatomical pathologies. Kramer's claims go well beyond the evidence in a way that could lead to precarious clinical assumptions about those experiencing intense sadness.

Although brain research has not as yet demonstrated that most cases of depressive disorder have an anatomical grounding, it does have some interesting implications for the anatomical basis of normal sadness. One important study asked volunteer participants with no history of depression to prepare scripts describing recent personal experiences of sadness.[54] They then gave positron emission tomography (PET) scans to the participants while they used these scripts to provoke a sad mood state. Participants who experienced provoked states of normal sadness showed increases in blood flow in limbic-paralimbic regions of the brain and diminished blood flow in prefrontal regions that are comparable to those found in studies of patients with clinical depression.[55] This result suggests that these regions are related to both normal sad moods and pathological depression.

States of normal sadness that can be provoked in laboratory settings are likely a pale reflection of sadness that arises in natural situations of actual major loss. The preceding findings thus imply that normal participants who are given a biological diagnostic or screening test for depression *while they are exposed to sadness stimuli* would likely score high on these measures because they show the biological markers that underlie the symptoms of normal sadness and pathological depression alike.

Conclusion

We have argued that if brain researchers fail to consider the context in which sadness develops, they are in danger of misdiagnosing the normally sad as having depressive disorders and of muddling their samples with a heterogeneous mix of disordered and normal participants. Normal sadness, no less than depressive disorder, has correlates with brain states and can include intense sadness symptoms; people experiencing sadness may have some of the same biological markers as the truly depressively disordered. Thus showing a biological substrate to a condition of intense sadness symptoms that satisfy *DSM* criteria is not enough to indicate whether that particular substrate or the condition itself is normal or disordered. Understanding the context in which brain activity occurs is an essential precondition for knowing whether brains are functioning in normal or abnormal ways. An enhanced understanding of how normal brains respond to situations that involve loss would provide an essential benchmark to compare with the possible brain dysfunctions that are connected to depressive disorders. Better defined research on the brain thus has the potential to more effectively distinguish and illuminate both abnormal and normal responses to loss.

9

The Rise of Antidepressant Drug Treatments

The *DSM-III*'s neutral stance toward the etiology of mental disorders meant that advocates of all treatment orientations were supposed to find equal value in its symptom-based classification system. In practice, however, pharmaceutical companies were best able to capitalize on the *DSM*'s focus on symptoms, which allowed them to broadly construe states of intense sadness as depressive disorder and thus to vastly increase the potential market for antidepressant medication. Several other developments helped propel an explosive growth in the use of these drugs, including the emergence of the selective serotonin reuptake inhibitors (SSRIs) in the late 1980s, the spread of managed care throughout the U.S. health care system in the 1990s, and the approval of direct-to-consumer (DTC) advertisements in 1997. This chapter considers the relationship between the *DSM* revolution and the roughly contemporaneous exponential growth of drug treatments for depression.

A Brief History of Drug Treatments for Sadness and Depression

The First Tranquilizers

For thousands of years, physicians have used medications to treat depression. Beginning with the ancient Greeks and Romans, doctors commonly prescribed purgative and laxative medicines that induced vomiting and evacuation of the bowels.[1] Richard Napier, the seventeenth-century physician mentioned in chapter 3, typically used sedatives and analgesics, as well as laxatives and purging concoctions, in his practice.[2] He prescribed opium for about 10% of his melancholic patients. By the nineteenth century opium, morphine, and other alkaloids had become common treatments for depression, joined by the barbiturate sedatives during the early twentieth century.[3]

During the 1950s specific drugs to treat distress over life problems emerged, beginning with the tranquilizer meprobamate (Miltown). The sedative and muscle relaxant qualities of Miltown made it effective for everyday tension and anxiety. It was immediately successful, and the demand for it and closely related drugs was, according to historian Edward Shorter, "greater than for any drug ever marketed in the United States."[4] Despite the misgivings of the American Psychiatric Association that these drugs were widely misused to alleviate "the routine tensions of everyday living," by 1956 1 in 20 Americans were taking some sort of tranquilizer.[5]

In the early 1960s, the benzodiazepines Librium and Valium were developed, quickly supplanting Miltown as the most successful drugs ever introduced in pharmaceutical history. Their effects were qualitatively similar to, but more potent than, Miltown. By 1969, Valium was the most prescribed medication in the United States. Surveys at the time indicated that between 15 and 25% of the population had ever used one of the tranquilizing drugs.[6] Research also showed that only about a third of the prescriptions for these drugs were written for people with diagnosed mental disorders, whereas most medications were given to those experiencing psychic distress, life crises, and psychosocial problems.[7]

Prescription drug use then, as it is now, was gender imbalanced, with women receiving about two of every three prescriptions.[8] Even the colloquial term for these medications, made famous by the Rolling Stones' hit song, "Mother's Little Helper," indicates their association with the normal misery of housewives, suggesting that "though she's not really ill" the pills help a mother to calm down, deal with her busy day, meet her husband's demands, and thus "minimize your plight."[9] Popular women's magazines, in particular, viewed these drugs as helpful in dealing with common problems such as sexual unresponsiveness, infidelity, troublesome children, or inability to attract a man.[10]

After their explosive growth in the 1950s and 1960s, a counterreaction to the antianxiety drugs set in. Some critics cited how these drugs numbed people's reactions to social problems and, in particular, how women used them to avoid confronting oppressive interpersonal situations.[11] Others worried about the use of these drugs to cope with daily life: "It is only now," wrote one psychiatrist, "that we are faced with the possible utilization of psychoactive drugs by a major portion of the population in what might be considered problems of daily living."[12] Likewise, Stanley Yolles, the director of the NIMH, expressed unease about whether "the chemical deadening of anxiety" was harmful and about whether "Western culture (would) be altered by widespread use of tranquilizers."[13] Still others expressed serious concerns about the addicting qualities, adverse side effects, and overdose potential of these drugs.

Numerous Congressional hearings at the time focused on the dangers and misuse of psychotropic medications, beginning with the well-known Kefauver hearings in 1960 and continuing through the 1970s. The use of the benzodiazepines for treating common problems of living was a specific concern. For example, during a hearing in 1971 Senator Gaylord Nelson asked the commissioner of the FDA: "Isn't there a very fundamental distinction between prescribing a drug to help the patient manage a serious problem of depression and tension and prescribing a drug to help the patient meet the ordinary . . . frustration of daily living?"[14] The commissioner of the FDA, Charles Edwards, responded by expressing the "growing concern" of his agency that "advertisements have also promoted their use in the treatment of symptoms arising from the stresses of everyday living, which cannot properly be defined as pathological."[15]

During the 1960s and 1970s the FDA took action against pharmaceutical companies' claims to treat problems of living. For example, in 1971, it requested that advertisers of psychotropic drugs refrain from promoting their use in coping with everyday life strains. This action evidently had some effect, and such general appeals disappeared from these ads for the rest of the decade.[16] The FDA also placed both meprobamate and the benzodiazepines on its list of "schedule IV" drugs in 1975, which meant restricting refills and initiating "special reporting requirements" for their use.[17] In 1980, FDA regulations specifically noted that "anxiety or tension associated with the stress of everyday life usually does not require treatment with an anxiolytic."[18]

The attitude of the popular press also sharply changed, from its initially favorable reception of these drugs when they were introduced toward a decidedly critical view. The proportion of articles in lay periodicals that took unfavorable attitudes toward tranquilizers more than doubled, from about a third in the 1950s to over two-thirds in the 1970s.[19] The climate had clearly turned against the widespread use of the benzodiazepines, and the craze for antianxiety drugs was tapering off by the time the *DSM-III* was published in 1980. Valium was still the largest selling prescription drug of any sort, but tranquilizer and benzodiazepine use had declined dramatically, from a peak of over 100 million prescriptions written in 1975 to slightly over 70 million in 1980, and it continued to decrease during the 1980s.[20]

The Rise of Antidepressants

The initial tranquilizing drugs were called *anxiolytics* because they targeted anxiety rather than depression. Drugs that were specifically targeted at depression also emerged in the 1950s, including monoamine oxidase inhibitors (MAOIs) and tricyclic antidepressants, such as imipramine (Tofranil) and amitriptyline (Elavil). Although by 1980 nearly 30 million prescriptions were being written for antidepressants, this was far fewer than the number for the anxiolytics.[21] At the time, depression was not viewed as a widespread problem, and conditions of normal misery were likely to be seen as problems of tension and anxiety.[22] Moreover, the tricyclics and especially the MAOIs had substantial side effects that limited their usefulness. Thus antidepressant drugs had a fairly small market niche, a situation that would quickly change over the next decade.

The SSRIs

There is no evidence that pharmaceutical companies had a role in developing *DSM-III* diagnostic criteria. Yet, serendipitously, the new diagnostic model was ideally suited to promoting the pharmaceutical treatment of the conditions it delineated. Since 1962, the FDA had required manufacturers to market drugs only for the relief of specific diseases rather than for more general purposes such as reduction of tension or distress stemming from problems in living (although, as noted earlier, advertisements sometimes violated these regulations). But because all of the diagnoses in the *DSM-III* were formulated as categorical disease entities, they provided many different targets for the products of pharmaceutical companies to treat.[23] The diagnosis of Major Depression, which used common symptoms such as sadness, lack of energy, or sleeplessness as indicators, was particularly well suited for expanding the market for psychotropic drugs because it inevitably encompassed many patients who formerly might have been thought to be suffering from problems of living. It would not take long for pharmaceutical companies to capitalize on this felicitous aspect of the *DSM-III*.

The *DSM-III* also unintentionally provided drug companies with a way out of the dilemma they faced in marketing their antianxiety medications. As noted, for many years anxiety, rather than depression, was viewed as the most common psychic problem resulting from the stresses of daily life. Drug companies typically marketed their products as treatments for anxiety disorders, and their products were generally viewed as antianxiety agents. In fact, there is a huge overlap between symptoms of anxiety and those of depression.[24] Indeed, as we saw in chapter 3, clinical theorists traditionally saw anxiety as an integral part of depressive conditions, but the *DSM-III* attempted to identify a pure depressive syndrome independent of anxiety. Which condition is emphasized largely depends on diagnostic fashions, the interests of various professional and advocacy groups, and economic costs and benefits.[25] By 1980, the balance of these factors was shifting away from anxiety because of the backlash against the anxiolytics. In this climate, the *DSM* diagnosis of MDD was more suitable than any of the various anxiety disorders for capturing the distress of persons seeking help from general physicians and outpatient psychiatrists. Subsequently, MDD gradually replaced anxiety as the diagnosis of choice in these venues.[26]

During the 1980s, this transformation accelerated when research on new drug treatments began to focus on the serotonin system and on the development of SSRIs to increase the amount of serotonin in the brain.[27] These new medications had fewer negative side effects and were safer than the earlier anxiolytics and antidepressants, so they required less monitoring through blood testing. The

SSRIs do not target a specific illness but instead act on a general neurochemical system that influences many brain functions in healthy, as well as ill, patients.[28] They are used to treat a variety of problems, including anxiety, panic, obsessive-compulsive disorder, eating problems, substance abuse, and attention-deficit disorder, as well as depression and general distress in nondisordered people. Moreover, although this issue remains controversial, they appear to influence temperament, unhappiness, and demoralization as well as depressive symptoms.[29]

Given that the FDA requires that a drug must be efficacious against a particular disease before it can be put on the market, the SSRIs could not be called "psychic energizers," "personality boosters," or "distress inhibitors," however accurate these terms might be in describing their effects. They could have easily been marketed as "antianxiety" medications, but when they were approved in the late 1980s they were marketed instead as "antidepressants" because of the negative associations that had developed around the anxiolytics.[30] By 2001, about two and a half times more people were using SSRIs than antianxiety medications, and their use was growing nearly five times as quickly as that of the anxiolytics.[31] The "antidepressant" label provided tremendous impetus for making depression, rather than anxiety, the primary target of pharmaceutical promotions.

In 1993, Peter Kramer's *Listening to Prozac: A Psychiatrist Explores Antidepressant Drugs and the Remaking of the Self* galvanized the formulation of life problems as problems of depression and their treatment with "antidepressant" medications. Kramer himself observed that the SSRIs work across a variety of conditions. "The same medications," he concludes, "are effective against panic anxiety, and they could as appropriately have been called anxiolytics. The term 'antidepressant' encourages us to attend arbitrarily to one use to which these drugs can be put."[32] Nevertheless, his use of the term *antidepressants* to characterize the SSRIs and his book's focus on depression helped associate both the drugs and the condition that they treat specifically with depression.

Kramer's book also helped create a mythic status for Prozac (his generic term for the SSRIs) by asserting that it not only alleviated particular symptoms but also influenced normal as well as disordered feelings and thus made people "better than well." For Kramer, the SSRIs had distinctly different effects from the earlier drugs such as Miltown, Valium, and Librium that were used to deal with life problems. Whereas these drugs relaxed and tranquilized people, drugs such as Prozac energized them and boosted their self-esteem. They did not so much blunt negative emotional responses to the world as act as agents of personality enhancement. Formerly depressed people became more energetic, outgoing, extroverted, and flexible. Prozac, for Kramer, seemed to transform personal identity more than to treat a disease.

What followed Kramer's wildly successful book was, in the historian Edward Shorter's words, "a media psychocircus of suggestion, as Prozac and its competitors were extended to the world public as a panacea for coping with life's problems even in the absence of psychiatric illness."[33] Reflecting the initial enthusiasm for Miltown and, then, Librium and Valium, the new drugs were regarded uncritically and were overvalued. The use of antidepressant drugs, specifically the SSRIs, soared while that of the antianxiety drugs plunged.[34] By 1994, Prozac had become the second best-selling drug in the world, followed closely by its siblings Paxil and Zoloft. Although Kramer and many others asserted that people took Prozac and related drugs to enhance their lives, only anecdotal support indicates that these drugs make people "better than well."[35] Actually, the great preponderance of evidence indicates that they are no more effective than older antidepressants; they are simply better tolerated, their side effects are more benign, and they lack the addictive nature and potential lethality of the antianxiety medications.[36] Moreover, the evidence remains uncertain regarding the degree to which they influence normal sadness. Whatever their true efficacy, the SSRIs entered the culture as the newest "wonder drugs" and were promoted with the promise not only of alleviating depression and attendant ills but also of enhancing the lives of their many potential users.

The Impact of Managed Care

The earlier antianxiety drugs were rarely promoted as stand-alone treatments but instead as adjuncts to psychotherapy and counseling.[37] The SSRIs, however, entered a very different organizational environment. By the 1990s, managed care rose to become a dominant mode of providing mental health treatment in both general medicine and psychiatry, and it is now a powerful social force promoting the use of medications to treat depression and other mental conditions. Managed care approaches, although diverse, generally rely on strategies that reduce health care expenditures by underwriting the least expensive possible treatments.[38]

Managed care also encourages the use of general physicians, who almost always prescribe medication, instead of mental health specialists who may be more likely to use alternatives. As a result, general physicians have increasingly supplanted psychiatrists as the primary source of prescriptions for antidepressant drugs.[39] Because medication therapy takes considerably less practitioner and patient time than most psychotherapy, it is more amenable to the cost/benefit logic of managed care organizations.[40] Most managed care plans, therefore, provide more generous benefits for pharmaceutical than for psychotherapeutic treatments and usually place no barriers on SSRI use.[41] Conversely, these plans usually place severe limits on payment for psychotherapies, which they view as less necessary and more wasteful than medication. Medication thus involves lower out-of-pocket costs for patients than psychotherapy does, which also influences patients themselves to prefer drug treatments.[42]

Under the pressures of managed care, "visits in office-based psychiatry became shorter, less often included psychotherapy, and more often included a medication prescription. The proportion of visits that were 10 minutes or less in length increased."[43] Indeed, unlike earlier drugs, the SSRIs are more rarely used in conjunction with other, more expensive forms of therapy and are likely to be the sole source of treatment. At the same time as the number of people treated for depression with medication is growing explosively, the proportion who get psychotherapy is gradually declining.[44] For example, by 1998 two-thirds of elderly persons treated for depression received only an antidepressant, whereas a little more than 10% obtained only psychotherapy.[45] Payment for long-term psychotherapy has almost disappeared.[46] In sum, managed care organizations have increasingly become the arbiters of appropriate and inappropriate treatments, reinforcing the ascendancy of medication as a response to emotional difficulties.[47]

The Impact of Direct-to-Consumer Advertisements

A further step in the expanding use of SSRIs came in 1997 when the FDA approved the use of direct-to-consumer (DTC) drug advertisements in popular media. DTC ads fundamentally changed patterns of information flow about drugs. In the past, pharmaceutical companies marketed their products directly to physicians, through advertisements that appeared only in medical and psychiatric journals. These ads asked their target audience of physicians and psychiatrists to identify problems in their patients, whereas DTC ads appeal directly to consumers themselves to self-identify symptoms of a given condition and "ask their doctors" about taking antidepressants and other medications. "By the end of the twentieth century," Edward Shorter notes, "these drugs had acquired such currency that, much as in the eighteenth century, patients began to view physicians as mere conduits to fabled new products rather than as counselors capable of using the doctor-patient relationship itself therapeutically."[48] By 2000, the pharmaceutical industry was spending over $2 billion annually on DTC advertisements.[49]

Given regulations restricting the marketing of drugs to the treatment of diseases rather than of everyday life problems and the consequent need to present simple but inclusive descriptions of disease entities to the general public, the DSM definition of MDD could hardly have been better suited for the purposes of DTC advertisements. Pharmaceutical companies could legitimately claim that they are conforming to the FDA regulations when they alert the public to the fact that "sadness," "fatigue," "sleeplessness," and the like are potential symptoms of a disease.

DTC ads, in fact, exploit the DSM's lack of contextual constraints by typically portraying people who have DSM symptoms yet who appear to be suffering not necessarily from mental disorders but from symptoms commonly associated with problems in relating to intimates, with difficulties in the workplace, or with challenges in accomplishing valued goals. For example, an ad for Paxil features a woman on one side and her husband and son on the other side, with a list of symptoms drawn from the MDD diagnosis separating the two sides. The ad implies that symptoms of depression are the cause, rather than the result, of the family's problems. Other ads portray people who are already taking antidepressants and have fulfilling interactions with families, friends, and workmates as a result. Moreover, they present generic models of attractive women (and, occasionally, men) that are designed to appeal to the broadest possible audience. The images of the DTC ads unambiguously, although implicitly, show how drugs are used to regulate normality, as well as disease.

DTC ads, therefore, capitalize on the symptom-based definition of depression to thoroughly blur the boundary between normal sadness and depressive disorder. Pharmaceutical companies can hardly be faulted for trying to sell their products to the greatest possible number of people. The DSM definition of depression supplies them with the perfect vehicle for creating a large demand for the SSRIs. The formulation of common symptoms as illnesses provides both a legitimate way for people to obtain prescriptions and a legal way for companies to advertise their products.

DTC advertisements have the additional consequence of circumventing the psychiatric profession. They urge consumers to "consult your doctor," not explicitly a mental health professional. As a result, the major growth in prescriptions for antidepressants has occurred within the primary medical care sector, not in the specialty mental health care sector.[50] The percentage of emotional disorders treated in the general medical sector grew from about one-third in 1990–1992 to about one-half in 2001–2003, an absolute increase of more than 150%.[51] "The increased rate of treatment," according to epidemiologist Ronald Kessler and colleagues, "may have been due to aggressive, direct-to-consumer marketing of new psychotropic medications."[52] General medicine, not specialty mental health services, is now the major arena for the treatment of emotional distress.

Three-quarters of the visits to ambulatory care for mental health or substance abuse problems now result in a prescription, usually for an SSRI, and often without any other type of treatment. Some evidence indicates that DTC ads are responsible for part of this increased use of antidepressants: rising rates of prescriptions for antidepressants follow periods of increased spending on DTC ads.[53] Moreover, research confirms that when patients mention to their doctors specific drugs they have seen advertised, the doctor is much more likely to prescribe that medication.[54] It is not clear whether people actually define and experience their emotions of sadness as depressive disorders or are simply taking advantage of the opportunity to obtain legal medications to regulate their emotions. There is no question, however, that DTC advertisements have become a major conduit by which pharmaceutical companies use the DSM criteria to reshape the way that many people frame and interpret their emotions of sadness.

The Triumph of Big Pharma

The result of the emergence of the SSRIs, of their use within the context of managed care, of their promotion via DTC ads, and of their greater safety with respect to overdosing and lesser side effects is their exponential growth in use since their initial marketing in the late 1980s. Persons treated for depression were four and a half times more likely to have received a psychotropic medication in 1997 than in 1987.[55] This trend substantially expanded during the mid-1990s. The number of people using SSRIs and other newer antidepressants almost doubled, from 7.9 million in 1996 to 15.4 million in 2001.[56] Especially notable is their rising use for children, adolescents, and the elderly, for whom prescription rates increased by between 200 and 300% during the 1990s.[57] Between 1996 and 2001, overall spending on antidepressants rose from $3.4 billion to $7.9 billion.[58] By 2000, Prozac, Zoloft, and Paxil were all among the eight most prescribed drugs of any sort, and the antidepressants were the best-selling category of drugs in the United States.[59] Nevertheless, it is worth noting that a considerable segment of the public still resists using drugs for life problems; 64% of respondents in a national survey in 1998 said they were unlikely to take psychiatric medication in response to troubles in personal life, and even when the question was framed in terms of treating specific symptoms that result from life problems ("feeling depressed, tired, having trouble sleeping and concentrating, and feelings of worthlessness"), 45% still said they were unlikely to take medication.[60]

That said, the influence of the pharmaceutical industry is considerable and now extends well beyond the specific promotion of drugs. It donates substantial amounts of money to patient and family advocacy groups that promote the view that depression is a chemical deficiency to be remedied through the use of drugs. These companies also sponsor widespread educational campaigns, such as National Depression Awareness Day, which offer free screening for depression in universities and hospitals. In addition, they provide 800 numbers and Internet screening sites that allow responders to make self-diagnoses of depression and that urge them to consult their physicians to obtain prescriptions for the companies' products. Drug companies also fund the screening efforts in primary medical care and schools that were the subject of chapter 6. Moreover, the pharmaceutical industry sponsors a considerable proportion of clinical research on depression; the discipline of psychiatry itself is now thoroughly enmeshed with the corporate culture of this industry.[61] Industry-academic collaborations are becoming increasing sources of funding for universities, academic medical centers, and hospitals.[62] The *DSM's* easily applied symptom-based definition facilitates these efforts, and they, in turn, reinforce the validity of the definition.

The use of pharmaceuticals to deal with everyday life problems preceded the *DSM-III.* In many ways, the legal drug culture surrounding the SSRIs continues the craze for Miltown in the 1950s and for Valium and Librium in the 1960s and 1970s. Yet never before has this culture been so heavily promoted through the mass media, embedded in central institutions, and embraced by policy makers. Previously, establishment psychiatrists and government officials were often openly critical of the overprescribing of these medications and, in particular, of their use for coping with problems of living. Now, however, the legitimacy that the *DSM* concept of depression accords to the widespread treatment of common symptoms of normal malaise has become so entrenched that these groups have come to accept a definition of depressive disorder that encompasses much normal sadness and to endorse the use of antidepressant medications to deal with such conditions.

As happened with the antianxiety medications in the 1970s, a backlash is now developing against the expanding use of antidepressants, especially for children and adolescents.[63] Drug companies now face stiffer requirements to disclose potentially harmful side effects and possible risks of suicidality from their products. Moreover, as during the 1970s, the media have grown more skeptical of the claims of limited risks and vast benefits from antidepressant medications. What impact this more critical climate will have on the actual use of these drugs remains to be seen.

Antidepressants and the Treatment of Normal Sadness

The relationship between *DSM* diagnosis and medication is complicated by the fact that antidepressant medications, and the SSRIs in particular, affect general aspects of brain functioning and, as noted, may be capable of having similar effects on both normal sadness and depressive disorder. The few studies that compare the changes that SSRIs produce in presumably healthy people with the changes experienced by those diagnosed with a depressive disorder find that the SSRIs work on the disordered and nondisordered alike.[64] Thus the psychic relief that results from medication does not necessarily indicate that what has been relieved is a disease condition. For example, grieving people who are not disordered report fewer symptoms after treatment with antidepressants.[65]

Few would argue that medication has no role in the response to depressive disorders; medications can dramatically alleviate the hopelessness that accompanies MDD, and they helped to facilitate the process of deinstitutionalization in the mental health system that allows many people to avoid extended periods of hospitalization. A more controversial question regards the use of medication for painful but normal emotions. The SSRIs raise serotonin levels in the synapses, so it is plausible that unhappiness and mood disorder alike often respond to them. "We are entering," as Peter Kramer claims, "an era in which medication can be used to enhance the functioning of the normal mind."[66] Assuming that the findings that SSRIs can influence normal emotions are confirmed, should these drugs be prescribed for people who experience normal misery, as well as for those with MDD? Legitimate arguments exist on both sides of this issue.

One position, embodied in official treatment guidelines, evidence-based medicine, and government position papers, regards medication treatment in unambiguously positive terms. The Surgeon General's Report on Mental Health, for example, claims that "antidepressant medications are effective across the full range of severity of major depressive episodes in major depressive disorder and bipolar disorder."[67] Moreover, a vast majority of U.S. psychiatrists favor using SSRIs as the first-line treatment for depression.[68] In this view, drug treatment has proven effectiveness for the relief of depressive symptoms, albeit with small risks of negative side effects and other undesirable consequences. Moreover, the monetary benefits of such treatment are viewed as far exceeding its costs.[69] In addition, drugs are viewed as capable of preventing mild conditions from becoming more severe. Mild disorders thus ought to be treated as vigorously as more severe ones, it is claimed, not just to prevent a substantial proportion of future serious cases but also to limit future outcomes such as hospitalization, work disability, and suicide attempts.[70]

Advocates of medications worry about the underuse of the antidepressants and try to find ways to motivate people to seek and use them. They want to encourage people to recognize that they have treatable illnesses, to seek medical care for their conditions, and to overcome the perceived stigma about taking medication.[71] Moreover, they are concerned that not only the public but also general physicians underrecognize depression and, therefore, underprescribe antidepressant medications.[72] For advocates, increasing awareness of and education about the benefits of psychotropic drugs can optimize the treatment of depression. Opposition to using medication reflects, in psychiatrist Gerald Klerman's term, "pharmacological Calvinism" that considers any drug that makes people feel good as something bad:

> Psychotherapeutically, the world is divided into the first class citizens, the saints who can achieve their cure or salvation by willpower, insight, psychoanalysis or by behavior modification, and the rest of the people, who are weak in their moral fiber and need a crutch, whether it is Thorazine, Miltown, or Compoz.[73]

What Klerman calls the "Calvinist" view of psychotropic medication leads a substantial proportion of the public to resist taking drugs because they associate their use with a moral weakness, despite the benefits they might receive from taking them.

Most advocates, following the *DSM*, simply assume that the conditions that drugs treat are depressive disorders and not normal sadness. Their position regarding the use of medication to treat normal sadness is, therefore, not explicit. Some advocates, however, are quite clear that drugs should be used to treat any form of suffering.[74] The pain arising from, for instance, the death of an intimate, the breakup of a romantic relationship, or the loss of a job is just as real as that stemming from a depressive disorder. The position of these advocates is that there is simply no good reason why people should tolerate the psychic pain from normal sadness as long as safe and effective means are available to palliate it. After all, few people would not want women to be able to use anesthesia to numb the normal pain that stems from childbirth. Advocates argue that if people think that SSRIs can brighten their lives, provide greater control over their emotions, and increase their self-esteem, as well as relieve the inevitable pain that arises from human existence, they should be able to use them, even in the absence of any disorder. The relief of suffering, in this view, is a greater value than any costs that might accrue from medicating normal sadness.

Challenges to this pro-medication position generally come from outside of the psychiatric profession, the clinical research community, and government agencies. One argument against medicating normal sadness is that it treats as pathological what is actually an inherent and valuable part of the human condition. For thousands of years, people have used religion, spirituality, and philosophy to understand how their unhappiness is tied into larger questions about life.[75] Such questioning allows people to comprehend how their emotions are related to basic aspects of human existence and to gain a deeper appreciation of their feelings than palliation through medication can provide. "At least part of the nagging worry about Prozac and its ilk," philosopher Carl Elliott laments, "is that for all the good they do, the ills that they treat are part and parcel of the lonely, forgetful, unbearably sad place where we live."[76] Using pills represents an escape from truly confronting life's problems. Quite aside from philosophical issues, there may be psychological benefits of normal sadness that treatment would nullify. We do not as yet fully understand why we are biologically designed to experience sadness in response to loss, and, until we do, it is possible that there are benefits of withdrawing into a sad state after a major loss that are not immediately apparent but that are nonetheless real and important to long-term psychological functioning.

Another argument, echoing criticisms made in the 1950s and 1960s, emphasizes that widespread antidepressant use leads people to accept, rather than resist, oppressive situations. From this perspective, psychotropic drug use promotes a view of the world that erroneously misconstrues social problems as personal problems. Prescribing a pill communicates that public issues—inegalitarian marriages, deplorable working conditions, inadequate finances, and the like—are private concerns of the individual to be treated with medication.[77] "Diseasing" normal sadness that arises over these concerns implies that medication is the appropriate way to deal with them, at the cost of ignoring other possible remedies. This process deflects attention away from developing policies that might change the conditions that give rise to sadness.[78] Indeed, in 1958, the Surgeon General, L. E. Burney, warned that "problems of daily living" cannot be "solved with a pill,"[79] a far cry from the attitude of recent surgeon generals.

Others raise the issue of whether normal emotions of sadness are a legitimate subject for public concern or, instead, a personal matter. The promotion of antidepressants sets forth a view of the self that is feeble and fragile and that requires the continuous intervention and protection of professional experts.[80] Private selves become increasingly available for public scrutiny and regulation through screening and subsequent medication. The detection of emotions and feelings is inevitably far more intrusive and coercive than is the detection of physical diseases that usually do require expert help.

Other critics do not question the political and cultural implications of antidepressant drugs so much as their effectiveness and safety. They contest the benign nature of the antidepressants and contend that the side effects of these medications, such as loss of sexual desire, nausea, diarrhea, and headaches, are more common and malignant than their advocates claim.[81] They also cite the heightened potential for suicidality, especially for young people during the initial stages of taking these drugs, although evidence for this claim is not well established.[82] Finally, they point to the potential for adverse effects from the long-term use of these medications. Although there is little doubt that the newer antidepressants are safer than their predecessors, there is still reason for concern over their widespread use.

Moreover, critics claim that advocates have grossly overinflated the effectiveness of these medications. Current guidelines promote the SSRIs as the first-line medications for moderate to severe depression.[83] The evidence, however, that antidepressant medications are more effective than placebo, as judged by randomized, double-blind placebo trials, is mixed. "Although many trials," one research team summarizes, "do find antidepressants are superior to placebo, many do not, including some of the largest and most well known landmark trials such as the Medical Research Council trial and the early National Institute for Mental Health trial."[84] A comprehensive review by the National Institute for Health and Clinical Excellence (NICE) in England suggests that SSRIs do not have clinically meaningful advantages over placebos across the entire range of severity of conditions. A report on this study concludes: "Given doubts about their benefits and concern about their risks, current recommendations for prescribing antidepressants should be reconsidered."[85] The evidence lends little support to the enthusiasm for prescribing medications.

Still less evidence exists for the effectiveness of antidepressants in treating nonpsychotic conditions that are not especially intense (sometimes called "mild" depression), many of which are undoubtedly cases of normal sadness. Even the fervor for antidepressant medication in the Surgeon General's report is somewhat mitigated for these cases. "With mild depressive episodes," the report concludes, "the overall response rate is about 70 percent, including a placebo rate of about 60 percent."[86] The effectiveness of antidepressants for mild conditions, in other words, exceeds that of placebos by only 10%. Indeed, from half to two-thirds of patients with mild depression improve with placebo alone. This might indicate that what was treated in the first place was not a disorder but normal sadness that naturally remits over time or through such ordinary interventions as interacting with and receiving the emotional support of others. Even some of the most vigorous advocates for treating mild cases of depression conclude: "Controlled treatment trials have provided no evidence that pharmacotherapy significantly improves mild disorders."[87] When compared with control groups who receive active placebos that mimic some of the side effects from antidepressants, no differences between antidepressants and placebos emerge.[88]

The evidence regarding the effectiveness of antidepressant medications, especially for mild depression, is thus ambiguous. Still, given their popularity, it is difficult to believe that the effectiveness of antidepressants is as limited and their negative side effects are as great as the critics claim. Many people find that antidepressants provide legal and generally safe ways to regulate their distressing emotions. Moreover, the results of clinical trials can be misleading. In practice, consumers and their physicians often try out several different drugs before one finally works.[89] In contrast, clinical trials might minimize the overall rate of effectiveness because they deal with one particular type of medication, which might not be effective for particular individuals in the trial although another, untested type might be. Indeed, recent multidrug trials designed to address this issue do seem to achieve higher rates of improvement.[90] So the fact that medication has little more effectiveness than placebos is perhaps less of a decisive criticism than is often believed. It is, however, difficult to find any compelling reasons why public policy ought to *encourage* the use of drugs to treat mild conditions, many of which are likely to be cases of normal sadness.

It is not easy to sort out the competing claims regarding antidepressant use. All of the considerations on both sides of the debate seem to have some merit, and there is no one general answer to the question of whether psychotropic medication should be prescribed for normal, negative emotions. Ultimately, consumers themselves have to integrate all these considerations and be the judges of whether they ought to use antidepressant medications to regulate their moods. Over the past few decades, the public's judgment has certainly swung in the direction of medication; tolerance for normal but painful emotions has declined, and many people in the modern world have come to value medication as a way to control their feelings.[91] If they find that their lives seem brighter when they are medicated, a belief in autonomy and free choice dictates that people should not be prevented from seeking that relief from a responsible physician. It should also not be forgotten that DTC ads do get many truly depressed people to seek help and to receive useful medications from their physicians.[92] The issue to keep in mind, we have argued, is that diagnosis should not be invalidly shaped to indicate disorder so as to bias such decisions.

Conclusion

Given how many issues regarding the appropriate role of antidepressant medication remain unresolved, the wisest course would involve caution and the avoidance of sweeping statements advocating or condemning their use. In the past, governmental officials were concerned about the possible dangers and overuse of psychotropic medications, as well as with the pharmaceutical industry's efforts at encouraging ever-wider segments of the population to take them. Numerous congressional hearings questioned the promotion of pharmaceuticals, especially for problems in living. In a vast turnabout, symptom-based diagnostic criteria now easily reconceptualize the "stresses of everyday living" as indications of disease. Surely, there is a sensible middle course.

What, for example, might the consequences be for DTC advertising if the criteria for Major Depression in the *DSM* were changed to more adequately distinguish normal sadness and depressive disorder? By way of comparison, in the 1960s the pharmaceutical company Sandoz marketed a new tranquilizer, Serentil, using an ad that explicitly promoted its use for general problems of living: "The newcomer in town who *can't* make friends. The organization man who *can't* adjust to altered status within his company. The woman who *can't* get along with her new daughter-in-law. The executive who *can't* accept retirement." The FDA forced Sandoz to withdraw the ad and publish a correction stating that it did not intend that Serentil be used for "everyday anxiety situations encountered in the normal course of living" but only for "certain disease states."[93] If the *DSM* were to create more restrictive standards for MDD, DTC advertisements for antidepressants would have to follow these criteria. The result would be to at least marginally lessen the appeal of drug use for normal life problems, if in fact that is a desirable goal.

But the sorts of debates that took place before 1980 regarding the wisdom of medicating normal distress have largely disappeared from psychiatry, although similar discussions continue in general medicine (e.g., whether normally short individuals should be administered growth hormones).[94] Instead, discussions more narrowly focus on issues of effectiveness, side effects, or whether alternative therapies to medication would be more desirable. This lack of discussion seems to be due to the fact that, when conditions are predefined as diseases, the consideration of what treatment is most appropriate is already skewed by the assumption that something is wrong within the individual. The question of whether interfering with normal mechanisms should be subject to a higher threshold than correcting dysfunctional mechanisms is defined out of existence, and medical thinking becomes correspondingly less nuanced.

Our analysis suggests the need for greater conceptual clarity by the diagnosing professional and for more fully informed consent by the patient. A fundamental part of informed consent is receiving an accurate diagnosis to the degree possible, and there is no more basic diagnostic distinction than that between a disorder and a normal emotional state in response to life circumstances that is likely to remit over time without intervention. Prognosis and decisions about the appropriateness of possible treatments depend on this distinction, and it is important for the professional to share this information with the patient in deciding on an informed course of action.

10

The Failure of the Social Sciences to Distinguish Sadness From Depressive Disorder

The field of psychiatry does not exist in a vacuum; it depends on other disciplines for much of the intellectual underpinnings of its clinical theory. One might thus expect that disciplines such as anthropology and sociology should be in good positions to help correct the confusion in psychiatric nosology about the distinction between depressive disorder and normal intense sadness. Anthropologists could identify universal emotional mechanisms that are part of human nature and elaborate the cultural variations in their expression, and they could pinpoint when these normal variations lead to mistaken labeling of disorder. Sociologists could demonstrate how stressful social arrangements often produce nondisordered sadness, which can sometimes be severe enough to meet *DSM* criteria, and could distinguish between the study of normal emotional responses to social stress and the study of mental disorder.

In fact, however, rather than offering the grounds for a critique of psychiatry's conflation of normal sadness and disorder, these disciplines have functioned as "enablers" of psychiatry's overinclusive definitions of disorder by themselves failing to draw the appropriate distinctions within their disciplinary domains. Anthropologists focus on the presumed cultural relativity of definitions of sadness and disorder, claiming that no definitions of these conditions are possible outside of each culture's particular value system. Sociologists interchangeably use concepts of distress and disorder without separating the two. This chapter examines how the failure of these disciplines to adequately distinguish ordinary sadness from depressive disorder has not only abandoned psychiatry to its conceptual challenges but has also caused these disciplines to descend into confusion in their own research.

Anthropology

The Role of Universal Concepts

As chapter 2 argued, both cultural values and the universal functional design of loss response mechanisms must enter into good definitions of normal sadness and depressive disorders. General experiences of loss, such as humiliating declines in social status, loss of valued attachments, and inability to achieve social goals, are universal. And the emotion of sadness and some of its associated symptoms, although subject to variation in their expressions, are also universal across cultures. But loss response mechanisms are programmed to react according to culturally defined ideas of status, valued attachments, or worthy goals, so distinctions between normal and disordered loss responses must take into account cultural systems of meaning. Culture also influences how people learn to express sadness and depression in appropriate ways.

Anthropologists are well positioned to study which aspects of loss responses are culturally influenced and which belong to the domain of human species-typical functioning. But instead they have helped perpetuate psychiatry's confusion by denying that a cogent distinction between normal and dysfunctional loss responses rooted in natural selection is even possible. This denial is to some extent an expression of an enduring resistance in anthropology to the very notion that there is a "human nature," because Eurocentric notions of normality have been used for oppressive purposes in the past to classify non-Western societies as inferior. But it is also an expression of a confused postmodernist perspective that regards more or less everything human as thoroughly culturally determined.

Anthropologists who study depression generally claim that the distinction between normality and disorder depends entirely on the value systems of particular cultural groups. Ruth Benedict's classic article, "Anthropology and the Abnormal," set the agenda for anthropological research about depression and other mental disorders, emphasizing that all definitions of normality and pathology derive from local concepts that cannot be generalized across cultures.[1] What some cultures view as disordered depression, Benedict argued, others view as normal sadness. For example, the Zuni of Arizona regard states of extreme passivity and fatalism, which Western psychiatrists might diagnose as Major Depression, as normal and even admirable expressions of a culturally defined personality style. For Benedict, all universal concepts of disorder and normality stem from ethnocentric Western norms that do not accurately reflect the indigenous behaviors to which they are applied. Instead, she claimed, local cultural definitions constitute what is normal or pathological in each society.

There are several weaknesses in Benedict's argument. It seems plain that the Zuni conditions she describes are indeed largely normal conditions that are rooted in philosophical attitudes and personality tendencies that the culture's meaning system shapes. Western psychiatrists who diagnosed these conditions as mentally disordered would be wrong. But Benedict did not carefully distinguish these salient conditions from other, less culturally explainable conditions that the Zuni themselves would consider to be true disorders. It is entirely possible for a condition in one culture to be considered normal but for a superficially similar condition in another culture to be considered disordered. This can occur if, in the first case, the condition arises from normal cultural shaping of meaning and expressive systems, whereas, in the other case, it is a product of a dysfunction in loss response mechanisms. For example, the appearance of extreme and chronic lack of pleasure that could be normal among the Zuni because of their cultural socialization could well indicate a depressive disorder in members of modern Western cultural groups that have experienced different socialization that would not normally lead to such feelings. But the fact that cultural norms must be taken into account in determining the normality-disorder distinction does not mean that such norms fully constitute this distinction because they are only one factor that shapes normal variation.

Benedict's assumptions persist as the central tenets of the *new cross-cultural psychiatry* that has dominated anthropological studies of mental illness since the 1970s. Centered around the work of Harvard anthropologist and psychiatrist Arthur Kleinman, this school has produced a great deal of insightful and detailed research about the culturally-specific aspects of depression, and it has developed cogent critiques of psychiatry's tendency to exaggerate the universal nature of depression. In particular, Kleinman's own careful cross-cultural scholarship, with its eloquent and illuminating rendering of the social and personal meanings behind patients' behaviors, has reshaped the understanding and study of cross-cultural psychiatry. Yet, in reacting against ethnocentrism, anthropologists working within Kleinman's paradigm have gone too far in the other direction by emphasizing cultural variability to the excessive exclusion of common, worldwide features of depression. This has consequently raised challenging conceptual questions about their entire approach. Many anthropologists refuse to use any distinction that is grounded in biological functioning, which is constant across cultures, to explain the huge differences in definitions and manifestations of depression in different societies.[2] Psychological functions such as thought, language, perception, and mood, they claim, stem much more from culture than from biology. Psychological systems, according to anthropologist Laurence Kirmayer, "are so malleable that they can be for almost anything. . . . Beyond a few relatively simple physiological functions, it is impossible to identify what psychological systems or functions are for in any universal sense."[3]

Anthropologists of depression thus emphasize cultural uniqueness. Culture refers to customs, symbols, beliefs, values, and norms that individuals within a group share but that are different among individuals in different groups. For anthropologists, such varying cultural rules *constitute* concepts of normality and pathology, making a universal definition of normal sadness or depressive disorder that is anchored in human nature impossible. Disorder, according to this view, just consists of whatever a culture defines as deviant or negative behavior. Assertions of common human standards of psychological functioning actually impose ethnocentric Western categories about appropriate or inappropriate behavior onto other cultures.[4] Claims about the natural functioning of sadness as an emotion and as a loss response mechanism, for example, involve taking cultural categories that Western psychiatrists and Western culture create and superimposing them on the products of another culture's definitions, rules, and expressions in which the Western categories do not apply.[5]

The anthropologist Gananeth Obeyesekere, for example, claims that Buddhists in Sri Lanka view symptoms of hopelessness, meaninglessness, and sorrow as part of a culturally recognized philosophy of life, not as an illness.[6] He asserts that Buddhists respond to loss by generalizing their despair from themselves to the world at large so that sadness takes on nonpathological meaning from Buddhist worldviews. Such extreme cultural variability in definitions of depression indicates, according to Obeyesekere, that it cannot be a universal disease category. What is considered to be depression must be described and analyzed within the terms of each particular cultural group.

The Sri Lankan Buddhists whom Obeyesekere describes certainly do not have depressive disorders, although they might meet DSM criteria for Major Depression. He is clearly talking about normal sadness, because the symptoms he describes develop and persist only as a function of the situation of loss and of philosophical views of life. Obeyesekere does not discuss cases of chronic deep sadness that arise for no philosophical or loss-event reason, which might properly be classified as a disorder. He offers no evidence that Sri Lankans themselves would not consider such conditions as disordered. Indeed, the history of Western accounts of depressive disorder is filled with disclaimers, similar to Obeyesekere's, that there are forms of philosophical depression, much like those the Sri Lankans cherish, that are not true disorders. The problem that Obeyesekere detects in trying to impose DSM criteria on Buddhist culture is not the imposition of invalid Western categories on a culture to which they do not apply. Rather, he detects the fact that the DSM definition of depressive disorder is invalid according to both Western and Buddhist views and that there is general agreement that proportionate reactions to loss or philosophical dispositions should not be labeled as depressive disorders. Western and Sri Lankan conceptualizations only *seem* to differ because of errors in the DSM's formulation of the Western view.

Instead of examining his data through the lens of a proper distinction between disorder and nondisorder, Obeyesekere uses the Sri Lankan example to deny the possibility of making *any* universal statements about the nature of mental disorder: "The *conception* of the disease (i.e., illness) *is* the disease. Or to put it differently, there are only illnesses and no diseases."[7] Here, *illness* is supposed to refer to culturally bound definitions of who is placed in the sick role, whereas *disease* is the notion of an objective pathology and the claim is that disease is nothing more than illness. But Obeyesekere's data show nothing of the sort; rather, they show that different cultures correctly recognize that sadness responses are normal, the *DSM*'s problems notwithstanding.

Catherine Lutz's work among the Ifaluk of Micronesia is another well-known anthropological study of depression. Lutz regards the concept of depression as a "specifically Western cultural category" and contrasts Ifaluk responses to loss with those found in Western medicine. She finds that Ifaluk whose intimates die or leave the island develop sadness that involves "excessive thinking/feeling about the missed person, loss of the desire to eat or engage in conversation or other activities, and sleepiness."[8] Lutz goes on to contrast Ifaluk symptoms with the presumably intrapsychic conditions that Western psychiatry features:

> These various interpretations for situations of loss all point to people as the primary object to which one can be attached and from which one can be separated. Unfocused or objectless loss responses are not spoken of, as far as I know. All [these] emotions are considered normal states.[9]

She concludes, "the cross-cultural investigation of depression might be replaced by the examination of indigenous definitions of situations of loss and the blocking of goals, and the social organization of responses to them."[10]

Lutz provides an excellent description of normal sadness among the Ifaluk. Her critique ought to focus on the overexpansive definitions of depressive disorder in Western psychiatry, which might mistakenly classify these responses as dysfunctions. Instead, like Obeyesekere, she uses her work to critique the possibility of using universal definitions and to advocate the study of purely local concepts. In fact, her analysis shows how the Ifaluk make the same sorts of distinctions between normal sadness and depressive disorder that people in many times and places typically do. She then uses the fact that the *DSM* has mistakenly abandoned such standards in its symptom-based emphasis to argue that Western medicine classifies as disorders conditions that the Ifaluk would not. But it is likely that if the same ethnographic methods were used in Western cultures to compare the opinions of ordinary people across cultures, Westerners would agree that the conditions Lutz describes are not disorders. Lutz's work shows not that universally applicable distinctions are impossible but that the relationship between loss and normal sadness has a universal element that current Western psychiatric definitions do not adequately capture.

Arthur Kleinman himself has conducted the best-known and most pathbreaking studies of cultural differences in the expression of depression. At times, Kleinman adopts the extreme position that depression "is a cultural category constructed by psychiatrists in the West to yield a homogeneous group of patients."[11] In some of his writings he regards Western psychiatric categories as examples of a category fallacy that mistakes culture-bound diagnoses for universal features of illness. In fact, Kleinman asserts that there are no culture-free entities but only culturally specific modes of explanation.[12]

More commonly, however, Kleinman makes a distinction between *disease* and *illness*.[13] For him, *disease* refers to abnormal physiological states that are aspects of the natural world. *Illness* refers to the actual lived experience of disease and encompasses the perceptions, interpretations, coping responses, and presentations that people give to various disease states. Diseases are universal somatic sensations; in contrast, cultural norms and meanings fundamentally shape illness, and so it varies widely in different social groups.

Through extensive observation and interviews in China, Kleinman concludes that the physiological symptoms that Chinese use to express depression are fundamentally different from the psychological presentations that Westerners make. Among Chinese patients, the major feature of depression lies in its physiological emphasis and corresponding lack of psychological symptoms. They present somatic complaints but, unlike Westerners, usually do not report feeling depressed. Furthermore, Chinese patients view their illnesses as physiological and reject the idea that they have any sort of mental disorder. Kleinman links the focus on physical symptoms and the denial of psychological symptoms to the values of Chinese culture. Chinese norms discourage verbal expression of intimate personal emotions and emphasize the fulfillment of social roles and interpersonal relationships. Expressions of feelings such as loneliness and sadness lead to stigma and embarrassment and indicate excessive self-absorption. In contrast, Chinese culture encourages expressions of physical complaints. Kleinman's studies lead him to assert that the central anthropological focus must be on illness rather than on disease:

> Depression experienced entirely as low back pain and depression experienced entirely as guilt-ridden existential despair are such substantially different forms of illness behaviour with different symptoms, patterns of help-seeking, course and treatment responses that though the disease in each instance may be the same, the illness rather than the disease is the determinant factor.[14]

In principle, we agree with Kleinman's distinction between disease as a universal underlying dysfunction and illness as the culturally shaped expression of a given dysfunction. The difficulties with his argument arise because he places almost exclusive emphasis on the "illness" aspect of disorder. There are several problems with such a focus. First, if there are indeed underlying common dysfunctions, then treatment presumably depends in large part on the science of identifying and intervening in such dysfunctions irrespective of their cultural presentation. Second, Kleinman labels various conditions as "depression" in China even as he claims that these conditions have little in common with Western-defined depression. This raises the question of what he sees across cultures that is the same and that thus makes all these conditions instances of the same disorder—depression. It would seem that either the context, such as loss, or some other shared characteristic must be at work to constitute such a concept and to lead Kleinman and others to infer a shared underlying dysfunction, but that assumption already suggests that there is something misleading in his antiuniversalist argument. In fact, every culture recognizes depression in forms that Westerners would recognize.

Third, however one identifies depressive states in general, Kleinman never takes seriously the question of how various cultures distinguish normal from disordered depressive conditions, because this would involve exploring how individuals infer underlying dysfunction that does not solely involve negative cultural presentations. He uses *illness* in a very broad way for unpleasant, subjective, culturally recognized experiences and then defines *disease* as whatever physiological state underlies an illness. This runs together normal negative emotions and disorder, thus obscuring distinctions that every culture makes.

Fourth, oddly for an anthropologist, Kleinman does not clearly distinguish what people are willing to say because it is socially desirable to say it from what people really feel or believe. Some cultural tendencies to publicly hide feelings suggest the possibility that observed differences are only superficial and hide the emotions that people actually experience.[15] This lack of refined distinctions between underlying experiences and their culturally shaped expression leads to the final problem.

Kleinman's central and signature point—that Chinese people experience psychosomatic symptoms of depression and not Western-style emotional symptoms—is questionable. A careful examination of his own data shows that, although his Chinese sample did not spontaneously characterize their depressive experiences by focusing on the same symptoms as Westerners, they in fact reported high rates of *DSM*-style symptoms when they were specifically asked about them. Moreover, subsequent empirical work shows that Chinese and Western samples generally experience much more similar symptoms than Kleinman claimed.[16] Thus his classic finding that Asian populations express their depression through an "idiom of distress" that focuses on somatic complaints rather than on mental *DSM* symptoms seems to be more a finding about how people tend to socially present themselves than about what people actually experience.[17]

To the degree that there remain differences in expression, the somatization of depression may occur because some cultures may not have linguistic terms to describe internal, emotional states, or they may have social norms against perceiving or talking about inner feelings. Moreover, whether or not the *expression* of depression differs across cultures, this research fails to address the fundamental question of whether different expressions of emotions are variants of normal sadness or of depressive disorders.

The Need to Balance Universal
and Cultural Factors

The study of cross-cultural variation in normal and disordered depressive conditions is a fertile field that yields surprising insights into the power of cultural meaning systems to shape human experience. Yet the contemporary focus in medical anthropology on such variation to the exclusion of underlying universal structures that are constraints on such experiences has had problematic consequences. Anthropologists who study depression have generally embraced a relativistic view according to which there is no way to apply a concept of disorder or normality beyond local cultural practices. Consequently, they often take the *DSM* symptom checklist itself as representative of the Western conception of depressive disorder, enabling them to easily demonstrate that other cultures' conception of normality includes conditions that we would place under the category of disorder and thus supporting a position of cultural relativity. Intellectually dominated by relativistic doctrines and fear of cultural ethnocentrism, anthropologists cannot step back and critique the *DSM*'s implicit assumptions about human nature from a perspective that is not itself culturally relative.

It is true that reality can be divided up in many different ways and that categories from one culture must not be imperialistically imposed on another. But it is equally true that no sensible cross-cultural understanding of disorder categories can ignore universals of human nature due to our common evolutionary heritage and the role these universals play in identifying normal and disordered conditions. Even if concepts are socially deployed structures, what the concepts refer to in the world need not be socially constructed. The review in chapter 2 showed the universality of sadness as an emotion and of some of the elements that determine how it is triggered; where universal emotion-generating mechanisms exist, one would also expect that there are some universal kinds of things that could go wrong with those mechanisms. Although culture shapes the particular ways that people express intense and even disordered sadness, *what* is being shaped is a more universal state. Great cultural variance in symptoms is compatible with a universal base around which symptomatic presentations diverge. Moreover, the study of variation in depression cannot adequately proceed without some notion of what is universal. For example, the claim that some cultures express depression through physiological symptoms and others through psychological symptoms depends on some underlying conception of depression that transcends its symptomatic expression.

The refusal to explore universal concepts of disorder and normality also prevents anthropologists from formulating compelling critiques of Western psychiatry. The view that all definitions of normality and pathology are culturally relative means that anthropologists have no definition of normality that transcends any particular diagnostic system and that would show the inadequacy of psychiatric diagnoses within that system. Until anthropologists recognize that proper specifications of what is culturally relative depend on notions of what is universal, they will not be able to develop strong concepts of either normality or disorder or strong theories of the factors that determine cultural expressions of depressive conditions. They thus severely limit their ability to derive substantive lessons from their studies for Western psychiatry or to provide a corrective to the excesses of Western diagnosis. Further development of the notion of "dysfunction" and study of how dysfunction interacts with cultural meanings could offer a welcome realization of the powerful insights from the "new cross-cultural anthropology" for making constructive critiques of psychiatric diagnosis.

Sociology

The Sociology of Stress

Sociologists should be in an excellent position to critique the overly inclusive *DSM* definition of mental disorder and to show the distinctiveness of sadness and depressive disorder. The major goal of the dominant sociological paradigm of mental health, the sociology of stress, is to assess the psychological consequences of stressful social arrangements.[18] To this end, sociologists examine how exposure to stressors, such as acute life events or chronic and persisting negative social conditions, affects health outcomes. The kinds of stressors that sociologists usually study—failing marriages, lost jobs, blocked social mobility, conflicts between work and family obligations, inequitable living conditions, and the like—lead to just the kind of distressed responses that nondisordered people should be expected to have to their social circumstances, although such stressors also can sometimes trigger disorder. Likewise, the natural thrust of sociological work points toward social conditions, rather than individual pathologies, as being the source of symptoms, which should provide a corrective to the psychiatric profession's pervasive medicalization of social problems.

Numerous sociological studies indicate that stressful social arrangements typically lead to distress that both emerges and fluctuates in accordance with social conditions.[19] Indeed, the three major general processes that predict high rates of distress correspond to the low positions in status hierarchies, losses of valued attachments, and the inability to achieve valued goals that chapter 2 indicated are the major sources of normal sadness.[20] Sociological research demonstrates the distressing mental health consequences not only of socioeconomic stratification but also of subordinate positions in familial and interpersonal hierarchies.[21] Low positions in status hierarchies expose people to the kinds of circumstances, such as inadequate financial resources, oppressive work and family conditions, and severe health problems in oneself and others that naturally produce distress. Moreover, research shows that such inferior statuses are far more likely to be the cause than the consequence of normal sadness.[22]

The second major source of distress stems from the loss of intimate attachments. Indeed, the three life events considered most stressful in samples of ordinary Americans are the death of a spouse, divorce, and marital separation.[23] Losses of valued attachments are powerful enough to produce intense distress among huge proportions—generally between one-third and one-half—of people who experience them.[24] Finally, the inability to achieve valued social goals is also associated with elevated levels of distress. Situations in which people cannot disengage from unreachable goals or feel their lives have not turned out in ways that they desire commonly produce nondisordered sadness. Examples are graduate students who cannot find jobs in their academic fields or faculty members who fail to get tenure.[25] Likewise, adults who do not attain goals they set for themselves in earlier stages of life report more distress than those whose attainments match their original aspirations.[26] Women who intensely desire to bear children but who are infertile also experience very high rates of distress.[27]

Studies from the sociology of stress do not just show how inequality, attachment loss, and failure to achieve goals commonly trigger distress; they also indicate that the severity and duration of the loss response are related to the degree of stressfulness found in the conditions of people's lives. The severity of symptoms is a direct function of the number and intensity of the chronic stressors and acute life events that people experience.[28] Likewise, distress persists as a function of the duration of economic and interpersonal stressors.[29] The conclusion is inescapable that the great majority of distress-inducing conditions that sociologists study appear to involve normal distress that arises because of social circumstances and endures roughly as long as those circumstances persist.

One might think that this body of research would sound an alarm about the potential medicalizing of what are really socially induced conditions of normal distress. To the contrary, sociologists have themselves accepted a *DSM*-like symptom-based approach that classifies a broad range of negative emotional reactions as disorders. They have thus supported and even extended the confusions of the *DSM* rather than drawn the necessary distinctions that would possibly correct the situation.

Most prevalence estimates in sociological studies stem from the Center for Epidemiological Studies measure of depression (CES-D), a scale developed during the 1970s to assess depression in community populations.[30] The CES-D contains a series of 20 standardized questions that ask how often a symptom occurred during the previous week. Responses are scored from 0 to 3 on the basis of their frequency over this time frame, and answers are summarized into a total number. The particular questions are:

1. I was bothered by things that usually don't bother me.
2. I did not feel like eating; my appetite was poor.
3. I felt that I could not shake off the blues even with help from my family or friends.

4. I felt that I was just as good as other people (reverse scored).
5. I had trouble keeping my mind on what I was doing.
6. I felt depressed.
7. I felt that everything I did was an effort.
8. I felt hopeful about the future (reverse scored).
9. I thought my life had been a failure.
10. I felt fearful.
11. My sleep was restless.
12. I was happy (reverse scored).
13. I talked less than usual.
14. I felt lonely.
15. People were unfriendly.
16. I enjoyed life (reverse scored).
17. I had crying spells.
18. I felt sad.
19. I felt that people disliked me.
20. I could not get "going."

Total scores are considered to lie on a continuum of pathology that ranges from mild to severe. Especially high scores, usually those of 16 and above, are considered to be probably comparable to treated cases of depression.

The CES-D, like the *DSM*, does not consider the context in which symptoms develop. In other respects, it is far easier to make a diagnosis of depression with the CES-D than with the *DSM*. Whereas the *DSM* requires either the presence of depressed mood or the inability to experience pleasure, the CES-D has no necessary symptom of depression. This means that a score of 16 can be reached in numerous ways, even when people do not have the cardinal markers of a depressed state. More important, the CES-D has far less stringent duration requirements than the *DSM*. The *DSM* requires that all symptoms persist for at least a 2-week period. In contrast, the CES-D gives some positive score when a symptom is present for even a single day over the preceding week. Given its nature, it is not surprising that the CES-D uncovers enormous prevalence rates. For example, more than half of bereaved participants, half of those who had undergone marital separations, and a third who became unemployed have CES-D scores that are considered to be comparable to treated cases of clinical depression.[31]

In addition, about one-third to two-thirds of adolescents report scores that are generally viewed as comparable to cases of clinical depression on the CES-D.[32] Four studies undertaken as part of the Oregon Adolescent Depression Project in the late 1980s found that between 39 and 60% of boys and 56 and 63% of girls met CES-D caseness criteria for clinical depression.[33] Another large study that used measures at two different points in time found that only about a third of adolescents were *not* depressed at either assessment.[34] Even studies that significantly raise CES-D criteria to 24 or higher still find that about 10% of all adolescents are depressed.[35]

The minimal duration requirement means that the CES-D is extraordinarily sensitive to such transitory yet commonly occurring phenomena as failing a test, losing a crucial game in sports, or discovering that a boyfriend or girlfriend is going out with someone else.[36] Indeed, the best predictor of high CES-D scores among adolescents is the breaking up of a romantic relationship, a nearly ubiquitous phenomenon in this age group. People who say they were bothered by things, had trouble concentrating, felt depressed, had restless sleep, were not happy, did not enjoy life, felt sad, and could not shake off the blues would be considered possible "cases" of depressive disorder even if symptoms disappeared a few days after such events took place.

Yet sociologists persistently fail to distinguish whether high scores on symptom scales stem from persons with chronic and recurrent conditions that fluctuate independently of social conditions or from those with transitory and situationally induced distress. Typical sociological articles interchangeably use terms such as *depression, distress, lack of well-being, mental illness,* or *mental disorder.* Common psychological consequences of stressful social arrangements are sometimes called *distress* and at other times (often in the same paragraph of the same article) *depression* or *mental disorder.* Instead of separating nondisordered distress that fluctuates as a function of external situations and is proportionate to these situations from depressive disorders that indicate the presence of an internal psychological dysfunction, sociologists have only perpetuated the confusion between these two conditions.

Consequently, lacking any delineation of disorder and distress, sociologists have failed to appreciate that current studies in the sociology of stress conflate two different domains of research. The first domain has nothing at all to do with mental disorder and instead concerns the consequences for normal distress of various stressors and positions within the social system. The second domain concerns the sociological determinants of genuine mental disorder to the degree that severe social stressors can cause or trigger such disorder. Traumatic external conditions can lead wartime combatants, victims of violent crimes, or Holocaust survivors, for example, to develop psychological dysfunctions.[37] Not just extreme conditions of trauma but also longstanding social stressors can produce lasting internal dysfunctions. Chronic poverty without prospects of redress, for example, can lead people to develop internalized and pervasive senses of hopelessness and helplessness, which often do not change even if their social circumstances do change for the better.[38]

However, the *typical* outcomes of the sorts of stressful social arrangements that sociologists usually study are not internal psychological dysfunctions but instead are natural responses that nondisordered people have to stressful conditions. They are the kinds of "expectable and culturally sanctioned response(s) to a particular event, for example the death of a loved one," that even the *DSM* specifically excludes from its definition of mental disorder.[39] They arise in exactly the types of situations—low and declining positions in status hierarchies, losses of attachments, and the failure to achieve desirable goals—that normally functioning loss response mechanisms were designed to deal with.[40] The failure of sociology to recognize these facts renders potentially confusing and ambiguous much of the research in the sociology of stress.

George Brown's Studies of Depression

George Brown, a British sociologist, is possibly the world's preeminent researcher on depression. His work has had more influence on psychiatry, especially in Great Britain, than that of any other social scientist. The sophisticated social model of depression that Brown has developed amply justifies his influence. His comprehensive approach includes an unusual combination of attention to subtle subjective meanings that influence emotional states and to methodologically sophisticated strategies of both qualitative and quantitative measurement. Brown's work exemplifies an all-too-rare kind of sociological research that combines exploration of human meaning with careful methodology and penetrating theory.

That said, we focus here on one area we consider to be a limitation of Brown's work, namely, its ambiguity about the distinction between disorder and nondisorder. Indeed, it is unclear exactly what set of conditions his model explains or is intended to explain. Most of the cases that Brown considers to be depressive disorders actually seem to be cases of normal sadness, although others are probably genuine disorders. In failing to adequately distinguish cases of normal sadness from disordered depression, Brown unnecessarily limits the usefulness of his very valuable model of depression and inadvertently contributes to the confusion pervading current approaches to the diagnosis of depressive disorder.

Brown's great achievement has been to develop a strong methodology for measuring the social causes of loss responses. Most research on the relationship between stressful life events and depressive symptoms relies on respondent reports of what stressful life events they have suffered and how stressful they were. Such respondent-based methods inherently confound the subjective mental states of individuals with the properties of the stressful events that they experience. Thus it is not surprising that such studies find relationships between the stressfulness of life events (as reported by the respondent) and the intensity of symptoms (as reported by the respondent); the respondent will be likely to recall events as highly stressful if he or she recalls them as leading to intense symptoms. Brown's system, in contrast, uses objective independent ratings of observers (which can be done blindly, without knowledge of the respondent's subsequent symptoms) about how much distress a particular individual would be expected to suffer, given the nature and context of the life events that he or she experiences, including their various likely meanings (e.g., humiliation or entrapment). The resulting system provides ratings of the stressfulness of life events that are not dependent on respondents' psychological condition or assessment. Brown, therefore, clearly separates the measurement of stressful life events from the resulting outcome measures while at the same time building a variety of subtle biographical and contextual variables into the objective assessment of the life events. This kind of methodological care and attention to the subtleties of meaning associated with various life events is unprecedented in depression research.

Brown's system could be especially valuable from our perspective because it can allow researchers to compare the proportionality of resulting sadness responses with the independent ratings of the severity of the stressors that triggered the responses. Such measures are precisely what is needed to begin to get at the notion of a "proportional" response and thus to examine the distinction between normal and disordered depressive conditions. This, however, is not the direction in which Brown's work evolved, and he does not draw such a distinction.

Rather, Brown presents his work as a study of depressive disorder in the community. His measure of depression is the Present State Exam (PSE), a structured clinical interview developed in the early 1970s. The PSE yields diagnoses of depression that are very similar to those that stem from *DSM* criteria, requiring the presence of depressed mood over the preceding month, as well as at least four of the following symptoms: hopelessness, suicidal ideas or actions, weight loss, early waking, delayed sleep, poor concentration, brooding, loss of interest, self-depreciation, and anergia (the failure to respond to a toxin). Brown sometimes uses the lowered criteria of depressed mood and at least one other symptom of the PSE to measure what he calls *borderline* cases of depression that are analogous to subthreshold or minor depression.[41] The major difference between the PSE and structured interviews based on *DSM* criteria is that the PSE does not ascertain lifetime histories of depression; Brown examines preceding-year episodes of depression exclusively.

Brown's studies uncover rates of depression in community samples that are even higher than in U.S. studies. For example, about 15% of working-class women in London have what Brown calls *clinical depression* over a 12-month period.[42] When he adds rates of borderline symptoms of depression and anxiety to cases that meet full criteria, he considers that about half of the community populations he studies have disorders.[43] Using the same methodology translated cross-culturally, Brown finds that rates of depression over the previous year fluctuate widely across societies, ranging (as noted in chapter 2) from a high of 30% in urban areas of Zimbabwe to a low of about 3% in rural Basque-speaking areas of Spain.[44] This great variation in rates across societies leads Brown to conclude that psychosocial, rather than biological, factors account for most cases of clinical depression.

Brown's initial research focused on the connection between loss events and the subsequent development of depression among urban working-class women. He found that severe life events among women who had lost mothers in childhood, who had three or more children living at home, who had no intimate, confiding relationships with husbands or boyfriends, and who were not employed accounted for the association between social class and depression.[45] This research indicated that severely threatening life events occurred shortly before depressive onsets in between 67 and 90% of cases.[46] Most of these events involved interpersonal difficulties, such as a woman's husband calling her an unfit mother, a boyfriend deciding he did not want an exclusive relationship, or a child leaving the mother's home to live with other relatives.[47]

Brown's subsequent work focused on the particular nature of losses. Those that involve core roles, important and consequential plans, or cherished ideas about oneself or an intimate are especially likely to lead to depression.[48] Two qualities, in particular, are related to subsequent depression among people who have suffered those types of losses.[49] First, *humiliating* losses that devalue people, undermine their self-esteem, and result in subordination lead to depression. Second, losses that are *entrapping* and so do not allow people to escape from the loss situation are depressing. Brown found that nearly 50% of women who had experienced events considered both humiliating and entrapping had depressive responses; such women were three times more likely to develop depression than those who solely suffered some loss event.[50]

Qualities of life events account not only for which women develop depression but also for which ones recover from it. What Brown calls "fresh start" events, such as finding a new boyfriend, obtaining a better job, or moving to better housing, affect the chronicity of depressive episodes.[51] Reducing the stressfulness of environments or experiencing positive events accounts for recovery or improvement. The course of depression is thus the mirror image of its onset: certain kinds of life events predict both the emergence and the length of depression.

Brown's approach to the majority of depressive reactions he describes is seemingly very compatible with the conceptualization of normal sadness that this book presents. He views depression as rooted in a common human nature, reflecting the fact that the human brain has evolved to deal with stressful life events.[52] Therefore, the capacity to develop depressive responses is universal.[53] He also stresses the role of particular kinds of losses as provoking most depressed conditions. Likewise, he regards cognitions associated with depressive states, such as helplessness and hopelessness, as fully understandable in the context of adverse social conditions, not as inappropriate.[54] As well, he indicates that "we humans have an uncanny tendency to adapt to adversity and deprivation" and stresses that many loss responses end when environmental conditions change.[55] Brown's emphasis on the findings that particular kinds of losses precede the onset of depression and that particular kinds of positive social changes predict recovery from it seems to indicate that he is studying normal sadness and not depressive disorder.

Brown's characterization of the conditions he studies, however, makes it clear that he considers them to be depressive disorders and not normal sadness.

He does distinguish a small minority of largely endogenous cases from the majority of depressive conditions that he studies: "Melancholic/psychotic depressive conditions as a whole are unlikely to form more than one-tenth of the total range of clinically relevant depression."[56] But Brown refers to the remaining 90% of conditions as *depressive disorders, clinically relevant depression,* or *neurotic depression,* irrespective of their further properties. He consistently says that his community samples suffer from *psychiatric disorders* that are the same as those found in patient populations and emphasizes that the conditions of the community members he has studied are comparable to those of treated psychiatric patients.[57] His justification for this claim is that his studies comparing community populations with treated patients find that provoking events precede the vast majority of cases in both settings.[58] Likewise, he finds that, for the most part, community members and patients share common symptoms. Granted that the two populations are similar in these respects, we have seen that this similarity alone does not ensure that both groups are equally disordered. Normal and disordered responses to stress can manifest similar symptoms, and some responses to severe stresses can be proportional and related to the ongoing presence of the stressor, while others may be disproportionate or continue despite changing circumstances. Moreover, it is entirely possible that the psychiatrically treated outpatient group contains a considerable number of nondisordered individuals reacting normally to extreme losses. The problem is that that Brown does not further pursue the question of which members of either group have disorders and which do not.

In one article, Brown does explicitly consider whether the conditions he studies are instances of *distress* or *disease,* and one might hope to find here some illumination of the disorder-versus-nondisorder distinction.[59] He finds that cases in the community that meet PSE criteria are comparable to cases found in clinical treatment. Except for the 10% of cases that are "melancholic/psychotic," particular types of losses usually precede depression in both community members and psychiatric outpatients, and both groups have symptoms of comparable severity and duration. Brown therefore rejects the notion that community members suffer from distress, whereas psychiatric outpatients have diseases, and he concludes instead that in both groups, "depression (is) basically a distress response."[60] But these assertions do not address the disorder status of the conditions because neither of Brown's terms corresponds to disorder or nondisorder. By *disease,* Brown means endogenous or biological conditions that have no social triggers, which presumably are disorders. By *distress,* he means all reactions with social triggers. However, as we have seen, a stressor can trigger a disordered reaction or a reaction that is initially normal but that eventually develops into a malfunction involving disproportionate duration or intensity in depressive response, so that what Brown calls "distress" encompasses both disordered and normal reactions to loss. Brown's demonstration that most cases in both community and clinical samples are distress, not disease, thus fails to address the distinction between nondisordered and dysfunctional responses. In fact, Brown himself considers his comparison to be between two kinds of depressive disorder (roughly corresponding to the traditional categories of "endogenous" and "reactive" depression); he calls cases of either kind that meet PSE criteria *psychiatric disorders*. Brown's study thus illustrates the kinds of challenging terminological obstacles to interpreting current literature that does not start with a cogent distinction between disorder and nondisorder built into the methodology.

The evidence in fact suggests that Brown's studies mix together disordered and nondisordered individuals with depressive symptoms and that it is likely that most of his cases reflect normal sadness. Most not only arise in response to certain kinds of loss events but also persist with proportionate intensity to social circumstances and end when these circumstances change. A minority of cases in Brown's studies, however, endure beyond the circumstances that brought them about and are not responsive to positive environmental changes. About a third of the people in his community samples who experience major improvements in their living situations remain depressed.[61] Although Brown's work commendably focuses on conditions triggered by carefully specified social situations, it neglects depressive conditions that become disengaged from environmental contexts and appear to be maintained by some internal dysfunction and thus are likely to be disordered.

We thus believe that Brown's greatest achievement has been to accurately measure and characterize the nature and causes of intense, mostly normal sadness, even if he does not call it that. Further, he has developed the most nuanced theory of the particular qualities of losses—severity, humiliation, and entrapment—that most powerfully produce normal sadness and has documented how such conditions persist only as long as environmental stressors remain. Although Brown presents his research as a study of depressive disorder, it seems instead to be primarily a landmark contribution to the study of normal sadness in extremely adverse and often unjust social circumstances. Brown's superb work illustrates how even the best social scientific studies have tended to accept and support rather than challenge the growing confusion within psychiatry about the distinction between disorder and normal negative emotion.

Conclusion

Anthropological and sociological studies have helped perpetuate the conflation of normal sadness and depressive disorder. Because they reject the possibility of developing any concepts of depression that transcend local understandings, anthropologists lack any grounds for saying that the definitions of Western psychiatry could be improved. Sociologists use terms such as *distress* and *depression* interchangeably, implying that all sadness responses are variants of mental disorders, and so they too are unable to challenge psychiatry's overexpansive definition of depressive disorder. George Brown has built a sophisticated theory of the circumstances under which sadness arises, yet he does not distinguish depressive conditions that arise from dysfunctions from those that are normal reactions. Part of the reason that an adequate distinction between normality and disorder eludes us is the failure of the social scientific disciplines that study depression to take an independent critical stance and to challenge the *DSM* diagnostic criteria.

11
Conclusion

In this final chapter, we tie up several loose ends of our argument. First, we consider the question: If the flaws in current diagnostic criteria are as compellingly clear as we argue that they are, then why haven't they been changed, or why can't they easily be changed? In addressing this question, we shift from the logic of diagnosis to the logic of powerful constituencies and vested interests that come into existence once a definition of disorder is in place. Second, we return to the evolutionary perspective on disorder that we presented in the first two chapters and that serves as the framework for much of our argument. The scholarly literature has posed many objections to this view. We review some of the most interesting objections and briefly explain why we think none of them places the evolutionary understanding of normal human functioning in doubt. Finally, this book is mainly an analysis and critique. However, many readers will be wondering what the solution to the problems we identify might be. So we offer some initial thoughts on strategies by which the approach to diagnosis of MDD might be changed to be more valid.

The Constituencies for Depressive Disorder

We have argued that there is an obvious logical problem with the current *DSM* definition of Major Depressive Disorder. We have documented how this problem has radiated throughout the mental health treatment and research establishment, as well as into the realm of public policy, to expand the domain of depressive disorder. Yet the definition is resilient; it has survived three revisions of the *DSM*, and there are few signs to suggest that changes in the MDD criteria are a high priority for the next revision, *DSM-V.* Assuming that our argument has merit, it seems reasonable to ask: What stands in the way of simply changing this definition and correcting a logical gap?

All else being equal, there are legitimate reasons for being conservative about changing diagnostic criteria. Perhaps the major one is that studies that use different criteria for sample selection cannot easily be scientifically compared and cannot yield cumulative knowledge, thus undermining the very point of having reliable, scientifically respectable standards in the first place. It is also true that many proposals exist to change criteria in the direction favored by one group or another, but these proposals are almost never based on an accumulation of valid research evidence that would scientifically warrant the change. Thus transforming criteria can become a matter of politics rather than science.

However, all else is not equal when it comes to the problem we have outlined; there is a compelling, clear, and major violation of validity that can be identified on general conceptual and theoretical grounds, and it should be fixed. It makes little sense to defend diagnostic continuity for research purposes when what is being preserved is known to be invalid and thus inadequate for scientific research to begin with. So if the standard reasons for resistance to change do not apply in this case, why aren't the criteria being changed?

Addressing this question moves us from the sphere of definitional concepts into the realm of power relations within society and among its institutions. The exploitation of a concept for purposes of power can be judged only against an understanding of how the concept could legitimately be deployed. Thus an understanding of the concept's logical structure, on which we have focused, is required. But it is social factors, more than purely logical issues that determine how a concept is actually exploited and deployed, even fallaciously at times, to serve broader interests.[1] For example, the concept of depression, as we have analyzed it, picks out clear instances of normal sadness and of depressive disorder. But this concept also contains a high degree of indeterminacy, ambiguity, and vagueness around its boundaries, allowing different groups to exploit it in ways that suit their own interests. In particular, a number of constituencies have found a symptom-based concept of depression that generates high rates of pathology to be advantageous.

The profession of medicine more broadly and of psychiatry in particular has been a major promoter and beneficiary of a definition that allows it to label and treat previously nonmedical problems as disorders. All professions strive to broaden the realm of phenomena subject to their control, and whenever the label of disease is attached to a condition, the medical profession has the primary claim to jurisdiction over it.[2] Symptom-based conceptions of mental disorder thus expand the range of conditions that can be the legitimate objects of psychiatric management.[3] Piggybacked on justifiable exercises of psychiatric power aimed at mental disorder, normal human emotions, once they have been classified as disorders, are generally subjected to technologies such as psychotropic medications or psychotherapy. These technologies have spread from the mental hospital or psychiatric clinic to the doctor's office, the school classroom, and the Internet self-help site.

For mental health clinicians, symptom-based measures of depression justify reimbursement from third-party insurers for the treatment of a broad range of patients who might not otherwise qualify, because insurers will pay to treat disorders but not problems of living. Individual clinicians are faced every day with patients seeking help for conditions that appear to be intense normal sadness but that satisfy the *DSM*'s criteria for disorder. Many clinicians will readily admit that a sizable proportion of their "depression" caseload consists of individuals who are psychiatrically normal but experiencing stressful life events. The result is a strange case of two "wrongs" seemingly making a "right": The *DSM* provides flawed criteria that do not adequately distinguish disorder from nondisorder; the clinician, who cannot be faulted for applying officially sanctioned *DSM* diagnostic criteria, knowingly or unknowingly misclassifies some normal individuals as disordered; and these two errors lead to the patient receiving desired treatment for which the therapist is reimbursed. Symptom-based diagnoses allow clinicians to rationalize such decisions when the alternative is refusal of treatment to those who are suffering.

Researchers, too, have much to gain from symptom-based diagnoses. The conflation of mental disorder and ordinary sadness legitimizes a broad interpretation of the mandated domain of the National Institute of Mental Health (NIMH), the major sponsor of research on mental illness. An expansive definition allows it to argue more persuasively for increased funding on the basis that depression is rampant in the population. In addition, in contrast to the 1960s, when the NIMH was concerned about the psychological consequences of social problems such as poverty, racism, and discrimination, in today's political climate support is far more likely to accrue to an agency that is devoted to preventing and curing a widespread disease than to one that confronts controversial social problems.[4]

Mental health researchers also have much to lose if criteria for depression should change. Symptom-based criteria are relatively easy to use. They reduce the cost and complexity of research studies and allow for higher research productivity. Enhanced reliability also confers enhanced scientific respectability. Moreover, the *DSM*'s criteria are used in virtually all of the thousands of recent depression studies on which researchers' careers are built, and any major reconceptualization of diagnostic criteria would cast into doubt the value of that past research. Adequately distinguishing normal sadness from depressive disorder could also possibly narrow opportunities for research funding, especially if the NIMH chose to focus its efforts on true disorder. Nevertheless, researchers certainly appreciate that reaching the goal of understanding the etiology and appropriate treatment of depressive disorder ultimately depends on using a valid definition of disorder as the basis for sample selection in their studies.

Symptom-based definitions are also useful for constructing estimates of the apparently huge social and economic costs of depression, which in turn can justify providing more resources for treating and preventing depression. The World Health Organization (WHO) is the major group responsible for disseminating *DSM* definitions of depression from the United States to a worldwide audience.

Its signature concern has been to publicize the immense costs of depression. Most literature about depression cites WHO projections that by 2020 depression will become the second leading cause of worldwide disability, behind only heart disease, and that depression is already the single leading cause of disability for people in midlife and for women of all ages.[5] This massive amount of disability lends a sense of urgency to policy efforts designed to respond to depressive illness. Peter Kramer, reviewing the WHO study, proclaims: "The most disabling illness! The costliest!" According to Kramer, "depression is the major scourge of humankind."[6] In fact, the claimed enormity of this burden and its useful rhetorical qualities result from the failure to distinguish depressive disorders from normal sadness.

The WHO calculations of disease burden are extremely complex but arise from two basic components: the number of people who suffer from a condition and the amount of disability and premature death the condition causes. The first component of burden, the frequency of the condition, derives from symptom-based definitions that estimate that 9.5% of women and 5.8% of men suffer from depression in a 1-year period. The second component, disability, is ordered into seven classes of increasing severity, stemming from the amount of time lived with a disease, weighted by the severity of the disease. The severity scores come from consensual judgments of health workers from around the world that are applied to all cases of the disease. Depression is placed in the second most severe category of illness, behind only extremely disabling and unremitting conditions such as active psychosis, dementia, and quadriplegia, and is considered comparable to the conditions of paraplegia and blindness. It is viewed as more severe than, for example, Down syndrome, deafness, below-the-knee amputation, and angina. This extreme degree of severity assumes that all cases of depression share the depth, chronicity, and recurrence that are characteristic of the conditions that health workers see in their practices. Yet, in contrast to the severity of the treated conditions that often comprise professional caseloads, a high proportion of individuals who meet symptom-based criteria in the community populations that provide the frequency estimates for depression have acute episodes with little impairment that remit after short periods.[7] The WHO severity ratings thus ignore the great heterogeneity of impairment in cases of depression and apply the most serious rating to all cases.

The conflation of normal sadness and depressive disorder leads to overestimates of both the severity and the prevalence components of disability ratings, accounting for the widely quoted WHO figures. Advocates, in turn, use this apparently scientific evidence that depression is a massive public health problem to argue for committing far more resources to combating such a disabling condition.

Family advocacy organizations, such as the National Alliance on Mental Illness (NAMI), which became an influential political movement during the 1980s, are another powerful force upholding symptom-based definitions of depression. They have at the top of their agenda the destigmatization of mental illness and the achievement of insurance reimbursement parity for mental disorder. Symptom-based diagnoses expand the notion of mental illness to such an extent that they encompass a large proportion of the population. This lowers the boundary between normality and abnormality and seemingly can help achieve a greater acceptability of mental illness in the broader society. In addition, advocacy groups argue that mental disorders, including depression, are biological disorders, just like physical disorders, and deserve to be treated equally with respect to reimbursement. Admitting that current *DSM* criteria fail to distinguish true depressive disorders from normal sadness reactions would certainly muddy this argument and appears to go against these groups' agendas.

Pharmaceutical companies, which earn enormous profits from the transformation of sadness into depressive disorder, are perhaps the most visible beneficiaries of the *DSM*'s symptom-based diagnoses. Consequently, these companies are now major sponsors of the activities of both the psychiatric profession and advocacy groups, who in turn emphasize the benefits of using medication as the frontline treatment for depression.[8] Ubiquitous advertisements for antidepressant medication, using *DSM* criteria, emphasize that individuals who experience such common symptoms as sadness, fatigue, sleep or appetite difficulties, and the like should consult their physicians to see whether they might have a depressive disorder, and such campaigns have been enormously successful.[9] Like clinicians, drug companies can legitimately explain that they are only using the criteria officially sanctioned by the psychiatric profession, even as their ads tend to further confuse the public about the boundary between normality and disorder.

Finally, perhaps the most important constituency for medicalized definitions of distress is afflicted individuals themselves, who find that recognizing their symptoms as those of treatable illnesses enables them to get medical help more easily and thus to regulate their painful emotions. Advertisements and other media messages reinforce an image of consumers enjoying desirable lifestyles because they use psychotropic drugs, reducing the gap between actual suffering and desired normality. Such individuals may genuinely benefit from medication or other treatment, and embracing a self-definition as the victim of an illness provides a socially acceptable account of one's problems and some release from responsibility for those problems.

Many constituencies, including professional groups, researchers, mental health advocates, and pharmaceutical companies, as well as many individuals who want control over their emotional pain, thus have an interest in keeping the current diagnostic standards for depression, making it difficult to change these criteria. In the long run, however, it is difficult to imagine that any enterprise that claims to be based on scientific principles can continue to be grounded in obviously invalid criteria such as those that presently exist for MDD. By mixing together normal and disordered individuals in research samples, such confused criteria also hinder scientific progress in understanding the etiology of disorder and how it might best be treated. Unreasonably broad definitions of psychological disorder also have the potential costs of stigmatizing the disadvantaged as mentally ill, replacing social policies with unwarranted medical treatment, and creating a one-dimensional public discourse that can undermine the capacity for making moral and political distinctions.

The very magnitude of the figures on the prevalence of depressive disorder, despite their rhetorical usefulness, can paralyze the will to respond to a problem of such seeming enormity. At present, some critics argue against reimbursement parity for mental health care because, by allowing every instance of normal unhappiness to qualify for treatment, it would break the health care bank. A more honest discussion of normal versus abnormal conditions and their appropriate rights to reimbursement might help to address some of these objections. As well, the advantages of treating the normally sad as having depressive disorders might be offset by the liabilities of creating in such people a sense of victimhood, a diminished sense of personal responsibility, and a view of themselves as passive sufferers of biochemical deficiency.[10] Ultimately, the transformation of sadness into depressive disorder has the questionable effect of shrinking the range of normal emotions and expanding pathology to ever-widening realms of human experience.

Objections to Our Position

Much of our argument rests on distinguishing disorder from normal human functioning according to evolutionary criteria for how human beings are biologically designed to behave. The resulting approach reflects the dominant tradition in the history of psychiatry, as we documented in chapter 3. But is it possible that our distinction between depressive disorder and normal sadness is nonetheless simply wrong? Indeed, a number of objections have been posed to various aspects of our position. Debates over the concept of disorder are common across many disciplines, so our consideration of such objections is not at all meant to be complete.

One set of objections asserts that *disorder* is inherently just a value-laden term denoting undesirable mental or behavioral conditions, with no factual component that might have a real referent in human nature. Objective distinctions between disorder and nondisorder, in this view, are impossible to make.[11] We do agree that "disorder" is, in part, a value-laden concept; a condition that does no harm cannot be considered a disorder, and the notion of harm has an intrinsic value component. In addition, as we have seen, different groups manipulate this concept to suit their own interests. However, although it might seem attractive to equate disorder with whatever is negative, disorders are just one kind of negative condition. The claim that "disorder" is solely a value concept, although common, makes no sense simply because there are many negatively evaluated mental states that no one considers to be disorders, from ignorance and lack of talent to lust for extramarital partners and male aggressiveness to a taste for fatty and sugary foods that may be harmful in our current environment.

Thus there must be something beyond the value judgment, specifically some factual criterion, that distinguishes disorders from the myriad other negative mental and behavioral conditions that are negatively evaluated but are not considered disorders. That criterion seems to be whether the individual's bio- logically designed mechanisms are functioning in the ways they were naturally selected for; if the condition is within human nature in this sense, then even if the condition is currently harmful, it is not a disorder.

A related objection is that whether we call any given condition a *mental disor- der* must be capricious and ultimately vacuous because no sharp natural bound- ary exists between disordered and normal conditions.[12] Instead, normality and abnormality are arrayed on a continuum. It follows, it is argued, that attempts to divide conditions into those that are dysfunctional and those that are normal are arbitrary and must rest on social values.[13]

It is a misconception to think that a scientific concept of disorder must set such precise boundaries. What is essential is that the concept and its opposite can be clearly applied to a range of important cases; vagueness along the boundary is not critical and indeed is to be expected because the defining features them- selves have vague boundaries. Continuous distributions in nature are completely compatible with objective concepts, although it is true that the fuzziness of the concept means that fixing an exact boundary for practical purposes will indeed be more likely to depend on social values and conventions than on objective facts. For example, there are real differences, rooted in biological facts, between chil- dren and adults, between being asleep and being awake, between normal and high blood pressure, and between the colors black and white, yet in every one of these cases intermediate cases exist that create a fuzziness or a continuum.

Another common critique is that definitions of disorder must be rooted ex- clusively in the actual social practices of some community. This objection holds that concepts of disorder are relative to particular times and places and cannot be universally valid. For example, anthropologists Laurence Kirmayer and Alan Young argue that:

> Inappropriateness has much more to do with socially defined norms and circumstances than with evolutionarily defined ones. The inappropriate- ness that distinguishes disordered or dysfunctional responses from nor- mal ones is recognized and defined in terms of social context; deciding what is inappropriate is a social judgment.[14]

As we have seen, there is some truth in the cultural view of depression. Local cultural values and practices do help define the meanings of situations and thus which circumstances will be perceived as falling within one of the categories that trigger sadness. Yet this cultural relativity is quite consistent with the fact that universal biological processes underlie sadness responses and shape their sensitivity to certain kinds of meanings.

The central flaw in this argument is that the concept of *inappropriate circumstances,* which is critical to distinctions between disordered and normal responses, is not a purely socially shaped judgment but is itself partly an evolutionarily grounded concept. Loss responses are evolutionarily selected to respond to a specific range of stimuli and not to respond outside that range; they are as much designed to not respond to the wrong stimuli as they are to respond to the right stimuli. Cultural values do enter into definitions of what particular losses are defined as inside or outside the appropriate range of loss stimuli and can suggest standards for how intense an expression of a sadness response is socially acceptable. Yet the *categories* that trigger sadness responses—losses of intimate attachments, low or declining social status, or the failure to achieve desired goals—are universal.

Moreover, when concepts of disorder are equated with whatever conditions are called *disorders* in a particular group, the possibility of scientifically evaluating and critiquing these concepts is lost. Also lost is the commonsense understanding that a culture could be *wrong* in its judgments about disorder. For example, the Victorians were wrong in believing that masturbation and female orgasm were disorders, and some ante-bellum Southerners were wrong in holding that runaway slaves were suffering from a mental disorder. But if disorders are just culturally relative conditions, then we cannot explain why these judgments were wrong, because those diagnoses did indeed express the values of their times.

The reason why they could be wrong is that there is an additional, factual claim being made when one asserts that a condition is a disorder, namely, a claim that the condition involves a failure of human biological design (e.g., women are designed not to experience orgasmic pleasure or slaves are designed to be subservient), and this factual claim turns out to be just plain false. That is, the diagnostic claims were based on incorrect theories about human nature. In placing issues of diagnostic judgment outside the scope of science, the cultural view leaves no grounds for claiming that any definition of depression is any better or worse than any other. It is thus not just wrong but counterproductive, because it undermines the ability to constructively critique and improve psychiatric diagnosis. Our approach, in contrast, aims to help the psychiatric profession develop more useful definitions that do not define every undesirable consequence of sadness as a disorder.

Another set of objections rejects the particular evolutionary standard that we use to ascertain disorder status. One of these types of objections accepts a biological approach in using the fitness of a behavior to establish whether it is healthy but objects that current fitness, not what the mechanism was selected for in the past, determines disorder status.[15] According to this view, maladaptive conditions in the present environment, not standards taken from evolutionary functioning, should provide the criteria for disordered conditions. Yet the past is relevant because it explains how we came to be the way we are and thus determines which of our features were biologically selected and thus part of human nature. The question of whether a mechanism's effect is adaptive at present is distinct from the question of whether the effect is part of the mechanism's design. Problematic mismatches between human nature and current social desirability such as adulterous longings, male aggressiveness, or becoming sad after losses are not in themselves disordered. For example, it may be fitness enhancing in our culture not to have tastes for fat and sugar, but that does not mean that people who have such tastes are disordered; that is how we were designed to be, due to conditions that existed when we were evolving. The explanatory role of the concept of disorder is such that dysfunctions of psychological mechanisms are properly defined against evolutionary, rather than contemporary, standards.

However, sometimes environmental conditions that are too different from what is evolutionarily expected can produce real depressive disorders because people were not naturally selected to function in such settings. Modern warfare, for example, leads many soldiers to develop mental disorders that persist far beyond the immediate combat situation because the human brain was not developed to function under such conditions. More commonly, however, problematic loss responses in a new environment are not disorders at all; rather, the relevant mechanisms are acting in designed ways in response to novel types of losses.[16]

A different objection is that depression serves no evolutionary function at all but instead is, in Steven Jay Gould's terms, a spandrel or exaptation.[17] The term *spandrel* stems from the triangular spaces below the domes of Gothic cathedrals that were not planned but that necessarily result from the way that the dome is mounted on surrounding arches. Spandrels are evolutionary accidents that are not themselves selected but are unintended consequences that have no evolutionary advantages. When spandrels are put to a later use, as when designers of cathedrals painted images of the apostles on them, they become exaptations that put the accidental structure to some purposive use. Depression, according to this thesis, is a spandrel that has never held any overt nor hidden benefits either in the past or at present.[18]

The objection that depression was never selected for its evolutionary benefits suffers from several confusions. First, we do not believe that *depressive disorders* were ever adaptive. They are dysfunctions of loss response mechanisms and so were never selected over the course of evolution as either adaptations or exaptations. The argument that symptoms must have been selected for their adaptive qualities at some point in evolutionary history applies only to normal sadness, not to depressive disorder. Second, any adaptive functions that intense sadness after losses might have had in evolutionary history need not be salient at present. Arguments that depression-like symptoms are not currently adaptive are irrelevant to whether they were selected to arise in appropriate circumstances at some point in the distant past.

As we argued in chapter 2, at least some forms of sadness in response to certain triggers were naturally selected, as seems evident from the cross-cultural universality and infant and nonhuman primate expression of such emotions. But, admittedly, universality by itself does not argue for the specific biological design of a particular response, for the simple reason that spandrels can be universal if they are invariable by-products of universal designed features. To take a biological example, pain during childbirth may be a universal feature that is a side effect of selection for optimal skull size of infants and may have no function. Philosopher Dominick Murphy and psychologist Robert Woolfolk, citing the presumed universal spandrel of the chin, argue that mental spandrels could exist and cause pathology without failure of function:

> The human chin is a famous spandrel. It has no function itself but is simply a by-product of the engineering requirements of speech, chewing, and respiration. If mental spandrels exist, then there are mental mechanisms that are the by-products of evolution but have themselves never possessed adaptive functions (in Wakefield's evolutionary sense) and, therefore, could not malfunction. Such mechanisms, however, could produce pathological behavior.[19]

Perhaps the most common argument about depression in this regard is that intense sadness responses were selected specifically for the attachment relationship in infancy, and all other such responses are a spandrel-like side effect having no function.[20]

In fact, there is evidence that sadness responses are not all alike and that they are fitted to the specific kind of loss, thus suggesting natural selection rather than an accidental by-product.[21] For example, pessimism, fatigue, and anhedonia are associated with the failure to achieve valued goals, whereas crying and emotional pain are related to attachment losses. Moreover, it seems inexplicable that the sorts of sadness responses commonly seen in humans and other primates to attachment and status losses, respectively, would come about as a spandrel, because the triggers are just too unalike. Until a more persuasive form of the spandrel account is provided, the ubiquity of sadness after specific kinds of losses is prima facie evidence that it is performing some naturally selected function, even though we can only speculate about what that function might have been.

A final type of objection to our position is that it has negative implications for treatment. Many people fear that using evolutionarily derived criteria for psychological disorders would lead to unnecessarily strict standards for entitlement to treatment that would deny needed professional help to many sufferers. "Such a definitional criterion for disorder," according to psychiatrist

John Sadler, "would be used bureaucratically to exclude people from care who otherwise might have a credible need."[22]

Such fears stem from a belief that there is a one-to-one mapping between dysfunctions and treatable conditions so that only dysfunctions would be reimbursable conditions.[23] Issues of who should be treated, however, are not reducible to which conditions are disorders. Physicians often treat conditions and provide procedures that have nothing to do with disorders (e.g., childbirth, contraception). This is in part a political issue regarding mandated reimbursement for services and in part an empirical issue having to do with what can help people. It is true that our analysis does encourage refocusing policies away from efforts that attempt to reach unrecognized and untreated cases of sadness toward treating recognized disorders. It also leads us to be skeptical about the benefits of widespread screening programs or direct-to-consumer advertising campaigns that encourage people with common symptoms to enter treatment, because their symptoms are more likely to indicate normal sadness than depressive disorder.

Yet it is also true that nondisordered sadness can cause enormous suffering and that medication or counseling can relieve many cases of painful, but normal, sadness, although the general transience and self-correcting nature of normal reactions complicates the judgment of whether or not to treat. When people desire professional help for such acute emotional pain, they deserve clinical attention as a matter of justice and compassion. However, just as administering painkillers during childbirth does not make this process a disorder, medicating or counseling people with normal sadness should not be confused with treating a disorder.

Some Directions for Solving the Problem

This book has focused on critiquing current overexpansive definitions of depression. We have tried to clarify the conceptually confused situation in which psychiatry and the social sciences find themselves in the study of depression. Once this situation is acknowledged, these fields can proceed to develop the methods necessary to make distinctions between normal and abnormal conditions. Although it is beyond the scope of this book to develop such detailed methods, it is worth outlining some promising ways to proceed. In this section we provide some preliminary suggestions regarding how criteria could be improved in ways that would distinguish depressive disorders from normal sadness. Each suggestion depends on using contextual criteria, as well as the presence of symptoms, to make diagnostic decisions. The particular ways that these criteria are incorporated will depend on the settings in which diagnoses are made, such as in clinical practice, in screening programs, or in community studies.

The *DSM* definition of Major Depressive Disorder is primarily designed for use in clinical practice. The bereavement exclusion found in the current manual, which states, "the symptoms are not better accounted for by Bereavement," provides one model for valid criteria in clinical settings.[24] There is no reason why a clause could not be added to this exclusion that would either expand it into a more general condition, such as "Bereavement or some other major life stressor," or provide further specific examples, such as "Bereavement, marital dissolution, the loss of a valued job, etc." An expanded exclusion clause of this nature would keep the clinician as the ultimate judge of whether a patient presents with normal sadness or depressive disorder. Because current clinical diagnoses are made for patients who have already judged themselves as needing mental health treatment, expansions in the exclusion clause will probably not have a major effect on diagnostic decisions. Nevertheless, such changes would enhance the validity and integrity of *DSM* diagnoses. In addition, the "V codes," discussed in chapter 5, could be expanded to contain conditions excluded from diagnoses of MDD that are "nondisordered but treatable" conditions.

Screening instruments for depression in general medical practice are applied in settings with intense time pressures and must be very brief. Incorporating contextual criteria into these instruments thus involves a challenge. On the one hand, many patients in general medical settings are likely to have normal sadness stemming from stressful events such as physical illness. On the other hand, screening instruments that use contextual criteria will consume more time, and they might be less reliable than current instruments and so might not be practical.

Contextual criteria could be incorporated into such instruments at two levels: in the questions used in the self-administered instruments and in the instructions for physicians interpreting the results of these instruments. The addition of a simple instruction on a self-administered depression screen—for instance, "Did these symptoms emerge after particularly stressful events such as . . ."—could provide the appropriate cues to respondents that symptoms of normal sadness need not indicate a depressive disorder. Indeed, early community studies used questions such as whether heart palpitations arise "when you are not exercising or working hard" that contextualized responses for particular symptoms.[25]

In addition, instructions to physicians about how to interpret the results of checklists could explicitly mention the need to attend to the context of reported symptoms and judge whether symptoms reflect a physical condition or the impact of medication or of stressful life events instead of a depressive disorder. Physicians should also be explicitly cautioned to use their diagnostic common sense rather than to unquestioningly follow *DSM*-style symptom scales. The physician could also be encouraged in appropriate cases to respond to positive screens that involve contextual triggers with "watchful waiting" rather than immediate medication. Using contextual criteria in these ways could lower the number of false-positive screens without adding much time to the clinical encounter.

Given the particular dangers of overmedicating adolescents, screening instruments in schools must be especially sensitive to the contextual nature of many adolescent symptoms. Screening in these settings does not involve the intense time pressures of a physician's office. Using media presentations of cases with normal problems of adjustment, as well as of depressive disorders, before the administration of scales could help provide a context for adolescents to use in framing their answers. Such techniques could help minimize the number of false positives in school settings, where they can potentially have the most harmful results.

Incorporating contextual criteria into community studies involves a different set of issues than in clinical practice, primary care, or schools. Unlike clinicians, who can use their judgment to distinguish culturally expectable symptoms from internal dysfunctions, epidemiologists and sociologists must use standardized scales in their research. Using clinical judgments to distinguish expectable and proportionate responses from disordered, disproportionate ones is not practical and would damage the reliability of judgments across interviewers that are necessary to obtain valid estimates of rates of disorders in community populations. It should, however, be possible to develop standardized, yet contextual, scales that relate the degree of stressfulness in people's lives to the consequent number of symptoms they report.

The key to adequately distinguishing whether symptoms indicate distress or disorder in survey research is to examine their *proportionality* to the severity and duration of stressfulness in people's actual lives. As noted, George Brown has developed objective measures of stressfulness that use the context and meaning of events to determine how much distress a typical person is likely to experience in given circumstances.[26] Recently, researchers have drawn on Brown's approach to develop standardized scales for use in survey research that assign quantitative scores to the content, severity, and threat level of stressful events that people experience.[27] These scores can be used to predict the likely amount of distress that an average respondent should display in a given situation. Those with disproportionately higher symptom levels than expected, given the degree of stressfulness of their situations, can be assumed to be the most likely group to have mental disorders. Although contextual criteria would be used in a different way in survey research than for diagnostic purposes, in each case they should result in fewer false-positive diagnoses and more valid estimates of the amount of depressive disorder.

Despite the challenges, a serious trial-and-error process of developing contextual criteria for clinical and research diagnoses of MDD should, in all likelihood, eventually yield criteria of satisfactory reliability and validity. However it is accomplished, resolving this challenge is critical for the future of depression research. Based on the data presented in chapter 2 and other circumstantial arguments, it is clear that the "false positives" problem for MDD diagnosis is sizable. But no one can say exactly how sizable it is, simply because none of the diagnostic instruments clinicians and researchers now use adequately discriminates disordered from nondisordered sadness, and therefore no research studies address the issue.[28] Only when valid diagnostic criteria are devised and corresponding research instruments are developed will the magnitude and implications of the current false positives problem become known. Depression research, including treatment research, will then enter a new era in which questions and answers about both depressive disorder and normal sadness can be asked and answered in a more refined way than they are today.

Conclusion

Psychiatry has made immense strides in recent decades and now has many powerful techniques at its disposal to uncover the causes of depressive disorders. In addition, available treatments for depression are far better than at any time in human history. Yet efforts at identifying disorders, specifying their causes, and providing effective treatments for them are all handicapped by the absence of a valid definition of depressive disorder. When the *DSM-III* was written, the challenge was to justify that psychiatry could be a legitimate part of medicine at all and not merely an instrument of social control. But times have changed. It is now generally accepted that there are genuine medical disorders of the mind; the problem is to understand the limits of the concept of disorder so that it does not engulf all the problems that life poses. Developing adequate criteria that distinguish disorders from normal sadness should be one of the major priorities for students of depression.

Sadness is an inherent part of the human condition, not a mental disorder. Thus to confront psychiatry's invalid definition of depressive disorder is also to consider a painful but important part of our humanity that we have tended to shunt aside in the modern medicalization of human problems. As science allows us to gain more control over our emotional states, we will inevitably confront the question of whether normal intense sadness has any redeeming features or should be banished from our lives. Such a momentous scientific and moral issue should not be spuriously resolved by using a semantic confusion in the *DSM* that mistakenly places states of intense sadness under the medical category of disorder. We can only adequately confront the complex and important concerns involved if we clearly differentiate normal sadness from mental disorder. We hope that by examining the consequences of the current failure to adequately draw such a distinction, this book may encourage mental health professionals to embrace the needed distinction and to start talking to each other and to their patients in a more nuanced way that yields improved understanding and treatment.

Notes

Chapter 1

1. Auden, 1947/1994.
2. Klerman, 1988; Blazer, 2005.
3. Miller, 1949/1996.
4. Dohrenwend, 2000.
5. McKinley, 1999.
6. Blazer, Kessler, McGonagle, & Swartz, 1994; Kessler, Berglund, Demler, Jin, Koretz, Merikangas, et al., 2003.
7. Kessler, Berglund, et al., 2003.
8. Roberts, Andrews, Lewinsohn, & Hops, 1990; Lavretsky & Kumar, 2002; Lewinsohn, Shankman, Gau, & Klein, 2004.
9. Klerman, 1988; Klerman & Weissman, 1989; Hagnell, Lanke, Rorsman, & Ojesjo, 1982.
10. Murphy, Laird, Monson, Sobel, & Leighton, 2000; Kessler et al., 2005; Blazer, 2005, pp. 114–115.
11. Olfson, Marcus, Druss, Elinson, Tanielian, & Pincus, 2002.
12. Olfson, Marcus, Druss, & Pincus, 2002.
13. Kessler, Berglund, et al., 2003.
14. Crystal, Sambamoorthi, Walkup, & Akincigil, 2003.
15. Horwitz, 2002, p. 4.
16. Pear, 2004.
17. Pear, 2004.
18. Croghan, 2001.
19. Murray & Lopez, 1996.
20. Greenberg, Stiglin, Finkelstein, & Berndt, 1993.
21. See also Blazer, 2005, pp. 28–29; McPherson & Armstrong, 2006. Citation counts stem from Medline searches.
22. Jackson, 1986.
23. Kirk & Kutchins, 1992; Horwitz, 2002.
24. Regier et al., 1998; Narrow, Rae, Robins, & Regier, 2002.
25. American Psychiatric Association (APA), 2000.
26. APA, 2000, p. 356.

27. APA, 2000, p. 356.
28. Watson, 2006.
29. Dobbs, 2006, pp. 51–52.
30. Solomon, 2001, p. 18.
31. Styron, 1990, pp. 17–18; p. 62.
32. Karp, 1996, pp. 3–6.
33. APA, 2000, p. xxxi.
34. APA, 2000, p. xxxi.
35. Wakefield, 1992.
36. E.g., Klein, 1978; Spitzer, 1999.
37. E.g. Fodor, 1983; Buss, 1999; Pinker, 1997.
38. Keller & Nesse, 2005.
39. Young, 2003.
40. Wakefield, 1992.
41. Buss, 1999.
42. Beck, 1967.
43. Post, 1992.
44. E.g. Jackson, 1986, Ch. 9; Mendels & Cochrane, 1968; Kendell, 1968.
45. Dohrenwend, 2000; Kirkpatrick et al., 2003; Marshall, Schell, Elliott, Berthold, & Chun, 2005.
46. Szasz, 1961; Scheff, 1966; Kirmayer & Young, 1999.
47. Archer, 1999.
48. Klerman, 1974; Coyne, 1976; Gilbert, 1992
49. Goodwin & Guze, 1996.
50. Post, 1992.
51. Coyne et al., 2000; Nesse, 2005.
52. Kramer, 2005.
53. Horwitz & Wakefield, 2006.
54. Murray & Lopez, 1996.
55. U.S. Department of Health & Human Services (USDHHS), 2001; World Health Organization (WHO), 2004.
56. Nesse, 2000.

Chapter 2

1. Shelley, 1824/1986.
2. Coleridge, 1805/1986.
3. Keller & Nesse, 2006.
4. Nesse, 2006.
5. Brown, 2002; Dohrenwend, 2000.
6. E.g., Turner, Wheaton, & Lloyd, 1995; Wheaton, 1999.
7. Grinker & Spiegel, 1945.
8. Kendler, Karkowski, & Prescott, 1999.
9. E.g., Coyne, 1992; Oatley & Bolton, 1985; Gilbert, 1992.
10. Turner, 2000.

11. Brown, 1993.
12. Homer, 1990, p. 468.
13. Kovacs, 1989, pp. 70–71; 84–85.
14. Clayton, 1982.
15. Clayton, 1998.
16. Clayton & Darvish, 1979; Zisook & Shuchter, 1991.
17. Bruce, Kim, Leaf, & Jacobs, 1990; Zisook, Paulus, Shuchter, & Judd, 1997; Zisook & Shuchter, 1991.
18. Leahy, 1992–1993; Sanders, 1979–1980.
19. Harris, 1991.
20. DeVries, Davis, Wortman, & Lehman, 1997.
21. Bonanno, et al., 2002; Aneshensel, Botticello, & Yamamoto-Mitani, 2004.
22. Wortman & Silver, 1989; Parkes & Weiss, 1983; Zisook & Shuchter, 1991.
23. Clayton & Darvish, 1979; Hays, Kasl, & Jacobs, 1994.
24. Archer, 1989; Carr et al., 2000; Nesse, 2005.
25. Wortman, Silver, & Kessler, 1993.
26. Bonanno et al., 2002; Carr, House, Wortman, Nesse, & Kessler, 2001.
27. Schulz et al., 2001.
28. Mancini, Pressman, & Bonanno, 2005.
29. Wortman & Silver, 1989; Lopata, 1973; Mancini et al., 2005.
30. Umberson, Wortman, & Kessler, 1992; Wortman et al., 1993.
31. Carr, 2004.
32. Zisook & Shuchter, 1991; Gallagher, Breckenridge, Thompson, & Peterson, 1983; Archer, 1999, pp. 98–100; Bonanno et al., 2002.
33. Clayton, 1982.
34. Zisook & Schuchter, 1991; Bonanno & Kaltman, 2001; Bonanno et al., 2002.
35. Clayton, 1982.
36. Bonanno et al., 2002.
37. Jackson, 1986.
38. Nesse, 2005.
39. Neimeyer, 2000; Schut, Stroebe, Van den Bout, & Terheggen, 2001.
40. Sloman, Gilbert, & Hasey, 2003.
41. Nesse, 2005.
42. APA, 2000, p. xxxi (italics added).
43. Kitson, Babri, & Roach, 1985; Ross, Mirowsky, & Goldstein, 1990; Waite, 1995.
44. Kessler et al., 1994; Simon, 2002.
45. Bruce et al., 1990.
46. Bruce, 1998.
47. Bruce, 1998, p. 228.
48. Radloff, 1977; Sweeney & Horwitz, 2001.
49. Wheaton, 1990.
50. Brown, 2002.
51. Brown, Harris, & Hepworth, 1995.
52. Myers, Lindenthal, & Pepper, 1971; Bloom, Asher, & White, 1978.

53. Booth & Amato, 1991.

54. Booth & Amato, 1991.

55. E.g., Gerstel, Reissman, & Rosenfield, 1985; Menaghan & Lieberman, 1986; Ross, 1995.

56. Brown, 1993; Simon, 2002.

57. Wade & Pevalin, 2004.

58. Dew, Bromet, & Schulberg, 1987; Kessler, House, & Turner, 1987; Tausig & Fenwick, 1999; Dooley, Prause, & Ham-Rowbottom, 2000; Grzywacz & Dooley, 2003.

59. Fenwick & Tausig, 1994; Kessler et al., 1987; Turner, 1995; Dew, Bromet, & Penkower, 1992; Dooley, Catalano, & Wilson, 1994.

60. Angel, Frisco, Angel, & Chiriboga, 2003.

61. Ganzini, McFarland, & Cutler, 1990.

62. Wheaton, 1990; Reynolds, 1997.

63. Kasl & Cobb, 1979; Dew et al., 1986.

64. Horwitz, 1984; Turner, 1995.

65. Kessler, Turner, & House, 1989; Price, Choi, & Vinokur, 2002; Dooley et al., 2000.

66. Cobb & Kasl, 1977; Kasl & Cobb, 1979.

67. Brooke, 2003.

68. Zaun, 2004.

69. Durkheim, 1897/1951.

70. Lee, 1999.

71. Merton, 1938/1968; Heckhausen & Schultz, 1995; Sloman et al., 2003.

72. Nesse, 2000.

73. Keller & Nesse, 2005.

74. Carr, 1997.

75. McEwan, Costello, & Taylor, 1987.

76. Cuisinier, Janssen, deGraauw, Bakker, & Hoogduin, 1996; Heckhausen, Wrosch, & Fleeson, 2001.

77. Mollica, Poole, & Tor, 1998; Mollica et al., 1999; Marshall, Schell, Elliott, Berthold, & Chun, 2005.

78. Clymer, 2002.

79. Dohrenwend, 1973.

80. Turner et al., 1995; McLeod & Nonnemaker, 1999.

81. Turner & Lloyd, 1999.

82. Ritsher, Warner, Johnson, & Dohrenwend, 2001; Johnson, Cohen, Dohrenwend, Link, & Brook, 1999; Lorant et al., 2003; Dohrenwend et al., 1992.

83. Costello, Compton, Keeler, & Angold, 2003, Table 3.

84. Dearing, Taylor, & McCartney, 2005; see also Epstein, 2003.

85. E.g., Kirmayer, 1994.

86. Darwin, 1872/1998.

87. Willner, 1991.

88. Harlow & Suomi, 1974; McKinney, 1986; Gilmer & McKinney, 2003.

89. Mineka & Suomi, 1978.

90. Harlow, Harlow, & Suomi, 1971; Harlow & Suomi, 1974; Suomi, 1991.

91. Kaufman & Rosenblum, 1966.

92. Sloman et al., 2003.

93. Harlow & Suomi, 1974; Gilmer & McKinney, 2003.

94. Shively, 1998.

95. Sapolsky, 1989.

96. Sapolsky, 1992; Price, Sloman, Gardner, Gilbert, & Rohde, 1994.

97. McGuire, Raleigh, & Johnson, 1983; Raleigh, McGuire, Brammer, & Yuwiler, 1984.

98. Shively, Laber-Laird, & Anton, 1997.

99. Berman, Rasmussen, & Suomi, 1994.

100. Sapolsky, 1989.

101. Sapolsky, 2005.

102. Bowlby, 1969/1982, 1973, 1980.

103. Harlow & Suomi, 1974.

104. Darwin, 1872/1998, p. 185.

105. Darwin, 1872/1998, p. 177.

106. Ekman & Friesen, 1971.

107. Ekman, 1973.

108. Ekman, Friesen, O'Sullivan, Chan, Diacoyanni-Tarlatzis, Heider, et al., 1987.

109. Ekman & Friesen, 1971.

110. Turner, 2000.

111. Pinker, 1997.

112. Brown, 2002.

113. Carr & Vitaliano, 1985, p. 255.

114. Broadhead & Abas, 1998.

115. Desjarlais, Eisenberg, Good, & Kleinman, 1995.

116. Schieffelin, 1985.

117. Manson, 1995.

118. Miller & Schoenfeld, 1973.

119. Archer, 1999.

120. Good, Good, & Moradi, 1985, p. 386.

121. Wikan, 1988, 1990.

122. Wikan, 1988, 1990.

123. E.g., Lutz, 1985; Schieffelin, 1985; Kleinman, 1986.

124. Kleinman, 1986.

125. Cheung, 1982.

126. Kleinman, 1986.

127. E.g., Kirmayer & Young, 1999; Kleinman & Good, 1985; Murphy & Woolfolk, 2001.

128. E.g., Brown & Harris, 1978; Pearlin, 1989; Aneshensel, 1992; Turner & Lloyd, 1999.

129. Brown, 2002.

130. Gaminde, Uria, Padro, Querejeta, & Ozamiz, 1993.

131. Broadhead & Abas, 1998.

132. E.g., House, Landis, & Umberson, 1988; Turner, 1999.

133. Schieffelin, 1985

134. Deut. 25:5; Stroebe & Stroebe, 1987.

135. E.g., Kirmayer, 1994.

136. E.g., Mernissi, 1987; Jones, 2006.

137. Nesse & Williams, 1994.

138. Nesse & Williams, 1994.

139. Tooby & Cosmides, 1990.

140. Lewis, 1934.

141. Turner, 2000.

142. Hagen, 1999, 2002.

143. Klerman, 1974; Coyne, 1976; Gilbert, 1992.

144. Archer, 1999.

145. Bowlby, 1973; Price, Sloman, Gardner, Gilbert, & Rohde, 1994; Turner, 2000.

146. Darwin, 1872/1998, p. 347.

147. Bowlby, 1980.

148. Archer, 1999.

149. Price et al., 1994.

150. Price et al., 1994; Stevens & Price, 2000; Sloman, Gilbert, & Hasey, 2004.

151. Price & Sloman, 1987; Stevens & Price, 2000.

152. Gilbert & Allan, 1998; Sloman et al., 2003.

153. Wenegrat, 1995.

154. Nesse, 2006.

155. Klinger, 1975; Gut, 1989; Nesse, 2000; Wrosch, Scheier, Carver, & Schulz, 2003.

156. Watson & Andrews, 2002.

157. Nesse, 2000, p. 17.

158. Keller & Nesse, 2005; Keller & Nesse, 2006.

159. Murphy & Stich, 2000.

160. Nesse, 2000.

161. Merton, 1938/1968.

Chapter 3

1. Jackson, 1986, p. ix.

2. Kendell, 1968.

3. Radden, 2000.

4. Merikangas & Angst, 1995; Kessler, Abelson, & Zhao, 1998.

5. Hippocrates, 1923–1931, vol. 1, p. 263.

6. Hippocrates, 1923–1931, vol. 4, p. 185.

7. Roccatagliata, 1986, pp. 163–164.

8. Jackson, 1986, p. 32.

9. Aristotle, 2000, p. 59.

10. Aristotle, 2000, p. 57.

11. Aristotle, 1931, vol. 7, 954.

12. Jackson, 1986.

13. Aristotle, 2000, p. 60.
14. Aristotle, 2000, p. 59.
15. Jackson, 1986, p. 33.
16. Jackson, 1986, p. 33.
17. Jackson, 1986, p. 33.
18. Jackson, 1986, p. 34.
19. Jackson, 1986, p. 39.
20. Jackson, 1986, p. 40.
21. Jackson, 1986, p. 40.
22. Jackson, 1986, p. 39.
23. Jackson, 1986, p. 41.
24. Jackson, 1986, p. 42.
25. Jackson, 1986, p. 42.
26. Lewis, 1934.
27. Jackson, 1986, p. 315.
28. Jackson, 1986, p. 57.
29. Jackson, 1986, pp. 60, 61.
30. Avicenna, 2000, p. 77.
31. Jackson, 1986, p. 87.
32. Hildegard of Bingen, 2000, p. 81.
33. Bright, 1586/2000, p. 120.
34. Jackson, 1986, pp. 85–86.
35. Jackson, 1986, p. 84.
36. Jackson, 1986, p. 91.
37. Burton, 1621/2001, p. 331.
38. Burton, 1621/2001, pp. 143–144.
39. Burton, 1621/2001, p. 137.
40. Burton, 1621/1948, 331.
41. Burton, 1621/2000, p. 132.
42. Burton, 1621/2001, pp. 145–146.
43. Burton, 1621/2001, pp. 357–358.
44. Burton, 1621/2001, pp. 358–359.
45. MacDonald, 1981, p. 159.
46. MacDonald, 1981, p. 159.
47. MacDonald, 1981, p. 159.
48. MacDonald, 1981, p. 149.
49. MacDonald, 1981, p. 78.
50. Jackson, 1986, p. 136.
51. Jackson, 1986, p. 136.
52. Jackson, 1986, p. 316.
53. Jackson, 1986, p. 130 (italics added).
54. Johnson, 1755/1805; Radden, 2000, p. 5.
55. Jackson, 1986, p. 118.
56. Jackson, 1986, p. 124.
57. Mather, 1724/2000, p. 163.
58. Kant, 1793/2000, p. 201.

59. Pinel, 1801/2000, p. 205.
60. Pinel, 1801/2000, p. 209.
61. Jackson, 1986, p. 153.
62. Rush, 1812/2000, p. 213.
63. Maudsley, 1868/2000, p. 252.
64. Maudsley, 1868/2000, p. 253.
65. Griesinger, 1867/2000, p. 226.
66. Griesinger, 1867/2000, p. 226.
67. Griesinger, 1867, p. 213; in Jackson, 1986, p. 161.
68. Griesinger, 1867, pp. 168–169; in Jackson, 1986, p. 165.
69. Jackson, 1986, p. 166.
70. Jackson, 1986, pp. 166–167.
71. Jackson, 1986, p. 166.
72. Jackson, 1986, pp. 167–168.
73. Jackson, 1986, p. 169.
74. Jackson, 1986, p. 167.
75. Jackson, 1986, p. 167.
76. Jackson, 1986, p. 167.
77. Jackson, 1986, p. 180.
78. Jackson, 1986, p. 181.
79. Jackson, 1986, p. 182.
80. Jackson, 1986, p. 184.
81. Jackson, 1986, p. 184.
82. Jackson, 1986, p. 179.
83. Jackson, 1986, p. 180.
84. Jackson, 1986, p. 174.
85. Jackson, 1986, pp. 174–175.
86. Jackson, 1986, pp. 176–177.

Chapter 4

1. Wilson, 1993.
2. Fenichel, 1945/1996.
3. Abraham, 1911.
4. Freud, 1917/1957.
5. E.g., Blashfield, 1982; Klerman, 1978.
6. Shorter, 1997, p. 100.
7. Shorter, 1997.
8. E.g., Grob, 1973; Scull, MacKenzie, & Hervey, 1997.
9. Shorter, 1992.
10. Grob, 1991b.
11. Dohrenwend & Dohrenwend, 1982.
12. Ghaemi, 2003.
13. Kraepelin, 1921/1976, p. 1.

14. Kraepelin, 1921/1976, p. 1.

15. Kraepelin, 1921/1976, p. 181.

16. Kraepelin, 1921/1976, p. 180.

17. Spitzer, 1982.

18. Kraepelin, 1907/1915, p. 68.

19. Kraepelin, 1904/1917, pp. 4–5.

20. Kraepelin, 1904/1917, pp. 199–200.

21. Kraepelin, 1904/1917, p. 7.

22. Kraepelin, 1904/1917, p. 65.

23. Jackson, 1986, p. 198.

24. Jackson, 1986, p. 198.

25. Jackson, 1986, p. 198.

26. Jackson, 1976, p. 201.

27. Grob, 1985.

28. Grob, 1991b.

29. APA, 1942, pp. 41–42.

30. APA, 1952.

31. Grob, 1991b.

32. APA, 1952, p. 25.

33. APA, 1952, pp. 33–34.

34. APA, 1968, p. 40.

35. Lewis, 1934.

36. Curran & Mallinson, 1941; Tredgold, 1941; Kendell, 1968.

37. E.g., Kiloh & Garside, 1963; Mendels & Cochrane, 1968; Eysenck, 1970; Paykel, 1971; Kiloh, Andrews, Neilson, & Bianchi, 1972; Klein, 1974; Akiskal, Bitar, Puzantian, Rosenthal, & Walker, et al., 1978.

38. E.g., Kiloh & Garside, 1963; Overall, Hollister, Johnson, & Pennington, 1966; Klein, 1974.

39. Akiskal et al., 1978.

40. Kiloh & Garside, 1963.

41. Overall et al., 1966; Hamilton & White, 1959; Paykel, 1971; Raskin & Crook, 1976.

42. Kiloh et al., 1972; Everitt, Gourlay, & Kendell, 1971.

43. E.g., Kiloh & Garside, 1963; Kendell, 1968.

44. Lewis, 1934.

45. Kadushin, 1969; Grob, 1991a; Lunbeck, 1994.

46. Akiskal et al., 1978, p. 757.

47. Andreason & Winokur, 1979.

48. Callahan & Berrios, 2005, p. 115.

49. Feighner et al., 1972.

50. Feighner et al., 1972, p. 57.

51. Woodruff, Goodwin, & Guze, 1974, p. 6.

52. Klerman, 1983; Spitzer, Williams, & Skodol, 1980.

53. Rosenthal, 1968, p. 32.

54. Mendels & Cochrane, 1968, p. 10; see also Mendels, 1968, p. 1353.

55. Lehmann, 1959, p. S3.

56. Woodruff, Goodwin, & Guze, 1974.
57. Woodruff, Goodwin, & Guze, 1974, p. 16.
58. Clayton, Halikas, & Maurice, 1971; 1972.
59. Goodwin & Guze, 1996.
60. Feighner, 1989.
61. Spitzer, Endicott, & Robins, 1978; Endicott & Spitzer, 1978.
62. Endicott & Spitzer, 1979.
63. Spitzer, Endicott, & Robins, 1978.
64. Spitzer et al., 1978.
65. Spitzer, Endicott, & Robins, 1975.
66. Spitzer et al., 1978.
67. Spitzer et al., 1978, p. 781; Spitzer et al., 1980, p. 154.
68. Klerman, 1983; Kendell, 1983; Wilson, 1993.
69. Spiegel, 2005.
70. Spitzer et al., 1975, p. 1190; Skodol & Spitzer, 1982.
71. Eysenck, Wakefield, & Friedman, 1983.
72. Szasz, 1961; Scheff, 1966.
73. Mayes & Horwitz, 2005.
74. Spitzer, 1978; Bayer & Spitzer, 1985.
75. Spitzer & Fleiss, 1974; Kirk & Kutchins, 1992.
76. Cooper et al., 1972, p. 100.
77. E.g., Temerlin, 1968.
78. Rosenhan, 1973, p. 250.
79. Spitzer, 1975.
80. Skodol & Spitzer, 1982; Spitzer & Fleiss, 1974.
81. Kirk & Kutchins, 1992.
82. Spitzer & Williams, 1988; Kirk & Kutchins, 1992, pp. 121–131.
83. Zimmerman, 1990, p. 974.
84. Clayton & Darvish, 1979.
85. Robert Spitzer, personal communication, December 13, 2005.
86. Woodruff et al., 1974.
87. Klein, 1974.
88. Healy, 2004.

Chapter 5

1. APA, 2000, p. 375.
2. APA, 2000, p. 356.
3. APA, 2000, p. 356.
4. Nesse, 2000.
5. Zimmerman, Chelminski, & Young, 2004.
6. APA, 2000, p. xxxi (italics added).
7. Wakefield, 1992.
8. APA, 2000, pp. 96–97.
9. APA, 2000, pp. 355–356.

10. APA, 2000, pp. 740–741.
11. APA, 2000, p. 679.
12. APA, 2000, p. 679.
13. APA, 2000, p. 683.
14. Medline search.
15. APA, 1994, pp. 720–721.
16. APA, 2000, p. 381.
17. APA, 2000, p. 5.
18. APA, 2000, p. 4.
19. Bayer & Spitzer, 1985.
20. Zimmerman & Spitzer, 1989.
21. Zimmerman, Coryell, & Pfohl, 1986; Zimmerman & Spitzer, 1989.

Chapter 6

1. Karp, 1996.
2. Grob, 1985.
3. Plunkett & Gordon, 1960.
4. Grob, 1991a, p. 13.
5. Appel & Beebe, 1946, p. 1471.
6. Grob, 1991a.
7. Grinker & Spiegel, 1945, p. 115.
8. Jones, 2000, 9.
9. Brill & Beebe, 1955; Shephard, 2000.
10. Grob, 1991a.
11. Menninger, 1948.
12. Herman, 1995.
13. Grinker & Spiegel, 1945.
14. E.g., Holmes & Rahe, 1967.
15. Grob, 1991a.
16. Menninger, 1948.
17. Grob, 1991a.
18. Srole et al., 1962/1978.
19. Leighton, Harding, Macklin, Macmillan, & Leighton, 1963.
20. Lapouse, 1967.
21. Dohrenwend & Dohrenwend, 1982.
22. APA, 1952, p. 133.
23. Murphy, 1986.
24. Srole et al., 1962/1978; Leighton et al., 1963; Plunkett & Gordon, 1960.
25. E.g., Langner, 1962; Macmillan, 1957.
26. Srole et al., 1962/1978, p. 197.
27. Leighton et al., 1963, p. 121.
28. Lapouse, 1967, p. 952.
29. Srole et al., 1962/1978, p. 478.
30. Dohrenwend & Dohrenwend, 1982.

31. Horwitz, 2002.
32. Bayer & Spitzer, 1985.
33. Robins & Regier, 1991.
34. Robins et al., 1984, p. 952.
35. Leaf, Myers, & McEvoy, 1991, p. 12.
36. Eaton & Kessler, 1985; Robins & Regier, 1991.
37. Kessler et al., 1994.
38. APA, 1987; Blazer et al., 1994.
39. Blazer et al., 1994.
40. Blazer et al., 1994; Kessler et al., 1994.
41. Weissman & Myers, 1978.
42. Robins et al., 1984.
43. Regier et al., 1998.
44. Karp, 1996, pp. 112–113.
45. Brugha, Bebbington, & Jenkins, 1999.
46. Wittchen, 1994; Wittchen, Ustun, & Kessler, 1999.
47. Wakefield, 1999.
48. Anthony et al., 1985; Helzer et al., 1985.
49. Wakefield, 1999.
50. E.g., Greenberg, Stiglin, Finkelstein, & Berndt, 1993; Hirschfeld et al., 1997; U.S. Department of Health and Human Services, 1999.
51. Frances, 1998; Kendler & Gardner, 1998; Lavretsky & Kumar, 2002.
52. APA, 1994, p. 350.
53. Coyne, 1994.
54. Kendler & Gardner, 1998.
55. Judd, Akiskal, & Paulus, 1997.
56. Coyne, 1994.
57. Kessler, Merikangas et al., 2003.
58. Kramer, 2005.
59. Wells et al., 1989.
60. Kessler, Zhao, Blazer, & Swartz, 1997; Mojtabai, 2001.
61. Kramer, 2005, p. 171.
62. Judd, Rapaport, Paulus, & Brown, 1994; Kessler et al., 1997.
63. Broadhead, Blazer, George, & Tse, 1990.
64. Judd et al., 1994.
65. Judd & Akiskal, 2000, p. 5.
66. Kramer, 2005.
67. Kendler & Gardner, 1998.
68. Judd, Paulus, Wells, & Rapaport, 1996.
69. Kessler et al., 1997; Mojtabai, 2001.
70. Kessler et al., 1997, p. 28.
71. Kessler, Merikangas, et al., 2003.
72. Judd et al., 1997.
73. Horwath et al., 1992.
74. Horwath et al., 1992, p. 821.
75. Kessler, Merikangas, et al., 2003.

76. Kessler, Merikangas, et al., 2003, p. 1121.
77. Judd et al., 1997.
78. Judd et al., 1994.
79. Kessler et al., 1997.
80. Lavretsky & Kumar, 2002.
81. Judd et al., 1994, p. 226.
82. Mirowsky & Ross, 1989.
83. Judd et al., 1994.
84. Eaton et al., 1997, p. 996.
85. Eaton, Neufeld, Chen, & Cai, 2000.
86. Lapouse, 1967, p. 952.
87. Wakefield & Spitzer, 2002.
88. Horvath et al., 1992; Kessler et al., 1997; Insel & Fenton, 2005.
89. Judd et al., 1997.
90. Broadhead et al., 1990.
91. Katon et al., 1995.
92. Eaton et al., 1997.
93. Grob, 1991a.
94. Mechanic, 2003.
95. Mechanic, 2003.
96. Coyne et al., 2000, p. 107.
97. Lapouse, 1967, p. 953.

Chapter 7

1. Santora & Carey, 2005; Spitzer, Kroenke, & Williams, 1999.
2. New Freedom Commission on Mental Health, 2003.
3. Kessler, Merikangas, et al., 2003.
4. U.S. Department of Health and Human Services (USDHHS), 1999.
5. Katon & Von Korff, 1990; Katon et al., 1997.
6. Donohue, Berndt, Rosenthal, Epstein, & Frank, 2004.
7. Pescosolido et al., 2000.
8. Burnam & Wells, 1990.
9. Burnam & Wells, 1990.
10. Mulrow et al., 1995.
11. Henkel et al., 2004.
12. Hough, Landsverk, & Jacobson, 1990.
13. Henkel et al., 2004.
14. Health United States, 2003.
15. Katon et al., 1997.
16. Wells et al., 1989; Katon et al., 1997.
17. Kessler, Merikangas, et al., 2003.
18. Wells, Schoenbaum, Unutzer, Lagomasino, & Rubenstein, 1999; Katon & Schulberg, 1992; Wang et al., 2005.

19. Hirschfeld et al., 1997.

20. Schulberg et al., 1985; Katon et al., 1997; Lowe, Spitzer, Grafe, Kroenke, Quenter, Zipfel, et al., 2004; Schwenk, Klinkman, & Coyne, 1998; Wells et al., 1989.

21. Hirschfeld et al., 1997; Wells et al., 1999; Kessler et al., 2003.

22. Katon et al., 1997.

23. Cleary, 1990; Spitzer et al., 1999.

24. Regier et al., 1988.

25. Attkisson & Zich, 1990.

26. Schulberg, 1990, p. 276.

27. Schulberg et al., 1985; Hough et al., 1990; Cleary, 1990.

28. Attkisson & Zich, 1990.

29. Hough et al., 1990, p. 151.

30. E.g., Tufts Health Plan, 2005; U.S. Preventive Services Task Force, 2002.

31. Sartorius, 1997.

32. U.S. Preventive Services Task Force, 2002.

33. WHO, 1998; Henkel et al., 2003.

34. Wells et al., 1989; Whooley, Avins, Miranda, & Browner, 1997; Henkel et al., 2004.

35. Coyne, Fechner-Bates, & Schwenk, 1994.

36. Rost et al., 2000.

37. Spitzer et al., 1994.

38. Spitzer et al., 1994.

39. Spitzer et al., 1999; Kroenke, Spitzer, & Williams, 2001.

40. Health United States, 2003, p. 235, Table 70.

41. Spitzer et al., 1999.

42. Russell, 1994.

43. Callahan & Berrios, 2005.

44. Schwenk, Coyne, & Fechner-Bates, 1996.

45. Edlund, Unutzer, & Wells, 2004.

46. Edlund et al., 2004.

47. Williams et al., 1999.

48. Olfson, Marcus, Druss, Elinson, et al., 2002.

49. Coyne et al., 2000; Moncrieff, Wessely, & Hardy, 2004.

50. Katon, Unutzer, & Simon, 2004, p. 1154.

51. Olfson, Marcus, Druse, Elinson, Tanielian, & Pincus, 2002.

52. Rost et al., 2001.

53. Pyne et al., 2004.

54. Coyne et al., 2000.

55. Katon et al., 2001; Rost, Nutting, Smith, Werner, & Duan, 2001; Pyne et al., 2004.

56. Katon et al., 2004.

57. Katon et al., 1997; Coyne et al., 2000.

58. Coyne, Klinkman, Gallo, & Schwenk, 1997.

59. Lewinsohn, Rohde, Seeley, Klein, & Gotlib, 2000.

60. Shugart & Lopez, 2002.

61. New Freedom Commission on Mental Health, 2003.

62. Peterson et al., 1993, p. 162.

63. New Freedom Commission on Mental Health, 2003.

64. Pringle, 2005.

65. Roberts, Attkisson, & Rosenblatt, 1998.

66. Lewinsohn, Hops, Roberts, Seeley, & Andrews, 1993.

67. Lewinsohn, Shankman, Gau, & Klein, 2004.

68. Petersen et al., 1993, p. 164.

69. Larson, Clore, & Wood, 1999; Monroe, Rohde, Seeley, & Lewinsohn, 1999.

70. Joyner & Udry, 2000.

71. Coyne, 1994, p. 34.

72. Roberts et al., 1990.

73. Rushton, Forcier, & Schectman, 2002.

74. Lucas, 2001, p. 448.

75. Pringle, 2005.

76. Shaffer et al., 2004.

77. Shaffer et al., 2004, p. 77.

78. Jensen & Weisz, 2002; Lewczyk et al., 2003.

79. Shaffer et al., 2004, p. 77.

80. Columbia University TeenScreen Program, 2003.

81. Shaffer et al., 2004, p. 78.

82. Fisher & Fisher, 1996; Vitiello & Swedo, 2004.

83. Ambrosini, 2000.

84. Treatment for Adolescents with Depression Study Team, 2004.

85. U.S. Preventive Services Task Force, 2002.

86. Healy, 2004.

87. Keller et al., 2001; Vitiello & Swedo, 2004; Whittington et al., 2004; Treatment for Adolescents with Depression Study Team, 2004.

88. Davey & Harris, 2005.

Chapter 8

1. Luhrmann, 2000; Blazer, 2005.

2. Bouchard, Lykken, McGue, Segal, & Tellegen, 1990; Alford, Funck, & Hibbing, 2005.

3. Archer, 1999.

4. Mayberg et al., 1999.

5. Mayberg et al., 1999

6. Kendler, Heath, Martin, & Eaves, 1986; Kendler et al., 1995; McGuffin, Katz, & Rutherford, 1991; Sullivan, Neale, & Kendler, 2000.

7. Cadoret, 1978.

8. Cadoret, O'Gorman, Heywood, & Troughton, 1985; von Knorring, Cloninger, Bohman, & Sigvardsson, 1983.

9. Sullivan et al., 2000.

10. Bouchard et al., 1990; DiLalla, Carey, Gottesman, & Bouchard, 1996; Bouchard & Loehlin, 2001.

11. Schildkraut, 1965.

12. Lacasse & Leo, 2005.

13. Healy, 1997, p. 156.

14. Schildkraut, 1965, p. 509.

15. Schidkraut, 1965, p. 517.

16. Valenstein, 1998, p. 99.

17. Valenstein, 1998, p. 101.

18. Schildkraut, 1965.

19. Valenstein, 1998; Lacasse & Leo, 2005.

20. McGuire, Raleigh, & Johnson, 1983; Raleigh, McGuire, Brammer, & Yuwiler, 1984.

21. Engh et al., 2006.

22. Gold, Goodwin, & Chrousos, 1988.

23. Anisman & Zacharko, 1992.

24. Valenstein, 1998, p. 135.

25. Sadock & Sadock, 2003.

26. Caspi et al., 2003.

27. Vedantam, 2003, p. A1.

28. Holden, 2003, p. 291.

29. Horwitz, 2005.

30. Monroe & Simons, 1991.

31. French, Old, & Healy, 2001.

32. Turner, 2003.

33. Caspi et al., 2003, p. 389.

34. Kendler et al., 2005; Eley et al., 2004; Gillespie et al., 2004; Surtees et al., 2006.

35. Mayberg et al., 1999.

36. Sapolsky, 2001.

37. Davidson, 2003.

38. Everdell, 1997, p. 131.

39. Davidson, 2003.

40. Rajkowska et al., 1999.

41. Kramer, 2005, 61.

42. Videbech & Ravnkilde, 2004.

43. Cotter, Mackay, Landau, Kerwin, & Everall, 2001.

44. Liotti, Mayberg, McGinnis, Brennan, & Jerabek, 2002.

45. Van Elst, Ebert, & Trimble, 2001; Davidson, 2003.

46. Kramer, 2005.

47. Sapolsky, 2001; Schatzberg, 2002; Davidson, 2003.

48. Rajkowska et al., 1999.

49. Rajkowska et al., 1999; Liotti et al., 2002.

50. Kramer, 2005, p. 7.

51. Kendler & Gardner, 1998.

52. Kramer, 2005, p. 171.

53. Valenstein, 1998.
54. Mayberg et al., 1999.
55. Mayberg et al., 1999, p. 679.

Chapter 9

1. Jackson, 1986.
2. MacDonald, 1983, p. 190.
3. Shorter, 1997.
4. Shorter, 1997, p. 316.
5. Grob, 1991a, p. 149; Shorter, 1997, p. 316.
6. Parry, Balter, Mellinger, Cisin, & Manheimer, 1973; Smith, 1985, pp. 46–47.
7. Shapiro & Baron, 1961; Raynes, 1979; Cooperstock & Leonard, 1979.
8. Cooperstock, 1978; Smith, 1985; Olfson & Klerman, 1993.
9. Jagger & Richards, 1967.
10. Metzl, 2003.
11. Healy, 1997, p. 226.
12. Gardner, 1971.
13. Smith, 1985, p. 179.
14. Smith, 1985, p. 187.
15. Smith, 1985, p. 189.
16. Smith, 1985, p. 127.
17. Shorter, 1997, p. 319.
18. Smith, 1985, p. 210.
19. Smith, 1985, p. 81.
20. Smith, 1985, pp. 31–32; Olfson & Klerman, 1993.
21. Smith, 1985, p. 32.
22. Healy, 1997.
23. Horwitz, 2002.
24. Merikangas, Prusoff, & Weissman, 1988.
25. Horwitz, 2002.
26. Healy, 1991; Olfson, Marcus, Druss, Elinson, et al., 2002.
27. Shorter, 1997.
28. Kramer, 1993, p. 64.
29. Kramer, 1993.
30. Healy, 1991.
31. Zuvekas, 2005.
32. Kramer, 1993, p. 176.
33. Shorter, 1997, p. 323.
34. Pincus et al., 1998.
35. Elliott, 2004a; Squier, 2004.
36. Mann, 2005.
37. Metzl, 2003.
38. Mechanic, 1998.

39. Wang et al., 2005.
40. Luhrmann, 2000.
41. Cutler, 2004.
42. Cutler, 2004.
43. Olfson, Marcus, & Pincus, 1999, p. 451.
44. Olfson, Marcus, Druss, & Pincus, 2002; Zuvekas, 2005.
45. Crystal, Sambamoorthi, Walkup, & Akincigil, 2003.
46. Zuvekas, 2005.
47. Conrad, 2005.
48. Shorter, 1997, p. 314.
49. Elliott, 2003, p. 102.
50. Olfson, Marcus, Druss, & Pincus, 2002.
51. Kessler et al., 2005.
52. Kessler et al., 2005, p. 2521.
53. Donohue et al., 2004.
54. Kravitz et al., 2005.
55. Olfson, Marcus, Druss, Elinson, et al., 2002.
56. Zuvekas, 2005.
57. Crystal et al., 2003; Thomas, Conrad, Casler, & Goodman, 2006.
58. Zuvekas, 2005.
59. Elliott, 2004a, p. 5.
60. Croghan et al., 2003.
61. Shorter, 1997.
62. Clarke, Shim, Mamo, Fosket, & Fishman, 2003.
63. Healy, 2004.
64. Knutson et al., 1998; Kramer, 1993.
65. Zisook, Schuchter, Pedrelli, Sable, & Deaciuc, 2001.
66. Kramer, 1993, p. 247.
67. USDHHS, 1999, p. 262.
68. Olfson & Klerman, 1993.
69. Greenberg et al., 1993; Frank, Busch, & Berndt, 1998.
70. Kessler, Merikangas, et al., 2003; Kramer, 2005.
71. Hirschfeld et al., 1997.
72. Hirschfeld et al., 1997.
73. Klerman as quoted in Smith, 1985, p. 89.
74. Kramer, 1993.
75. Dworkin, 2001.
76. Elliott, 2004b, p. 129.
77. Conrad, 1992.
78. Furedi, 2004.
79. Smith, 1985, p. 73.
80. Furedi, 2004.
81. Glenmullen, 2000.
82. Healy, 2004.
83. Mann, 2005, p. 1827.
84. Moncrieff & Kirsch, 2005, p. 156.

85. Moncrieff & Kirsch, 2005, p. 158.
86. USDHHS, 1999, p. 262.
87. Kessler et al., 2005, p. 2520.
88. Moncrieff et al., 2004.
89. Hamburg, 2000.
90. Trivedi et al., 2006.
91. Conrad, 2005.
92. Cutler, 2004.
93. Smith, 1985; Elliott, 2003, xv–xvi.
94. Conrad, 2007.

Chapter 10

1. Benedict, 1934.
2. Kirmayer & Young, 1999.
3. Kirmayer, 1994, p. 19.
4. Kleinman, 1988.
5. Kirmayer, 1994; Kirmayer & Young, 1999.
6. Obeyesekere, 1985.
7. Obeyesekere, 1985, p. 136, italics in original.
8. Lutz, 1985, p. 85.
9. Lutz, 1985, p. 86.
10. Lutz, 1985, p. 92.
11. Kleinman, 1977, p. 3.
12. Kleinman, 1988.
13. Kleinman, 1986.
14. Kleinman, 1987, p. 450.
15. Cheung, 1982.
16. Cheung, 1982.
17. Kleinman, 1986.
18. Pearlin, 1989; Aneshensel, 1992.
19. E.g. Aneshensel & Phelan, 1999; Horwitz & Scheid, 1999.
20. Horwitz, 2007.
21. Aneshensel, 1992; McLeod & Nonnemaker, 1999; Mirowsky & Ross, 2003; Turner & Lloyd, 1999; Turner, Wheaton & Lloyd, 1995.
22. E.g., Dohrenwend et al., 1992; Ritsher, Warner, Johnson, & Dohrenwend, 2001; Johnson, Cohen, Dohrenwend, Link, & Brook, 1999; Lorant et al., 2003.
23. Holmes & Rahe, 1967.
24. Radloff, 1977.
25. Nesse, 2000.
26. Carr, 1997.
27. McEwan, Costello, & Taylor, 1987.
28. Turner & Lloyd, 1999; Turner, 2003; Turner & Avison, 2003.
29. Pearlin, 1999.

30. Radloff, 1977; Radloff & Locke, 1986.

31. Radloff, 1977.

32. Roberts, Andrews, Lewinsohn, & Hops, 1990; Roberts, Lewinsohn, & Seeley, 1991; Roberts, Roberts, & Chen, 1997.

33. Roberts et al., 1990.

34. Roberts et al., 1990.

35. Rushton et al., 2002.

36. Coyne, 1994.

37. E.g., Mollica, Poole, & Tor, 1998; Mollica et al., 1999; Marshall et al., 2005; Dohrenwend, 2000; Schwartz, Dohrenwend, & Levav, 1994.

38. Seligman, 1975; Sapolsky, 1998.

39. APA, 1994, p. xxi.

40. Price, Sloman, Gardner, Gilbert, & Rohde, 1994; Bowlby, 1980; Nesse, 2000.

41. Brown, 1993.

42. Brown, 2002.

43. Brown, Craig & Harris, 1985, p. 616.

44. Brown, 2002.

45. Brown & Harris, 1978.

46. Brown, Bifulco & Harris, 1987; Brown, 1998.

47. Brown, Harris & Hepworth, 1995.

48. Brown, 2002.

49. Brown et al., 1987, p. 34.

50. Brown et al., 1995.

51. Brown, Adler, & Bifulco, 1988.

52. Brown, 1998, p. 368.

53. Brown, 2002.

54. Brown, 1998, p. 367.

55. Brown, 1998, p. 366.

56. Brown, 1998, p. 361.

57. Brown, Harris, Hepworth, & Robinson, 1994.

58. Brown et al., 1995.

59. Brown et al., 1985.

60. Brown et al., 1985, p. 620.

61. Brown et al., 1988, p. 492.

Chapter 11

1. Foucault, 1965, 1979.

2. Friedson, 1970; Abbott, 1988; Conrad, 2004.

3. Horwitz, 2002.

4. Kirk, 1999.

5. Murray & Lopez, 1996.

6. Kramer, 2005, p. 155, p. 153.

7. Blazer, 2005, p. 31; Spijker, deGraaf, Bijl, Beekman, Ormel, & Nolen, 2003.

8. Valenstein, 1998.

9. Donohue et al., 2004.

10. Karp, 1996.

11. E.g., Campbell-Sills & Stein, 2005; Richters & Hinshaw, 1999.

12. Lilienfeld & Marino, 1999, p. 401.

13. Kirmayer & Young, 1999.

14. Kirmayer & Young, 1999, p. 450.

15. Lilienfeld & Moreno, 1995; Richters & Hinshaw, 1999.

16. Cosmides & Tooby, 1999.

17. Gould & Lewontin, 1979.

18. Kramer, 2005.

19. Murphy & Woolfolk, 2001.

20. Archer, 1999.

21. Keller & Nesse, 2005.

22. Sadler, 1999, p. 436.

23. Cosmides & Tooby, 1999.

24. APA, 2000, p. 356.

25. Langner, 1962.

26. Brown, 2002.

27. Almeida, Wethington, & Kessler, 2002; Coyne, Thompson, & Pepper, 2004; Wethington & Serido, 2004.

28. See, however, Wakefield, Schmitz, First, & Horwitz, 2007.

References

Abbott, A. (1988). The system of the professions. Chicago: University of Chicago Press.

Abraham, K. (1953). Notes on the psycho-analytical investigation and treatment of manic-depressive insanity and allied conditions. In *Selected papers of Karl Abraham* (D. Bryan & A. Strachey, Trans; pp. 137–156). London: Hogarth Press. (Original work published 1911)

Akiskal, H. S., Bitar, A. H., Puzantian, V. R., Rosenthal, T. L., & Walker, P.W. (1978). The nosological status of neurotic depression. *Archives of General Psychiatry, 35,* 756–766.

Alford, J. R., Funck, C. L., & Hibbing, J. R. (2005). Are political orientations genetically transmitted? *American Political Science Review, 99,* 153–167.

Almeida, D. M., Wethington, E., & Kessler, R. C. (2002). The daily inventory of stressful events: An interview-based approach for measuring daily stressors. *Assessment, 9,* 41–55.

Ambrosini, P. (2000). A review of pharmacotherapy of major depression in children and adolescents. *Psychiatric Services, 51,* 627–633.

American Psychiatric Association. (1942). *Statistical manual for the use of hospitals for mental diseases.* Utica, NY: State Hospitals Press.

American Psychiatric Association. (1952). *Diagnostic and statistical manual of mental disorders.* Washington, DC: Author.

American Psychiatric Association. (1968). *Diagnostic and statistical manual of mental disorders* (2nd ed.). Washington, DC: Author.

American Psychiatric Association. (1980). *Diagnostic and statistical manual of mental disorders* (3rd ed.). Washington, DC: Author.

American Psychiatric Association. (1987). *Diagnostic and statistical manual of mental disorders* (3rd ed., revised). Washington, DC: Author.

American Psychiatric Association. (1994). *Diagnostic and statistical manual of mental disorders* (4th ed.). Washington, DC: Author.

American Psychiatric Association. (2000). *Diagnostic and statistical manual of mental disorders* (4th ed., text rev.). Washington, DC: Author.

Andreason, N. C., & Winokur, G. (1979). Newer experimental methods for classifying depression. *Archives of General Psychiatry, 36,* 447–452.

Aneshensel, C. S. (1992). Social stress: Theory and research. *Annual Review of Sociology, 18*, 15–38.

Aneshensel, C. S., Botticello, A. L., & Yamamoto-Mitani, N. (2004). When caregiving ends: The course of depressive symptoms after bereavement. *Journal of Health and Social Behavior, 45*, 422–441.

Aneshensel, C. S., & Phelan, J. C. (Eds.). (1999). *Handbook of the sociology of mental health*. New York: Kluwer/Plenum.

Angel, R. J., Frisco, M., Angel, J. L., & Chiriboga, D. (2003). Financial strain and health among elderly Mexican-origin individuals. *Journal of Health and Social Behavior, 44*, 536–551.

Anisman, H., & Zacharko, R. M. (1992). Depression as a consequence of inadequate neurochemical adaptation in response to stressors. *British Journal of Psychiatry, 160*, 36–43.

Anthony, J. C., Folstein, M. F., Romanoski, A. J., von Korff, M. R., Nestadt, G. R., Chahal, R., et. al. (1985). Comparison of lay diagnostic interview schedule and a standardized psychiatric diagnosis. *Archives of General Psychiatry, 42*, 667–675.

Appel, J. W., & Beebe, G. W. (1946). Preventive psychiatry. *Journal of the American Medical Association, 131*, 1469–1475.

Archer, J. (1989). Why help friends when you can help sisters and brothers? *Behavioral and Brain Sciences, 12*, 519–520.

Archer, J. (1999). *The nature of grief: The evolution and psychology of reactions to loss*. New York: Routledge.

Aristotle. (1931). Problemata. In J. A. Smith & W. D. Ross (Eds.), *The works of Aristotle translated into English: Vol. 7*. Oxford, UK: Clarendon Press.

Aristotle. (2000). Brilliance and melancholy. In J. Radden (Ed.), *The nature of melancholy: From Aristotle to Kristeva* (pp. 55–60). New York: Oxford University Press.

Attkisson, C. C., & Zich, J. M. (Eds.). (1990). *Depression in primary care: Screening and detection*. New York: Routledge.

Auden, W. H. (1994). *The age of anxiety*. Cutchoque, NY: Buccaneer Books. (Original work published 1947)

Avicenna. (2000). Black bile and melancholia. In J. Radden (Ed.), *The nature of melancholy: From Aristotle to Kristeva* (pp. 75–78). New York: Oxford University Press.

Bayer, R., & Spitzer, R. L. (1985). Neurosis, psychodynamics, and *DSM-III:* History of the controversy. *Archives of General Psychiatry, 42*,187–196.

Beck, A. T. (1967). *Depression: Causes and treatment*. Philadelphia: University of Pennsylvania Press.

Benedict, R. (1934). Anthropology and the abnormal. *Journal of General Psychology, 10*, 59–80.

Berman, C. M., Rasmussen, K. L. R., & Suomi, S. J. (1994). Responses of free-ranging rhesus monkeys to a natural form of social separation. *Child Development, 65*, 1028–1041.

Blazer, D. G. (2005). *The age of melancholy: Major depression and its social origins*. New York: Routledge.

Blazer, D. G., Kessler, R. C., McGonagle, K. A., & Swartz, M. S. (1994). The prevalence and distribution of major depression in a national community sample: The National Comorbidity Survey. *American Journal of Psychiatry, 151*, 979–986.

Blashfield, R. K. (1982). Feighner et al., invisible colleges, and the Matthew effect. *Schizophrenia Bulletin, 8,* 1–8.

Bloom, B. L., Asher, S. J., & White, S. W. (1978). Marital disruption as a stressor: A review and analysis. *Psychological Bulletin, 85,* 867–894.

Bonanno, G. A., & Kaltman, S. (2001). The varieties of grief experience. *Clinical Psychology Review, 21,* 705–734.

Bonanno, G. A., Wortman, C. B., Lehman, D. R., Tweed, R. G., Haring, M., Sonnega, J., et al. (2002). Resilience to loss and chronic grief: A prospective study from preloss to 18 months postloss. *Journal of Personality and Social Psychology, 83,* 1150–1164.

Booth, A., & Amato, P. (1991). Divorce and psychological stress. *Journal of Health and Social Behavior, 32,* 396–407.

Bouchard, T. J., & Loehlin, J. C. (2001). Genes, evolution, and personality. *Behavior Genetics, 31,* 243–273.

Bouchard, T. J., Lykken, D. T., McGue, M., Segal, N. O., & Tellegen, A. (1990). Sources of human psychological differences: The Minnesota study of identical twins reared apart. *Science, 250,* 223–228.

Bowlby, J. (1973). *Attachment and loss: Vol. 2. Separation: Anxiety and anger.* New York: Basic Books.

Bowlby, J. (1980). *Attachment and loss: Vol. 3. Loss: Sadness and depression.* London: Hogarth Press.

Bowlby, J. (1982). *Attachment and loss: Vol 1. Attachment.* New York: Basic Books. (Original work published 1969)

Bright, T. (2000). Melancholy. In J. Radden (Ed.), *The nature of melancholy: From Aristotle to Kristeva* (pp. 119–128). New York: Oxford University Press.

Brill, N. Q., & Beebe, G. W. (1955). *A follow-up study of war neuroses.* Washington, DC: U.S. Veterans Administration.

Broadhead, J., & Abas, M. (1998). Life events, difficulties, and depression amongst women in an urban setting in Zimbabwe. *Psychological Medicine, 28,* 39–50.

Broadhead, W. E., Blazer, D. G., George, L. K., & Tse, C. K. (1990). Depression, disability days, and days lost from work in a prospective epidemiologic survey. *Journal of the American Medical Association, 264,* 2524–2528.

Brooke, J. (2003, August 4). Indicted Hyundai executive plunges to death in Seoul. *The New York Times,* p. A6.

Brown, G. W. (1993). Life events and affective disorder: Replications and limitations. *Psychosomatic Medicine, 55,* 248–259.

Brown, G. W. (1998). Loss and depressive disorders. In B. P. Dohrenwend (Ed.), *Adversity, stress, and psychopathology* (pp. 358–370). New York: Oxford University Press.

Brown, G. W. (2002). Social roles, context and evolution in the origins of depression. *Journal of Health and Social Behavior, 43,* 255–276.

Brown, G. W., Adler, Z., & Bifulco, A. (1988). Life events, difficulties and recovery from chronic depression. *British Journal of Psychiatry, 152,* 487–498.

Brown, G. W., Bifulco, A., & Harris, T. O. (1987). Life events, vulnerability and onset of depression: Some refinements. *British Journal of Psychiatry, 150,* 30–42.

Brown, G. W., Craig, T. K. J., & Harris, T. O. (1985). Depression: Distress or disease? Some epidemiological considerations. *British Journal of Psychiatry, 147,* 612–622.

Brown, G. W., & Harris, T. O. (1978). *The social origins of depression.* London: Tavistock.

Brown, G. W., Harris, T. O., & Hepworth, C. (1995). Loss, humiliation, and entrapment among women developing depression. *Psychological Medicine, 25,* 7–21.

Brown, G. W., Harris, T. O., Hepworth, C., & Robinson, R. (1994). Clinical and psychosocial origins of chronic depressive episodes: II. A patient enquiry. *British Journal of Psychiatry, 165,* 457–465.

Bruce, M. L. (1998). Divorce and psychopathology. In B. P. Dohrenwend (Ed.), *Adversity, stress, and psychopathology* (pp. 219–232). New York: Oxford University Press.

Bruce, M. L., Kim, K., Leaf, P. J., & Jacobs, S. (1990). Depressive episodes and dysphoria resulting from conjugal bereavement in a prospective community sample. *American Journal of Psychiatry, 157,* 608–611.

Brugha, T. S., Bebbington, P. E., & Jenkins, R. (1999). A difference that matters: Comparisons of structured and semi-structured psychiatric diagnostic interviews in the general population. *Psychological Medicine, 29,* 1013–1020.

Burnam, M. A., & Wells, K. B. (1991). Use of a two-stage procedure to identify depression: The Medical Outcomes Study. In C. Attkisson & J. Zich (Eds.), *Depression in primary care: Screening and detection* (pp. 98–116). New York: Routledge.

Burton, R. (1948). *The anatomy of melancholy* (F. Dell & P. Jordon-Smith, Eds.). New York: Tudor. (Original work published 1621)

Burton, R. (2000). *The anatomy of melancholy.* In J. Radden (Ed.), *The nature of melancholy: From Aristotle to Kristeva* (pp. 131–155). New York: Oxford University Press. (Original work published 1621)

Burton, R. (2001). *The anatomy of melancholy.* New York: New York Review Books. (Original work published 1621)

Buss, D. M. (1999). *Evolutionary psychology: The new science of mind.* Boston: Allyn & Bacon.

Cadoret, R. J. (1978). Evidence for genetic inheritance of primary affective disorder in adoptees. *American Journal of Psychiatry, 135,* 463–466.

Cadoret, R. J., O'Gorman, T. W., Heywood, E., & Troughton, E. (1985). Genetic and environmental factors in major depression. *Journal of Affective Disorders, 9,* 155–164.

Callahan, C., & Berrios, G. E. (2005). *Reinventing depression: A history of the treatment of depression in primary care 1940–2004.* New York: Oxford University Press.

Campbell-Sills, L., & Stein, M. B. (2005). Justifying the diagnostic status of social phobia: A reply to Wakefield and others. *Canadian Journal of Psychiatry, 50,* 320–323.

Carr, D. S. (1997). The fulfillment of career dreams at midlife: Does it matter for women's mental health? *Journal of Health and Social Behavior, 38,* 331–344.

Carr, D. S. (2004). Gender, pre-loss marital dependence and older adults' adjustment to widowhood. *Journal of Marriage and the Family, 66,* 220–235.

Carr, D. S., House, J. S., Kessler, R. C., Nesse, R. M., Sonnega, J., & Wortman, C. S. (2000). Marital quality and psychological adjustment to widowhood among older adults: A longitudinal analysis. *Journal of Gerontology: Social Sciences, 55B*(4), S197–S207.

Carr, D. S., House, J. S., Wortman, C. S., Nesse, R. M., & Kessler, R. C. (2001). Psychological adjustment to sudden and anticipated spousal death among the older widowed. *Journal of Gerontology: Social Sciences, 56B,* S237–S248.

Carr, J. E. & Vitaliano, P. P. (1985). The theoretical implications of converging research on depression and the culture-bound syndromes. In A. Kleinman & B. Good (Eds.), *Culture and depression,* (pp. 244–266). Berkeley: University of California Press.

Caspi, A., Sugden, K., Moffitt, T. E., Taylor, A., Craig, I. W., Harrington, H., et al. (2003). Influence of life stress on depression: Moderation by a polymorphism in the 5-HTT gene. *Science, 301,* 386–389.

Cheung, F. M. (1982). Psychological symptoms among Chinese in urban Hong Kong. *Social Science and Medicine, 16,* 1339–1344.

Clarke, A. E., Shim, J. K., Mamo, L., Fosket, J. R., & Fishman, J. R. (2003). Biomedicalization: Technoscientific transformations of health, illness, and U.S. biomedicine. *American Sociological Review, 68,* 161–195.

Clayton, P. J. (1982). Bereavement. In E. S. Paykel (Ed.), *Handbook of affective disorders* (pp. 15–46). London: Churchill Livingstone.

Clayton, P. J. (1998). The model of stress: The bereavement reaction. In B. P. Dohrenwend (Ed.), *Adversity, stress, and psychopathology* (pp. 96–110). New York: Oxford University Press.

Clayton, P. J., & Darvish, H. S. (1979). Course of depressive symptoms following the stress of bereavement. In J. E. Barrett, R. M. Rose, & G. Klerman (Eds.), *Stress and mental disorder* (pp. 121–136). New York: Raven Press.

Clayton, P. J., Halikas, J. A., & Maurice, W. L. (1971). The bereavement of the widowed. *Diseases of the Nervous System, 32,* 597–604.

Clayton, P. J., Halikas, J. A., & Maurice, W. L. (1972). The depression of widowhood. *British Journal of Psychiatry, 120,* 71–78.

Cleary, P. D. (1990). Methodological issues associated with the use of depression screening scales in primary care settings. In C. Attkisson & J. Zich (Eds.), *Depression in primary care: Screening and detection* (pp. 169–180). New York: Routledge.

Clymer, A. (2002, May 19). Emotional ups and downs after 9/11 traced in report. *The New York Times,* A35.

Cobb, S., & Kasl, S. (1977). *Termination: The consequences of job loss.* Cincinnati, OH: National Institute of Occupational Safety and Health.

Coleridge, S. T. (1986). Dejection: An ode. In M. H. Abrams, E. T. Donaldson, A. David, H. Smith, B. K. Lewalski, R. M. Adams, et al. (Eds.), *Norton anthology of English literature* (5th ed., pp. 374–380). New York: Norton. (Original work published 1805)

Columbia University TeenScreen Program. (2003). *Getting started guide.* New York: Author.

Conrad, P. (1992). Medicalization and social control. *Annual Review of Sociology, 18,* 209–232.

Conrad, P. (2005). The shifting engines of medicalization. *Journal of Health and Social Behavior, 46,* 3–14.

Conrad, P. (2007). *The medicalization of society.* Baltimore: Johns Hopkins University Press.

Cooper, J., Rendell, R., Burland, B., Sharpe, L., Copeland, J., & Simon, R. (1972). *Psychiatric diagnosis in New York and London.* London: Oxford University Press.

Cooperstock, R. (1978). Sex differences in psychotropic drug use. *Social Science and Medicine, 12B,*179–186.

Cooperstock, R., & Leonard, H. (1979). Some social meanings of tranquillizer use. *Sociology of Health and Illness, 1,* 331–347.

Cosmides, L., & Tooby, J. (1999). Toward an evolutionary taxonomy of treatable conditions. *Journal of Abnormal Psychology, 108,* 453–464.

Costello, E. J., Compton, S. N., Keeler, G., & Angold, A. (2003). Relationships between poverty and psychopathology: A natural experiment. *Journal of the American Medical Association, 290,* 2023–2029.

Cotter, D., Mackay, D., Landau, S., Kerwin, R., & Everall, I. (2001). Reduced glial cell density and neuronal size in the anterior cingulate cortex in major depressive disorder. *Archives of General Psychiatry, 58,* 545–553.

Coyne, J. C. (1976). Depression and the response of others. *Journal of Abnormal Psychology, 85,* 186–193.

Coyne, J. C. (1992). A critique of cognitions as causal entities with particular reference to depression. *Cognitive Therapy and Research, 6,* 3–13.

Coyne, J. C. (1994). Self-reported distress: Analog or ersatz depression? *Psychological Bulletin, 116,* 29–45.

Coyne, J. C., Fechner-Bates, S., & Schwenk, T. L. (1994). Prevalence, nature, and comorbidity of depressive disorders in primary care. *General Hospital Psychiatry, 16,* 267–276.

Coyne, J. C., Klinkman, M. S., Gallo, S. M., & Schwenk, T. L. (1997). Short-term outcomes of detected and undetected depressed primary care patients and depressed psychiatric patients. *General Hospital Psychiatry, 19,* 333–343.

Coyne, J. C., Thompson, R., Palmer, S. C., Kagee, A., & Maunsell, E. (2000). Should we screen for depression? Caveats and potential pitfalls. *Applied and Preventive Psychology, 9,* 101–121.

Coyne, J. C., Thompson, R., & Pepper, C. M. (2004). The role of life events in depression in primary medical care versus psychiatric settings. *Journal of Affective Disorders, 82,* 353–361.

Croghan, T. W. (2001). The controversy over increasing spending for antidepressants. *Health Affairs, 20,* 129–135.

Croghan, T. W., Tomlin, M., Pescosolido, B. A., Schnittker, J., Martin, J., Lubell, K., et al. (2003). American attitudes toward and willingness to use psychiatric medications. *Journal of Nervous and Mental Disease, 191,* 166–174.

Crystal, S., Sambamoorthi, U., Walkup, J. T., & Akincigil, A. (2003). Diagnosis and treatment of depression in the elderly Medicare population: Predictors, disparities, and trends. *Journal of the American Geriatric Society, 51,* 1718–1728.

Cuisinier, M., Janssen, H., deGraauw, C., Bakker, S., & Hoogduin, C. (1996). Pregnancy following miscarriage: Course of grief and some determining factors. *Journal of Psychosomatic Obstetrics and Gynecology, 17,* 168–174.

Curran, D., & Mallinson, W. P. (1941). Depressive states in war. *British Medical Journal, 1,* 305–309.

Cutler, D. M. (2004). *Your money or your life: Strong medicine for America's health care system.* New York: Oxford University Press.

Darwin, C. R. (1998). *The expression of the emotions in man and animals.* London: HarperCollins. (Original work published 1872)

Davey, M., & Harris, G. (2005, March 26). Family wonders if Prozac prompted school shootings. *The New York Times,* p. A7.

Davidson, R. J. (2003). Darwin and the neural bases of emotion and affective style. *Annals of the New York Academy of Sciences, 1000,* 316–336.

Dearing, E., Taylor, B. A., & McCartney, K. (2005). Implications of family income dynamics for women's depressive symptoms three years after childbirth. *American Journal of Public Health, 94,* 1372–1377.

De Fleury, M. (1900). *Medicine and the mind* (S. B. Collins, Trans.). London: Downey.

Desjarlais, R., Eisenberg, L., Good, B., & Kleinman, A. (1995). *World mental health: Problems and priorities in low-income countries.* New York: Oxford University Press.

DeVries, B., Davis, C. G., Wortman, C. B., & Lehman, D. R. (1997). Long-term psychological and somatic consequences of later life parental bereavement. *Omega, 35,* 97–117.

Dew, M. A., Bromet, E. J., & Penkower, L. (1992). Mental health effects of job loss in women. *Psychological Medicine, 22,* 751–764.

Dew, M. A., Bromet, E. J., & Schulberg, H. C. (1987). A comparative analysis of two community stressors: Long-term mental health effects. *American Journal of Community Psychology, 15,* 167–184.

DiLalla, D. L., Carey, G., Gottesman, I. I., & Bouchard, T. J. (1996). Heritabilility of MMPI personality indicators of psychopathology in twins reared apart. *Journal of Abnormal Psychology, 105,* 491–499.

Dobbs, D. (2006, April 2). A depression switch? *The New York Times Magazine,* pp. 50–55.

Dohrenwend, B. P. (2000). The role of adversity and stress in psychopathology: Some evidence and its implications for theory and research. *Journal of Health and Social Behavior, 41,* 1–19.

Dohrenwend, B. P., & Dohrenwend, B. S. (1982). Perspectives on the past and future of psychiatric epidemiology. *American Journal of Public Health, 72,* 1271–1279.

Dohrenwend, B. P., Levav, I., Shrout, P. E., Schwartz, S., Naveh, G., Link, B. G., et al. (1992). Socioeconomic status and psychiatric disorders: The causation-selection issue. *Science, 255,* 946–952.

Dohrenwend, B. S. (1973). Life events as stressors: A methodological inquiry. *Journal of Health and Social Behavior, 14,* 167–175.

Donohue, J. M., Berndt, E. R., Rosenthal, M., Epstein, A. M., & Frank, R. G. (2004). Effects of pharmaceutical promotion on adherence to the treatment guidelines for depression. *Medical Care, 42,* 1176–1185.

Dooley, D., Catalano, R., & Wilson, G. (1994). Depression and unemployment: Panel findings from the Epidemiologic Catchment Area study. *American Journal of Community Psychology, 22,* 745–765.

Dooley, D., Prause, J., & Ham-Rowbottom, K. A. (2000). Underemployment and depression: Longitudinal relationships. *Journal of Health and Social Behavior, 41,* 421–437.

Durkheim, E. (1951). *Suicide: A study in sociology.* New York: Free Press. (Original work published 1897)

Dworkin, R. W. (2001). The medicalization of unhappiness. *Public Interest, 144,* 85–101.

Eaton, W. W., Anthony, J. C., Gallo, J., Cai, G., Tien, A., Romanoski, A., et al. (1997). Natural history of diagnostic interview schedule/*DSM-IV* major depression. *Archives of General Psychiatry, 54,* 993–999.

Eaton, W. W., & Kessler, L. G. (1985). *Epidemiological field methods in psychiatry: The NIMH Epidemiologic Catchment Area project.* Orlando, FL: Academic Press.

Eaton, W. W., Neufeld, K., Chen, L., & Cai, G. (2000). A comparison of self-report and clinical diagnostic interviews for depression: DIS and SCAN in the Baltimore ECA followup. *Archives of General Psychiatry, 57,* 217–222.

Edlund, M. J., Unutzer, J., & Wells, K. B. (2004). Clinician screening and treatment of alcohol, drug, and mental problems in primary care: Results from Healthcare for Communities. *Medical Care, 42,* 1158–1166.

Ekman, P. (1973). *Darwin and facial expression: A century of research.* San Diego: Academic Press.

Ekman, P., & Friesen, W. V. (1971). Constants across cultures in the face and emotion. *Journal of Personality and Social Psychology, 17,* 124–129.

Ekman, P., Friesen, W. V., O'Sullivan, M., Chan, A., Diacoyanni-Tarlatzis, I., Heider, K., et al. (1987). Universals and cultural differences in the judgments of facial expressions of emotion. *Journal of Personality and Social Psychology, 53,* 712–717.

Eley, T. C., Sugden, K., Corsico, A., Gregory, A. M., Sham, P., McGuffin, P., et al. (2004). Gene-environment interaction analysis of serotonin system markers with adolescent depression. *Molecular Psychiatry, 9,* 908–915.

Elliott, C. (2003). *Better than well: American medicine meets the American dream.* New York: Norton.

Elliott, C. (2004a). Introduction. In C. Elliott & T. Chambers (Eds.), *Prozac as a way of life* (pp. 1–20). Chapel Hill: University of North Carolina Press.

Elliott, C. (2004b). Pursued by happiness and beaten senseless: Prozac and the American dream. In C. Elliott & T. Chambers (Eds.), *Prozac as a way of life* (pp. 127–142). Chapel Hill: University of North Carolina Press.

Endicott, J., & Spitzer, R. L. (1978). A diagnostic interview: The Schedule for Affective Disorders and Schizophrenia. *Archives of General Psychiatry, 35,* 837–844.

Endicott, J., & Spitzer, R. L. (1979). Use of the research diagnostic criteria and the Schedule for Affective Disorders and Schizophrenia to study affective disorders. *American Journal of Psychiatry, 136,* 52–56.

Engh, A. E., Beehner, J. C., Bergman, T. J., Whitten, P. L., Hoffmeier, R. R., Seyfarth, R. M., et al. (2006). Behavioural and hormonal responses to predation in female chacma baboons (*Papio hamadryas ursinus*). *Proceedings of the Royal Society of London. Series B, Biological Sciences, 273*, 707–112.

Epstein, H. (2003, October 12). Enough to make you sick? *The New York Times Magazine, 74*–81.

Everdell, W. R. (1997). *The first moderns.* Chicago: University of Chicago Press.

Everitt, B. S., Gourlay, A. J., & Kendell, R. E. (1971). An attempt at validation of traditional psychiatric syndromes by cluster analysis. *British Journal of Psychiatry, 119*, 399–412.

Eysenck, H. J. (1970). The classification of depressive illness. *British Journal of Psychiatry, 117*, 241–250.

Eysenck, H., Wakefield, J., & Friedman, A. (1983). Diagnosis and clinical assessment: The *DSM-III. Annual Review of Psychology, 34*, 167–193.

Feighner, J. P. (1989, October 23). The advent of the "Feighner Criteria." *Citation Classics, 43*, 14.

Feighner, J. P., Robins, E., Guze, S. B., Woodruff, R. A., Winokur, G., & Munoz, R. (1972). Diagnostic criteria for use in psychiatric research. *Archives of General Psychiatry, 26*, 57–63.

Fenichel, O. M. (1996). *The psychoanalytic theory of neurosis.* New York: Norton. (Original work published 1945)

Fenwick, R., & Tausig, M. (1994). The macroeconomic context of job stress. *Journal of Health and Social Behavior, 35*, 266–282.

Fisher, R. L. & Fisher, S. (1996). Antidepressants for children: Is scientific support necessary? *Journal of Nervous and Mental Disease, 184*, 99–108.

Fodor, J. A. (1983). *The modularity of mind.* Cambridge, MA: MIT Press.

Foucault, M. (1965). *Madness and civilization: A history of insanity in the Age of Reason* (R. Howard, Trans.). New York: Pantheon.

Foucault, M. (1979). *Discipline and punish: The birth of the prison.* New York: Vintage.

Frances, A. (1998). Problems in defining clinical significance in epidemiological studies. *Archives of General Psychiatry, 55*, 119.

Frank, R. G., Bush, S. H., & Berndt, E. R. (1998). Measuring prices and quantities of treatment for depression. *American Economic Review, 88*, 106–111.

Freidson, E. (1970). *Profession of medicine: A study of the sociology of applied knowledge.* New York: Harper.

French, S., Old, A., & Healy, J. (2001). *Health care systems in transition: New Zealand.* Copenhagen, Denmark: World Health Organization.

Freud, S. (1957). Mourning and melancholia. In J. Strachey (Ed. & Trans.), *Standard edition of the complete works of Sigmund Freud* (Vol. 14; pp. 237–258). London: Hogarth Press. (Original work published 1917)

Fulford, K. W. M. (1999). Nine variations and a coda on the theme of an evolutionary definition of dysfunction. *Journal of Abnormal Psychology, 108*, 412–421.

Furedi, F. (2004). *Therapy culture.* New York: Routledge.

Gallagher, D. E., Breckenridge, J. N., Thompson, L. W., & Peterson, J. A. (1983). Effects of bereavement on indicators of mental health in elderly widows and widowers. *Journal of Gerontology, 38*, 565–571.

Gaminde, I., Uria, M., Padro, D., Querejeta, I., & Ozamiz, A. (1993). Depression in three populations in the Basque country: A comparison with Britain. *Social Psychiatry and Psychiatric Epidemiology, 28,* 243–251.

Ganzini, L., McFarland, B. H., & Cutler, D. (1990). Prevalence of mental disorders after catastrophic financial loss. *Journal of Nervous and Mental Disease, 178,* 680–685.

Gardner, E. (1971). Psychoactive drug utilization. *Journal of Drug Issues, 1,* 295–300.

Gerstel, N., Reissman, C. K., & Rosenfield, S. (1985). Explaining the symptomatology of separated and divorced women and men. *Social Forces, 64,* 84–101.

Ghaemi, S. N. (2003). *The concepts of psychiatry: A pluralist approach to the mind and mental illness.* Baltimore: Johns Hopkins University Press.

Gilbert, P. (1992). *Depression: The evolution of powerlessness.* New York: Guilford Press.

Gilbert, P., & Allan, S. (1998). The role of defeat and entrapment (arrested flight) in depression: An exploration of an evolutionary view. *Psychological Medicine, 28,* 585–598.

Gillespie, N. A., Whitfield, J. B., Williams, D., Heath, A. C., & Martin, N.G. (2004). The relationship between stress life events, the serotonin transporter (5-HTTLPR) genotype and major depression. *Psychological Medicine, 35,* 101–111.

Gilmer, W. S., & McKinney, W. T. (2003). Early experience and depressive disorders: Human and non-human primate studies. *Journal of Affective Disorders, 7,* 97–113.

Glenmullen, J. (2000). *Prozac backlash.* New York: Simon & Schuster.

Gold, P. W., Goodwin, F. K., & Chrousos, G. P. (1988). Clinical and biochemical manifestations of depression: Relation to the neurobiology of stress. *New England Journal of Medicine, 319,* 413–420.

Good, B., Good, M. J., & Moradi, R. (1985). The interpretation of Iranian depressive illness. In A. Kleinman & B. Good (Eds.), *Culture and depression* (pp. 369–428). Berkeley: University of California Press.

Goodwin, D. W., & Guze, S. B. (1996). *Psychiatric diagnosis* (5th ed.). New York: Oxford University Press.

Gould, S. J., & Lewontin, R. C. (1979). The spandrels of San Marco and the Panglossian paradigm: A critique of the adaptationist paradigm. *Proceedings of the Royal Society of London. Series B, Biological Sciences, 205,* 581–598.

Greenberg, P. E., Stiglin, L. E., Finkelstein, S. N., & Berndt, E. R. (1993). The economic burden of depression in 1990. *Journal of Clinical Psychiatry, 54,* 405–418.

Griesinger, W. (2000). Hypochondriasis and melancholia. In J. Radden (Ed.), *The nature of melancholy: From Aristotle to Kristeva* (pp. 223–229). New York: Oxford University Press. (Original work published 1867)

Grinker, R. R., & Spiegel, J. P. (1945). *War neuroses.* Philadelphia: Blakiston.

Grob, G. N. (1973). *Mental institutions in America: Social policy to 1875.* New York: Free Press.

Grob, G. N. (1985). The origins of American psychiatric epidemiology. *American Journal of Public Health, 75,* 229–236.

Grob, G. N. (1991a). *From asylum to community: Mental health policy in modern America.* Princeton, NJ: Princeton University Press.

Grob, G. N. (1991b). Origins of *DSM-I:* A study of appearance and reality. *American Journal of Psychiatry, 148,* 421–431.

Grzywacz, J. G., & Dooley, D. (2003). "Good jobs" to "bad jobs": Replicated evidence of an employment continuum from two large surveys. *Social Science and Medicine, 56,* 1749–1760.

Gut, E. (1989). *Productive and unproductive depression.* New York: Basic Books.

Hagen, E. H. (1999). The functions of postpartum depression. *Evolution and Human Behavior, 20,* 325–359.

Hagen, E. H. (2002). Depression as bargaining: The case postpartum. *Evolution and Human Behavior, 23,* 323–336.

Hagnell, O., Lanke, J., Rorsman, B., & Ojesjo, L. (1982). Are we entering an age of melancholy? *Psychological Medicine, 12,* 279–289.

Hamburg, S. R. (2000). Antidepressants are not placebos. *American Psychologist, 55,* 761–762.

Hamilton, M., & White, J. M. (1959). Clinical syndromes in depressive states. *Journal of Mental Science, 105,* 985–998.

Harlow, H. F., Harlow, M. K., & Suomi, S. J. (1971). From thought to therapy: Lessons from a primate laboratory. *American Scientist, 59,* 538–549.

Harlow, H. F., & Suomi, S. J. (1974). Induced depression in monkeys. *Behavioral Biology, 12,* 273–296.

Harris, E. S. (1991). Adolescent bereavement following the death of a parent: An exploratory study. *Child Psychiatry and Human Development, 21,* 267–281.

Hays, J. C., Kasl, S. V., & Jacobs, S. C. (1994). The course of psychological distress following threatened and actual conjugal bereavement. *Psychological Medicine, 24,* 917–927.

Health United States. (2003). Washington, DC: National Center for Health Statistics.

Healy, D. (1991). The marketing of 5-Hydroxytryptamine: Depression or anxiety? *British Journal of Psychiatry, 158,* 737–742.

Healy, D. (1997). *The anti-depressant era.* Cambridge, MA: Harvard University Press.

Healy, D. (2004). *Let them eat Prozac.* New York: New York University Press.

Heckhausen, J., & Schulz, R. (1995). A life-span theory of control. *Psychological Review, 102,* 284–304.

Heckhausen, J., Wrosch, C., & Fleeson, W. (2001). Developmental regulation before and after a developmental deadline: The sample case of "biological clock" for child-bearing. *Psychology and Aging, 16,* 400–413.

Helzer, J. E., Robins, L. N., McEvoy, L. T., Spitznagel, E. L., Stoltzman, R. K., Farmer, A., et al. (1985). A comparison of clinical and diagnostic interview schedule diagnoses: Reexamination of lay-interviewed cases in the general population. *Archives of General Psychiatry, 42,* 657–666.

Henkel, V., Mergl, R., Coyne, J. C., Kohnen, R., Moller, H., & Hegerl, U. (2004). Screening for depression in primary care: Will one or two items suffice? *European Archives of Psychiatry and Clinical Neuroscience, 254,* 215–223.

Henkel, V., Mergl, R., Kohnen, R., Maier, W., Moller, H., & Hegerl, U. (2003). Identifying depression in primary care: A comparison of different methods in a prospective cohort study. *British Medical Journal, 326,* 200–201.

Herman, E. (1995). *The romance of American psychology: Political culture in the age of experts.* Berkeley: University of California Press.

Hildegard of Bingen. (2000). Melancholia in men and women. In J. Radden (Ed.), *The nature of melancholy: From Aristotle to Kristeva* (pp. 81–85). New York: Oxford University Press.

Hippocrates. (1923–1931). *Works of Hippocrates* (Vols. 1–4, W. H. S. Jones & E. T. Withington, Eds. & Trans.). Cambridge, MA: Harvard University Press.

Hirschfeld, R. M., Keller, M. B., Panico, S., Arons, B. S., Barlow, D., Davidoff, F., et al. (1997). The National Depressive and Manic-Depressive Association consensus statement on the undertreatment of depression. *Journal of the American Medical Association, 277,* 333–340.

Holden, C. (2003). Getting the short end of the allele. *Science, 301,* 291–293.

Holmes, T. H., & Rahe, R. H. (1967). The social readjustment rating scale. *Journal of Psychosomatic Research, 11,* 213–218.

Homer. (1990). *The iliad* (R. Fagles, Trans.). New York: Viking.

Horwath, E., Johnson, J., Klerman, G. L., & Weissman, M. M. (1992). Depressive symptoms as relative and attributable risk factors for first-onset major depression. *Archives of General Psychiatry, 49,* 817–823.

Horwitz, A. V. (1984). The economy and social pathology. *Annual Review of Sociology, 10,* 95–119.

Horwitz, A. V. (2002). *Creating mental illness.* Chicago: University of Chicago Press.

Horwitz, A. V. (2005). Media portrayals and health inequalities: A case study of characterizations of gene x environment interactions. *Journal of Gerontology, 60B,* 48–52.

Horwitz, A. V. (2007). Classical sociological theory, evolutionary theory, and mental health. In B. Pescosolido, W. Avison, & J. McLeod (Eds.), *Mental health/social mirror* (pp. 67–93). New York: Springer.

Horwitz, A. V., & Scheid, T. L. (Eds.). (1999). *A handbook for the study of mental health: Social contexts, theories, and systems.* New York: Cambridge University Press.

Horwitz, A. V., & Wakefield, J. C. (2006). The epidemic of mental illness: Clinical fact or survey artifact? *Contexts, 5,* 19–23.

Hough, R. L., Landsverk, J. A., & Jacobson, G. F. (1990). The use of psychiatric screening scales to detect depression in primary care patients. In C. Attkisson & J. Zich (Eds.), *Depression in primary care: Screening and detection* (pp. 139–154). New York: Routledge.

House, J. S., Landis, K. R., & Umberson, D. (1988). Social relationships and health. *Science, 241,* 540–545.

Insel, T. R., & Fenton, W. S. (2005). Psychiatric epidemiology: It's not just about counting anymore. *Archives of General Psychiatry, 62,* 590–592.

Jackson, S. W. (1986). *Melancholia and depression: From Hippocratic times to modern times.* New Haven, CT: Yale University Press.

Jagger, M. & Richards, K. (1967). Mother's little helper [Recorded by the Rolling Stones]. On *Flowers* [Album]. New York: ABKCO.

Jamison, K. R. (1996). *An unquiet mind.* New York: Vintage Books.

Jensen, A. L., & Weisz, J. R. (2002). Assessing match and mismatch between practitioner-generated and standardized interview-generated diagnoses for clinic-referred children and adolescents. *Journal of Counseling and Clinical Psychology, 70,* 158–168.

Johnson, J. G., Cohen, P., Dohrenwend, B. P., Link, B. G., & Brook, J. S. (1999). A longitudinal investigation of social causation and social selection processes involved in the association between socioeconomic status and psychiatric disorders. *Journal of Abnormal Psychology, 108,* 490–499.

Johnson, S. (1805). *Dictionary of the English language in which the words are deduced from their originals, and illustrated in their different significations by examples from the best writers* (9th ed., Vols. 1–4). London: Longman, Hurst, Rees, & Orme. (Original work published 1755)

Jones, A. (2006). *Kabul in winter: Life without peace in Afghanistan.* New York: Metropolitan Books.

Jones, F. D. (2000). Military psychiatry since World War II. In R. W. Menninger & J. C. Nemiah (Eds.), *American psychiatry after World War II: 1944–1994* (pp. 3–36). Washington, DC: American Psychiatric Press.

Joyner, K., & Udry, J. R. (2000). You don't bring me anything but down: Adolescent romance and depression. *Journal of Health and Social Behavior, 41,* 369–391.

Judd, L. J., & Akiskal, H. S. (2000). Delineating the longitudinal structure of depressive illness: Beyond thresholds and subtypes. *Pharmacopsychiatry, 33,* 3–7.

Judd, L. J., Akiskal, H. S., & Paulus, M. P. (1997). The role and clinical significance of subsyndromal depressive symptoms (SSD) in unipolar major depressive disorder. *Journal of Affective Disorders, 45,* 5–18.

Judd, L. L., Paulus, M. P., Wells, K. B., & Rapaport, M. H. (1996). Socioeconomic burden of subsyndromal depressive symptoms and major depression in a sample of the general population. *American Journal of Psychiatry, 153,* 1411–1417.

Judd, L. L., Rapaport, M. H., Paulus, M. P., & Brown, J. L. (1994). Subsyndromal symptomatic depression: A new mood disorder? *Journal of Clinical Psychiatry, 55,* 18–28.

Kadushin, C. (1969). *Why people go to psychiatrists.* New York: Atherton Press.

Kant, I. (2000). Illnesses of the cognitive faculties. In J. Radden (Ed.), *The nature of melancholy: From Aristotle to Kristeva* (pp. 197–201). New York: Oxford University Press. (Original work published 1793)

Karp, D. A. (1996). *Speaking of sadness.* New York: Oxford University Press.

Kasl, S. V., & Cobb, S. (1979). Some mental health consequences of plant closing and job loss. In L. A. Ferman & J. P. Gordus (Eds.), *Mental health and the economy* (pp. 255–300). Kalamazoo, MI: Upjohn.

Katon, W., Rutter, C., Ludman, E. J., Von Korff, M., Lin, E., Simon, G., et al. (2001). A randomized trial of relapse prevention of depression in primary care. *Archives of General Psychiatry, 58,* 241–247.

Katon, W., & Schulberg, H. (1992). Epidemiology of depression in primary care. *General Hospital Psychiatry, 14,* 237–247.

Katon, W., Unutzer, J., & Simon, G. (2004). Treatment of depression in primary care: Where we are, where we can go. *Medical Care, 42,* 1153–1157.

Katon, W., & Von Korff, M. (1990). Caseness criteria for major depression: The primary care clinician and the psychiatric epidemiologist. In C. Attkisson & J. Zich

(Eds.), *Depression in primary care: Screening and detection* (pp. 43–61). New York: Routledge.

Katon, W., Von Korff, M., Lin, E., Unutzer, J., Simon, G., Walker, E., et al. (1997). Population-based care of depression: Effective disease management strategies to decrease prevalence. *General Hospital Psychiatry, 19,* 169–178.

Katon, W., Von Korff, M., Lin, E., Walker, E., Simon, G. E., Bush, T., et al. (1995). Collaborative management to achieve treatment guidelines: Impact on depression in primary care. *Journal of the American Medical Association, 273,* 1026–1031.

Kaufman, I. C., & Rosenblum, L. A. (1966). A behavioral taxonomy for *M. Nemistrinet* and *M. Radiata:* Based on longitudinal observations of family groups in the laboratory. *Primates, 7,* 205–258.

Keller, M. B., Ryan, N. D., Strober, M., Klein, R. G., Kutcher, S. P., Birmaher, B., et al. (2001). Efficacy of paroxetine in the treatment of adolescent major depression. *Journal of the American Academy of Child and Adolescent Psychiatry, 40,* 762–772.

Keller, M. C., & Nesse, R. M. (2005). Is low mood an adaptation? Evidence for subtypes with symptoms that match precipitants. *Journal of Affective Disorders, 86,* 27–35.

Keller, M. C. & Nesse, R. M. (2006). The evolutionary significance of depressive symptoms: Different adverse situations lead to different depressive symptoms patterns. *Journal of Personality and Social Psychology, 91,* 316–330.

Kendell, R. E. (1968). *The classification of depressive illness.* London: Oxford University Press.

Kendell, R. E. (1983). *DSM-III:* A major advance in psychiatric nosology. In R. L. Spitzer, J. B. Williams, & A. E. Skodol (Eds.), *International perspectives on DSM-III* (pp. 55–68). Washington DC: American Psychiatric Press.

Kendler, K. S., & Gardner, C. O. (1998). Boundaries of major depression: An evaluation of *DSM-IV* criteria. *American Journal of Psychiatry, 155,* 172–177.

Kendler, K. S., Heath, A. C., Martin, N. G., & Eaves, L. J. (1986). Symptoms of anxiety and depression in a volunteer twin population: The etiological role of genetic and environmental factors. *Archives of General Psychiatry, 43,* 213–221.

Kendler, K. S., Karkowski, L. M., & Prescott, C. A. (1999). Causal relationship between stressful life events and the onset of major depression. *American Journal of Psychiatry, 156,* 837–841.

Kendler, K. S., Kessler, R. C., Walters, E. E., MacLean, C., Neale, M. C., Heath, A. C., et al. (1995). Stressful life events, genetic liability, and onset of an episode of major depression in women. *American Journal of Psychiatry, 152,* 833–842.

Kendler, K. S., Kuhn, J. W., Vittum, J., Prescott, C. A., & Riley, B. (2005). The interaction of stressful life events and a serotonin transporter polymorphism in the prediction of episodes of major depression: A replication. *Archives of General Psychiatry, 62,* 529–535.

Kessler, R. C., Abelson, J. M., & Zhao, S. (1998). The epidemiology of mental disorders. In J. B. W. Williams & K. Ell (Eds.), *Advances in mental health research: Implications for practice* (pp. 3–24). Washington, DC: NASW Press.

Kessler, R. C., Beglund, P., Demler, O., Jin, R., Koretz, D., Merikangas, K. R., et al. (2003). The epidemiology of major depressive disorder: Results from the

National Comorbidity Survey replication. *Journal of the American Medical Association, 289,* 3095–3105.

Kessler, R. C., Demler, O., Frank, R. G., Olfson, M., Pincus, H.A., Walters, E. E., et al. (2005). Prevalence and treatment of mental disorders, 1990–2003. *New England Journal of Medicine, 352,* 2515–2523.

Kessler, R. C., House, J. S., & Turner, J. B. (1987). Unemployment and health in a community sample. *Journal of Health and Social Behavior, 28,* 51–59.

Kessler, R. C., McGonagle, K. A., Zhao, S., Nelson, C. B., Hughes, M., Eshelman, S., et al. (1994). Lifetime and 12-month prevalence of *DSM-III-R* psychiatric disorders in the United States. *Archives of General Psychiatry, 51,* 8–19.

Kessler, R. C., Merikangas, K. R., Beglund, P., Eaton, W. W., Koretz, D. S., & Walters, E. E. (2003). Mild disorders should not be eliminated from the *DSM-V. Archives of General Psychiatry, 60,* 1117–1122.

Kessler, R. C., Turner, J. B., & House, J. S. (1989). Unemployment, reemployment, and emotional functioning in a community sample. *American Sociological Review, 54,* 648–657.

Kessler, R. C., Zhao, S., Blazer, D. G., & Swartz, M. (1997). Prevalence, correlates, and course of minor depression and major depression in the National Comorbidity Survey. *Journal of Affective Disorders, 45,* 19–30.

Kiloh, L. G., Andrews, G., Neilson, M., & Bianchi, G. N. (1972). The relationship of the syndromes called endogenous and neurotic depression. *British Journal of Psychiatry, 121,* 183–196.

Kiloh, L. G., & Garside, R. F. (1963). The independence of neurotic depression and endogenous depression. *British Journal of Psychiatry, 109,* 451–463.

Kirk, S. A. (1999). Instituting madness: The evolution of a federal agency. In C. A. Aneshensel & J. C. Phelan, *Handbook of the sociology of mental health* (pp. 539–562). New York: Plenum.

Kirk, S. A. & Kutchins, H. (1992). *The selling of DSM: The rhetoric of science in psychiatry.* New York: Aldine de Gruyter.

Kirkpatrick, D. G., Ruggiero, K. J., Acierno, R., Saunders, B. E., Resnick, H. S., & Best, C. L. (2003). Violence and risk of PTSD, major depression, substance abuse/dependence, and comorbidity: Results from the National Survey of Adolescents. *Journal of Consulting and Clinical Psychology, 71,* 692–700.

Kirmayer, L. J. (1994). Rejoinder to Professor Wakefield. In S. A. Kirk & S. D. Einbinder (Eds.), *Controversial issues in mental health* (pp. 7–20). Boston: Allyn & Bacon.

Kirmayer, L. J., & Young, A. (1999). Culture and context in the evolutionary concept of mental disorder. *Journal of Abnormal Psychology, 108,* 446–452.

Kitson, G. C., Babri, K. B., & Roach, M. J. (1985). Who divorces and why: A review. *Journal of Family Issues, 6,* 255–293.

Klein, D. F. (1974). Endogenomorphic depression. *Archives of General Psychiatry, 31,* 447–454.

Klein, D. F. (1978). A proposed definition of mental illness. In R. Spitzer & D. F. Klein (Eds.), *Critical issues in psychiatric diagnosis* (pp. 41–71). New York: Raven Press.

Kleinman, A. (1977). Depression, somatization and the new cross-cultural psychiatry. *Social Science and Medicine, 11,* 3–10.

Kleinman, A. (1986). *Social origins of distress and disease: Depression, neurasthenia and pain in modern China.* New Haven, CT: Yale University Press.

Kleinman, A. (1987). Anthropology and psychiatry. *British Journal of Psychiatry, 151,* 447–454.

Kleinman, A. (1988). *Rethinking psychiatry: From cultural category to personal experience.* New York: Free Press.

Kleinman, A., & Good, B. (1985). Introduction: Culture and depression. In A. Kleinman & B. Good (Eds.), *Culture and depression* (pp. 1–33). Berkeley: University of California Press.

Klerman, G. L. (1971). A reaffirmation of the efficacy of psychoactive drugs. *Journal of Drug Issues, 1,* 312–320.

Klerman, G. L. (1974). Depression and adaptation. In R. J. Friedman & M. M. Katz (Eds.), *The psychology of depression* (pp. 127–145). Washington, DC: Winston.

Klerman, G. L. (1978). The evolution of a scientific nosology. In J. C. Shershow (Ed.), *Schizophrenia: Science and practice.* Cambridge, MA: Harvard University Press.

Klerman, G. L. (1983). The significance of *DSM-III* in American psychiatry. In R. L. Spitzer, J. B. Williams, & A. E. Skodol (Eds.), *International perspectives on DSM-III* (pp. 3–24). Washington, DC: American Psychiatric Press.

Klerman, G. L. (1988). The current age of youthful melancholia: Evidence for increase in depression among adolescents and young adults. *British Journal of Psychiatry, 152,* 4–14.

Klerman, G. L., & Weissman, M. M. (1989). Increasing rates of depression. *Journal of the American Medical Association, 261,* 2229–2235.

Klinger, E. (1975). Consequences of commitment to and disengagement from incentives. *Psychological Review, 82,* 1–25.

Knutson, B., Wolkowitz, O. M., Cole, A.W., Chan, T., More, E. A., Johnson, R. C., et al. (1998). Selective alteration of personality and social behavior by serotonergic intervention. *American Journal of Psychiatry, 155,* 373–379.

Kovacs, M. G. (Trans.). (1989). *The epic of Gilgamesh.* Stanford, CA: Stanford University Press.

Kraepelin, E. (1915). *Clinical psychiatry: A text-book for students and physicians abstracted and adapted from the seventh German edition of Kraepelin's* Lehrbuch der Psychiatrie (2nd ed., A. Ross Diefendorf, Ed. & Trans.). New York: Macmillan. (Original work published 1907)

Kraepelin, E. (1917). *Lectures on clinical psychiatry* (3rd English ed., T. Johnstone, Ed. & Trans.). New York: Wood. (Original work published 1904)

Kraepelin, E. (1976). *Manic-depressive insanity and paranoia* (R. M. Barclay, Trans.). New York: Arno Press. (Original work published 1921)

Kramer, P. D. (1993). *Listening to Prozac: A psychiatrist explores antidepressant drugs and the remaking of the self.* New York: Viking.

Kramer, P. D. (2005). *Against depression.* New York: Viking.

Kravitz, R. L., Epstein, R. M., Feldman, M. D., Franz, C. E., Azari, R., Wilkes, M. S., et al. (2005). Influence of patients' requests for direct-to-consumer advertised antidepressants: A randomized controlled trial. *Journal of the American Medical Association, 293,* 1995–2002.

Kroenke, K., Spitzer, R. L., & Williams, J. B. W. (2001). The PHQ-9: Validity of a brief depression severity measure. *Journal of General Internal Medicine, 16,* 606–613.

Kuhn, R. (1958). The treatment of depressive states with G22355 (imipramine hydrochloride). *American Journal of Psychiatry, 115,* 459–464.

Lacasse, J. R., & Leo, J. (2005). Serotonin and depression: A disconnect between the advertisements and the scientific literature. *PLoS Medicine, 2,* e392.

Langner, T. S. (1962). A twenty-two item screening score of psychiatric symptoms indicating impairment. *Journal of Health and Social Behavior, 3,* 269–276.

Lapouse, R. (1967). Problems in studying the prevalence of psychiatric disorder. *American Journal of Public Health, 57,* 947–954.

Larson, R. W., Clore, G. L., & Wood, G. A. (1999). The emotions of romantic relationships: Do they wreak havoc on adolescents? In W. Furman, B. B. Brown, & C. Feiring (Eds.), *The development of romantic relationships in adolescence* (pp. 19–49). New York: Cambridge University Press.

Lavretsky, H., & Kumar, A. (2002). Clinically significant non-major depression: Old concepts, new insights. *American Journal of Geriatric Psychiatry, 20,* 239–255.

Leaf, P. J., Myers, J. K., & McEvoy, L. T. (1991). Procedures used in the Epidemiologic Catchment Area study. In L. Robins & D. Regier (Eds.), *Psychiatric disorders in America* (pp. 11–32). New York: Free Press.

Leahy, J. M. (1992–1993). A comparison of depression in women bereaved of a spouse, child, or a parent. *Omega, 26,* 207–217.

Lee, S. (1999). Diagnosis postponed: Shenjing Shuairuo and the transformation of psychiatry in post-Mao China. *Culture, Medicine, and Psychiatry, 23,* 349–380.

Lehmann, H. E. (1959). Psychiatric concepts of depression: Nomenclature and classification. *Canadian Psychiatric Association Journal, 4,* S1–S12.

Leighton, D. C., Harding, J. S., Macklin, D. B., Macmillan, A. M., & Leighton, A. H. (1963). *The character of danger.* New York: Basic Books.

Lewczyk, C. M., Garland, A. F., Hurlbert, M. S., Gearity, J., & Hough, R. L. (2003). Comparing DISC-IV and clinical diagnoses among youths receiving public mental health services. *Journal of the American Academy of Child and Adolescent Psychiatry, 42,* 349–356.

Lewinsohn, P. M., Hops, H., Roberts, R. E., Seeley, J. R., & Andrews, J. A. (1993). Adolescent psychopathology: I. Prevalence and incidence of depression and other *DSM-III-R* disorders in high school students. *Journal of Abnormal Psychology, 102,* 133–144.

Lewinsohn, P. M., Rohde, P., Seeley, J. R., Klein, D. N., & Gotlib, I. H. (2000). Natural course of adolescent major depressive disorder in a community sample. *American Journal of Psychiatry, 157,* 1584–1591.

Lewinsohn, P. M., Shankman, S. A., Gau, J. M., & Klein, D. N. (2004). The prevalence and co-morbidity of subthreshold psychiatric conditions. *Psychological Medicine, 34,* 613–622.

Lewis, A. J. (1934). Melancholia: A clinical survey of depressive states. *Journal of Mental Science, 80,* 1–43.

Lewis, A. J. (1967). Melancholia: A historical review. In *The state of psychiatry: Essays and addresses* (pp. 71–110). London: Routledge & Kegan Paul.

Lilienfeld, S. O., & Marino, L. (1995). Mental disorder as a Roschian concept: A critique of Wakefield's "harmful dysfunction" analysis. *Journal of Abnormal Psychology, 104,* 411–420.

Lilienfeld, S. O., & Marino, L. (1999). Essentialism revisited: Evolutionary theory and the concept of mental disorder. *Journal of Abnormal Psychology, 108,* 400–411.

Liotti, M., Mayberg, H. S., McGinnis, S., Brennan, S. L., & Jerabek, P. (2002). Unmasking disease-specific cerebral blood flow abnormalities: Mood challenge in patients with remitted unipolar depression. *American Journal of Psychiatry, 159,* 1830–1840.

Lopata, H. Z. (1973). *Widowhood in an American city.* Cambridge, MA: Schenkman.

Lorant, V., Deliege, D., Eaton, W., Robert, A., Philippot, P., & Ansseau, M. (2003). Socioeconomic inequalities in depression: A meta-analysis. *American Journal of Epidemiology, 157,* 98–112.

Lowe, B., Spitzer, R. L., Grafe, K., Kroenke, K., Quenter, A., Zipfel, S., et al. (2004). Comparative validity of three screening questionnaires for *DSM-IV* depressive disorders and physicians' diagnoses. *Journal of Affective Disorders, 78,* 131–140.

Lucas, C. P., Zhang, H., Fisher, P. W., Shaffer, D., Regier, D. A., Narrow, W. E., et al. (2004). The DISC Predictive Scales (DPS): Efficiently screening for diagnoses. *Journal of the American Academy of Child and Adolescent Psychiatry, 40,* 443–449.

Luhrmann, T. M. (2000). *Of 2 minds: The growing disorder in American psychiatry.* New York: Alfred A. Knopf.

Lunbeck, E. (1994). *The psychiatric persuasion: Knowledge, gender, and power in modern America.* Princeton, NJ: Princeton University Press.

Lutz, C. (1985). Depression and the translation of emotional worlds. In A. Kleinman & B. Good (Eds.), *Culture and depression* (pp. 63–100). Berkeley: University of California Press.

MacDonald, M. (1981). *Mystical bedlam: Madness, anxiety, and healing in seventeenth-century England.* New York: Cambridge University Press.

Macmillan, A. M. (1957). The Health Opinion Survey: Technique for estimating prevalence of psychoneurotic and related types of disorder in communities. *Psychological Reports, 3,* 325–339.

Mancini, A., Pressman, D., & Bonanno, G. A. (2005). Clinical interventions with the bereaved: What clinicians and counselors can learn from the CLOC study. In D. S. Carr, R. M. Nesse, & C. B. Wortman (Eds.), *Late life widowhood in the United States* (pp. 255–278). New York: Springer.

Mann, J. J. (2005). The medical management of depression. *New England Journal of Medicine, 353,* 1819–1834.

Manson, S. M. (1995). Culture and major depression: Current challenges in the diagnoses of mood disorders. *Psychiatric Clinics of North America, 18,* 487–501.

Marshall, G. N., Schell, T. L., Elliott, M. N., Berthold, S. M., & Chun, C. (2005). Mental health of Cambodian refugees 2 decades after resettlement in the United States. *Journal of the American Medical Association, 294,* 571–579.

Mather, C. (2000). How to help melancholicks. In J. Radden (Ed.), *The nature of melancholy: From Aristotle to Kristeva* (pp. 161–165). New York: Oxford University Press. (Original work published 1724)

Maudsley, H. (2000). Affectivity in mental disorder. In J. Radden (Ed.), *The nature of melancholy: From Aristotle to Kristeva* (pp. 239–258). New York: Oxford University Press. (Original work published 1868)

Mayberg, H. S., Liotti, M., Brannan, S. K., McGinnis, S., Mahurin, R. K., Jerabek, P. A., et al. (1999). Reciprocal limbic-cortical function and negative mood: Converging PET findings in depression and normal sadness. *American Journal of Psychiatry, 156,* 675–682.

Mayes, R. & Horwitz, A.V. (2005). *DSM-III* and the revolution in the classification in mental illness. *Journal of the History of Behavioral Sciences, 41,* 249–267.

McEwan, K. L., Costello, C. G., & Taylor, P. J. (1987). Adjustment to infertility. *Journal of Abnormal Psychology, 96,* 108–116.

McGuffin, P., Katz, R., & Rutherford, J. (1991). Nature, nurture and depression: A twin study. *Psychological Medicine, 21,* 329–335.

McGuire, M., Raleigh, M. J., & Johnson, C. (1983). Social dominance in adult male vervet monkeys: General considerations. *Social Science Information, 22,* 89–123.

McKinley, J. (1999, February 28). Get that man some Prozac. *The New York Times,* E5.

McKinney, W. T. (1986). Primate separation studies: Relevance to bereavement. *Psychiatric Annals, 16,* 281–287.

McLeod, J. D., & Nonnemaker, J. M. (1999). Social stratification and inequality. In C. S. Aneshensel & J. C. Phelan, *Handbook of the sociology of mental health* (pp. 321–344). New York: Kluwer/Plenum.

McPherson, S., & Armstrong, D. (2006). Social determinants of diagnostic labels in depression. *Social Science and Medicine, 62,* 50–58.

Mechanic, D. (1998). Emerging trends in mental health policy and practice. *Health Affairs, 17,* 82–98.

Mechanic, D. (2003). Policy challenges in improving mental health services: Some lessons from the past. *Psychiatric Services, 54,* 1227–1232.

Menaghan, E. G., & Lieberman, M. A. (1986). Changes in depression following divorce: A panel study. *Journal of Marriage and the Family, 48,* 319–328.

Mendels, J. (1968). Depression: The distinction between syndrome and symptom. *American Journal of Psychiatry, 114,* 1349–1354.

Mendels, J., & Cochrane, C. (1968). The nosology of depression: The endogenous-reactive concept. *American Journal of Psychiatry, 124,* 1–11.

Menninger, W. C. (1948). *Psychiatry in a troubled world: Yesterday's war and today's challenge.* New York: Macmillan.

Merikangas, K. R., & Angst, J. (1995). Comorbidity and social phobia: Evidence from clinical, epidemiological, and genetic studies. *European Archives of Psychiatry and Clinical Neurosciences, 244,* 297–303.

Merikangas, K. R., Prusoff, B. A., & Weissman, M. M. (1988). Parental concordance for affective disorders: Psychopathology in offspring. *Journal of Affective Disorders, 15,* 279–290.

Mernissi, F. (1987). *Beyond the veil: Male-female dynamics in modern Muslim society* (Rev. ed.). Bloomington: Indiana University Press.

Merton, R. K. (1968). Social structure and anomie. In *Social theory and social structure* (pp. 185–214). New York: Free Press. (Original work published 1938)

Metzl, J. M. (2003). *Prozac on the couch: Prescribing gender in the era of wonder drugs.* Durham, NC: Duke University Press.

Miller, A. (1996). *Death of a salesman.* New York: Penguin. (Original work published 1949)

Miller, S. I., & Schoenfeld, L. (1973). Grief in the Navajo: Psychodynamics and culture. *International Journal of Social Psychiatry, 19,* 187–191.

Mineka, S., & Suomi, S. J. (1978). Social separation in monkeys. *Psychological Bulletin, 85,* 1376–1400.

Mirowsky, J., & Ross, C. E. (1989). Psychiatric diagnosis as reified measurement. *Journal of Health and Social Behavior, 30,* 11–24.

Mirowsky, J., & Ross, C. E. (2003). *Social causes of psychological distress* (2nd ed.). New York: Aldine de Gruyter.

Mojtabai, R. (2001). Impairment in major depression: Implications for diagnosis. *Comprehensive Psychiatry, 42,* 206–212.

Mollica, R. F., McInnes, K., Sarajlic, N., Lavelle, J., Sarajlic, I., & Massagli, M. P. (1999). Disability associated with psychiatric comorbidity and health status in Bosnian refugees living in Croatia. *Journal of the American Medical Association, 282,* 433–439.

Mollica, R. F., Poole, C., & Tor, S. (1998). Symptoms, functioning and health problems in a massively traumatized population. In B. P. Dohrenwend (Ed.), *Adversity, stress, and psychopathology* (pp. 34–51). New York: Oxford University Press.

Moncrieff, J., & Kirsch, I. (2005). Efficacy of antidepressants in adults. *British Medical Journal, 331,* 155–159.

Moncrieff, J., Wessely, S., & Hardy, R. (2004). Active placebos versus antidepressants for depression. *Cochrane Database of Systematic Reviews, 1.*

Monroe, S. M., Rohde, P., Seeley, J. R., & Lewinsohn, P. M. (1999). Life events and depression in adolescence: Relationship loss as a prospective risk factor for first onset of major depressive disorder. *Journal of Abnormal Psychology, 108,* 606–614.

Monroe, S. M., & Simons, A. D. (1991). Diathesis-stress theories in the context of life stress research: Implications for the depressive disorders. *Psychological Bulletin, 110,* 406–425.

Mulrow, C. D., Williams, J. W., Jr., Gerety, M. B., Ramirez, G., Montiel, O. M., & Kerber, C. (1995). Case-finding instruments for depression in primary care settings. *Annals of Internal Medicine, 122,* 913–921.

Muncie, W. (1939). *Psychobiology and psychiatry: A textbook of normal and abnormal behavior.* St. Louis, MO: Mosby.

Murphy, D., & Stich, S. (2000). Darwin in the madhouse: Evolutionary psychology and the classification of mental disorders. In P. Caruthers & A. Chamberlain (Eds.), *Evolution and cognition* (pp. 62–92). Cambridge, UK: Cambridge University Press.

Murphy, D., & Woolfolk, R. L. (2001). The harmful dysfunction analysis of mental disorder. *Philosophy, Psychiatry, and Psychology, 7,* 241–252.

Murphy, J. M. (1986). The Stirling County study. In M. M. Weissman, J. K. Myers, & C. E. Ross (Eds.), *Community surveys of psychiatric disorders* (pp. 133–154). New Brunswick, NJ: Rutgers University Press.

Murphy, J. M., Laird, N. M., Monson, R. R., Sobol, A. M., & Leighton, A. H. (2000). A 40-year perspective on the prevalence of depression: The Stirling County study. *Archives of General Psychiatry, 57,* 209–215.

Murray, C. J. L., & Lopez, A. D. (Eds.). (1996). *The global burden of disease.* Cambridge, MA: World Health Organization.

Myers, J. K., Lindenthal, J. J., & Pepper, M. P. (1971). Life events and psychiatric impairment. *Journal of Nervous and Mental Disease, 152,* 149–157.

Narrow, W. E., Rae, D. S., Robins, L. N., & Regier, D. A. (2002). Revised prevalence estimates of mental disorders in the United States: Using a clinical significance criterion to reconcile 2 surveys' estimates. *American Journal of Psychiatry, 59,* 115–123.

Neimeyer, R. A. (2000). Searching for the meaning of meaning: Grief therapy and the process of reconstruction. *Death Studies, 24,* 541–558.

Nesse, R. M. (2000). Is depression an adaptation? *Archives of General Psychiatry, 57,* 14–20.

Nesse, R. M. (2005). An evolutionary framework for understanding grief. In D. S. Carr, R. M. Nesse, & C. B. Wortman (Eds.), *Late life widowhood in the United States* (pp. 195–226). New York: Springer.

Nesse, R. M. (2006). Evolutionary explanations for mood and mood disorders. In D. J. Stein, D. J. Kupfer, & A. F. Schatzberg (Eds.), *American Psychiatric Publishing textbook of mental disorders* (pp. 159–175). Washington DC: American Psychiatric.

Nesse, R. M. & Williams, G. C. (1994). *Why we get sick.* New York: Random House.

New Freedom Commission on Mental Health. (2003). *Achieving the promise: Transforming mental health care in America* (DHHS Publication No. SMA-03–3832). Rockville, MD: U.S. Department of Health and Human Services.

Oatley, K., & Bolton, W. (1985). A social theory of depression in reaction to life events. *Psychological Review, 92,* 372–388.

Obeyesekere, G. (1985). Depression, Buddhism and the work of culture in Sri Lanka. In A. Kleinman & B. Good (Eds.), *Culture and depression* (pp. 134–152). Berkeley: University of California Press.

Olfson, M., & Klerman, G. R. (1993). Trends in the prescription of anti-depressants by office-based psychiatrists. *American Journal of Psychiatry, 150,* 571–577.

Olfson, M., Marcus, S. C., Druss, B., Elinson, L., Tanielian, T., & Pincus, H. A. (2002). National trends in the outpatient treatment of depression. *Journal of the American Medical Association, 287,* 203–209.

Olfson, M., Marcus, S. C., Druss, B., & Pincus, H. A. (2002). National trends in the use of outpatient psychotherapy. *American Journal of Psychiatry, 159,* 1914–1920.

Olfson, M., Marcus, S. C., & Pincus, H. A. (1999). Trends in office-based psychiatric practice. *American Journal of Psychiatry, 156,* 451–457.

Overall, J. E., Hollister, L. E., Johnson, M., & Pennington, V. (1966). Nosology of depression and differential response to drugs. *Journal of the American Medical Association, 195,* 162–164.

Parkes, C. M. & Weiss, R. S. (1983). *Recovery from bereavement.* New York: Basic Books.

Parry, H., Balter, M., Mellinger, G., Cisin, I., & Manheimer, D. (1973). National patterns of psychotherapeutic drug use. *Archives of General Psychiatry, 28,* 769–783.

Paykel, E. S. (1971). Classification of depressed patients: A cluster analysis derived grouping. *British Journal of Psychiatry, 118,* 275–288.

Pear, R. (2004, December 3). Americans relying more on prescription drugs, report says. *The New York Times,* A22.

Pearlin, L. I. (1989). The sociological study of stress. *Journal of Health and Social Behavior, 30,* 241–257.

Pearlin, L. I. (1999). Stress and mental health: A conceptual overview. In A. V. Horwitz & T. L. Scheid (Eds.), *A handbook for the study of mental health: Social contexts, theories, and systems* (pp. 161–175). New York: Cambridge University Press.

Pescosolido, B. A., Martin, J. K., Link, B. G., Kikuzawa, S., Burgos, G., Swindle, R., et al. (2000). *Americans' views of mental health and illness at century's end: Continuity and change.* Bloomington: Indiana Consortium for Mental Health Services Research.

Peterson, A. C., Compas, B. E., Brooks-Gunn, J., Stemmler, M., Ey, S., & Grant, K. E. (1993). Depression in adolescence. *American Psychologist, 48,* 155–168.

Pincus, H. A., Tanielian, T. L., Marcus, S. C., Olfson, M., Zarin, D. A., Thompson, J., et al. (1998). Prescribing trends in psychotropic medications: Primary care, psychiatry, and other medical specialities. *Journal of the American Medical Association, 279,* 526–531.

Pinel, P. (2000). Melancholia. In J. Radden (Ed.), *The nature of melancholy: From Aristotle to Kristeva* (pp. 203–210). New York: Oxford University Press. (Original work published 1801)

Pinker, S. (1997). *How the mind works.* New York: Norton.

Plunkett, R. J., & Gordon, J. E. (1960). *Epidemiology and mental illness.* New York: Basic Books.

Post, R. M. (1992). Transduction of psychosocial stress into the neurobiology of recurrent affective disorder. *American Journal of Psychiatry, 149,* 999–1010.

Price, J. S., & Sloman, L. (1987). Depression as yielding behavior: An animal model based upon Schjelderup-Ebbe's pecking order. *Ethology and Sociobiology, 8,* 85s–98s.

Price, J. S., Sloman, L., Gardner, R., Gilbert, P., & Rohde, P. (1994). The social competition hypothesis of depression. *British Journal of Psychiatry, 164,* 309–335.

Price, R. H., Choi, J. N., & Vinokur, A. D. (2002). Links in the chain of adversity following job loss. *Journal of Occupational Health Psychology, 7,* 302–312.

Pringle, E. (2005). *TeenScreen: Angel of mercy or pill-pusher.* Retrieved Dec. 22, 2005, from http://www.opednews.com/pringleEvelyn_041405_teenscreen.htm

Pyne, J. M., Rost, K. M., Farahati, F., Tripathi, S. P., Smith, J., Williams, D. K., et al. (2004). One size fits some: The impact of patient treatment attitudes on the cost-effectiveness of a depression primary-care intervention. *Psychological Medicine, 34,* 1–16.

Radden, J. (Ed.). (2000). *The nature of melancholy: From Aristotle to Kristeva.* New York: Oxford University Press.

Radloff, L. S. (1977). The CES-D scale: A self-report depression scale for research in the general population. *Applied Psychological Measurement, 3,* 249–265.

Radloff, L. S. & Locke, B. Z. (1986). The Community Mental Health Assessment Survey and the CES-D scale. In M. M. Weissman, J. K. Myers, & C. E. Ross (Eds.), *Community surveys of psychiatric disorders* (pp. 177–189). New Brunswick, NJ: Rutgers University Press.

Rajkowska, G., Miguel-Hidalgo, J. J., Wei, J., Pittman, S. D., Dilley, G., Overholser, J., et al. (1999). Morphometric evidence for neuronal and glial prefrontal cell pathology in major depression. *Biological Psychiatry, 45,* 1085–1098.

Raleigh, M. J., McGuire, M. T., Brammer, G. L., & Yuwiler, A. (1984). Social and environmental influences on blood serotonin concentrations in monkeys. *Archives of General Psychiatry, 41,* 405–410.

Raskin, A., & Crook, T. H. (1976). The endogenous-neurotic distinction as a predictor of response to antidepressant drugs. *Psychological Medicine, 6,* 59–70.

Raynes, N. (1979). Factors affecting the prescribing of psychotropic drugs in general practice consultations. *Psychological Medicine, 9,* 671–679.

Regier, D. A., Hirschfeld, R. M., Goodwin, F. K., Burke, J. D., Lazar, J. B., & Judd, L. L. (1988). The NIMH Depression Awareness, Recognition, and Treatment program: Structure, aims, and scientific basis. *American Journal of Psychiatry, 145,* 1351–1357.

Regier, D. A., Kaelber, C. T., Rae, D. S., Farmer, M. E., Knauper, B., Kessler, R. C., et al. (1998). Limitations of diagnostic criteria and assessment instruments for mental disorders. *Archives of General Psychiatry, 55,* 109–115.

Reynolds, J. R. (1997). The effects of industrial employment conditions on job-related distress. *Journal of Health and Social Behavior, 38,* 105–116.

Richters, J. E., & Hinshaw, S. P. (1999). The abduction of disorder in psychiatry. *Journal of Abnormal Psychology, 108,* 438–446.

Ritsher, J. E. B., Warner, V., Johnson, J. G., & Dohrenwend, B. P. (2001). Intergenerational longitudinal study of social class and depression: A test of social causation and social selection models. *British Journal of Psychiatry, 178,* S84–S90.

Roberts, R. E., Andrews, J. A., Lewinsohn, P. M., & Hops, H. (1990). Assessment of depression in adolescents using the Center for Epidemiologic Studies Depression scale. *Psychological Assessment: A Journal of Consulting and Clinical Psychology, 2,* 122–128.

Roberts, R. E., Attkisson, C. C., & Rosenblatt, A. (1998). Prevalence of psychopathology among children and adolescents. *American Journal of Psychiatry, 155,* 715–725.

Roberts, R. E., Lewinsohn, P. M., & Seeley, J. R. (1991). Screening for adolescent depression: A comparison of depression scales. *Journal of the Academy of Child and Adolescent Psychiatry, 30,* 58–66.

Roberts, R. E., Roberts, C. R., & Chen, Y. R. (1997). Ethnocultural differences in prevalence of adolescent depression. *American Journal of Community Psychology, 25,* 95–110.

Robins, L. N., Helzer, J. E., Weissman, M. M., Orvaschel, H., Gruenberg, E., Burke, J. D., et al. (1984). Lifetime prevalence of specific psychiatric disorders in three sites. *Archives of General Psychiatry, 41,* 949–956.

Robins, L. N., & Regier, D. A. (Eds.). (1991). *Psychiatric disorders in America: The Epidemiological Catchment Area study.* New York: Free Press.

Roccatagliata, G. (1986). *A history of ancient psychiatry.* Westport, CT: Greenwood Press.

Rogers, T. (1691). *A discourse concerning trouble of mind, and the disease of melancholy.* London: Parkhurst, Cockerill.

Rosenhan, D. L. (1973). On being sane in insane places. *Science, 179,* 250–258.

Rosenthal, S. H. (1968). The involutional depressive syndrome. *American Journal of Psychiatry, 124,* 21–35.

Ross, C. E. (1995). Reconceptualizing marital status as a continuum of attachment. *Journal of Marriage and the Family, 57,* 129–140.

Ross, C. E., Mirowsky, J., & Goldstein, K. (1990). The impact of the family on health: The decade in review. *Journal of Marriage and the Family, 52,* 1059–1078.

Rost, K., Nutting, P., Smith, J., Coyne, J. C., Cooper-Patrick, L., Rubenstein, L. (2000). The role of competing demands in the treatment provided primary care patients with major depression. *Archives of Family Medicine, 9,* 150–154.

Rost, K., Nutting, P., Smith, J., Werner, J., & Duan, N. (2001). Improving depression outcomes in community primary care practice. *Journal of General Internal Medicine, 16,* 143–149.

Rush, B. (2000). Hypochondriasis or tristimania. In J. Radden (Ed.), *The nature of melancholy: From Aristotle to Kristeva* (pp. 211–217). New York: Oxford University Press. (Original work published 1812)

Rushton, J. L., Forcier, M., & Schectman, R. M. (2002). Epidemiology of depressive symptoms in the national longitudinal study of adolescent health. *Journal of the American Academy of Child and Adolescent Psychiatry, 41,* 199–205.

Russell, L. B. (1994). *Educated guesses: Making policy about medical screening tests.* Berkeley: University of California Press.

Sadler, J. Z. (1999). Horsefeathers: A commentary on "Evolutionary versus prototype analyses of the concept of disorder." *Journal of Abnormal Psychology, 108,* 433–438.

Sadock, B. J., & Sadock, V. A. (2003). *Kaplan and Sadock's synopsis of psychiatry* (9th ed.). Philadelphia: Lippincott, Williams & Wilkins.

Sanders, C. M. (1979–1980). A comparison of adult bereavement in the death of a spouse, child and parent. *Omega, 10,* 303–322.

Santora, M., & Carey, B. (2005, April 13). Depressed? New York screens for people at risk. *The New York Times,* A1, A16.

Sapolsky, R. M. (1989). Hypercortisolism among socially subordinate wild baboons originates at the CNS level. *Archives of General Psychiatry, 46,* 1047–1051.

Sapolsky, R. M. (1992). Cortisol concentrations and the social significance of rank instability among wild baboons. *Psychoneuroendocrinology, 17,* 701–709.

Sapolsky, R. M. (1998). *Why zebras don't get ulcers: An updated guide to stress, stress-related disease and coping.* New York: Freeman.

Sapolsky, R. M. (2001). Depression, antidepressants, and the shrinking hippocampus. *Proceedings of the National Academy of Sciences of the USA, 98,* 12320–12322.

Sapolsky, R. M. (2005). The influence of social hierarchy on primate health. *Science, 308,* 648–652.

Sartorius, N. (1997). Psychiatry in the framework of primary health care: A threat or boost to psychiatry? *American Journal of Psychiatry, 154,* 67–72.

Savage, G. (1884). *Insanity and allied neuroses: Practical and clinical.* London: Cassell.

Schatzberg, A. F. (2002). Major depression: Causes or effects? *American Journal of Psychiatry, 159,* 1077–1079.

Scheff, T. J. (1966). *Being mentally ill: A sociological theory.* Chicago: Aldine.

Schieffelin, E. J. (1985). The cultural analysis of depressive affect: An example from New Guinea. In A. Kleinman & B. Good (Eds.), *Culture and depression* (pp. 101–133). Berkeley: University of California Press.

Schildkraut, J. J. (1965). The catecholamine hypothesis of affective disorders: A review of supporting evidence. *Journal of Neuropsychiatry and Clinical Neuroscience, 7,* 524–533.

Schulberg, H. C. (1990). Screening for depression in primary care: Guidelines for future practice and research. In C. Attkisson & J. Zich (Eds.), *Depression in primary care: Screening and detection* (pp. 267–278): New York: Routledge.

Schulberg, H. C., Saul, M., McClelland, M., Ganguli, M., Christy, W., & Frank, R. (1985). Assessing depression in primary medical and psychiatric practice. *Archives of General Psychiatry, 42,* 1164–1170.

Schulz, R., Beach, S. R., Lind, B., Martire, L. M., Zdaniuk, B., Hirsch, C., et al. (2001). Involvement in caregiving and adjustment to death of a spouse: Findings from the caregiver health effects study. *Journal of the American Medical Association, 285,* 3123–3129.

Schut, H., Stroebe, M. A., Van den Bout, J., & Terheggen, M. (2001). The efficacy of bereavement interventions: Determining who benefits. In M. Stroebe, R. O. Hansson, W. Strobe, & H. Schut (Eds.), *Handbook of bereavement research: Consequences, coping, and care* (pp. 705–737). Washington, DC: American Psychological Association.

Schwartz, S., Dohrenwend, B. P., & Levav, I. (1994). Nongenetic familial transmission of psychiatric disorders? Evidence from children of Holocaust survivors. *Journal of Health and Social Behavior, 35,* 385–403.

Schwenk, T. L., Coyne, J. C., & Fechner-Bates, S. (1996). Differences between detected and undetected patients in primary care and depressed psychiatric patients. *General Hospital Psychiatry, 18,* 407–415.

Schwenk, T. L., Klinkman, M. S., & Coyne, J. C. (1998). Depression in the family physician's office: What the psychiatrist needs to know. *Journal of Clinical Psychiatry, 59,* 94–100.

Scull, A. T., MacKenzie, C., & Hervey, N. (1997). *Masters of Bedlam.* Princeton, NJ: Princeton University Press.

Seligman, M. E. P. (1975). *Helplessness: On depression, development and death.* San Francisco: Freeman.

Shaffer, D., Scott, M., Wilcox, H., Maslow, C., Hicks, R., Lucas, C. P., et al. (2004). The Columbia Suicide Screen: Validity and reliability of a screen for youth suicide and depression. *Journal of the American Academy of Child and Adolescent Psychiatry, 43,* 71–79.

Shapiro, S., & Baron, S. (1961). Prescriptions for psychotropic drugs in a noninstitutional population. *Public Health Reports, 76,* 481–488.

Shelley, P. B. (1986). A dirge. In M. H. Abrams, E. T. Donaldson, A. David, H. Smith, B. K. Lewalski, R. M. Adams, et al. (Eds.), *Norton anthology of English literature* (5th ed., p. 755). New York: Norton. (Original work published 1824)

Shephard, B. (2000). *A war of nerves: Soldiers and psychiatrists in the twentieth century.* Cambridge, MA: Harvard University Press.

Shively, C. A. (1998). Social subordination stress, behavior, and central monoaminergic function in female Cynomolgus monkeys. *Biological Psychiatry, 44,* 882–891.

Shively, C. A., Laber-Laird, K., & Anton, R. F. (1997). Behavior and physiology of social stress and depression in female Cynomolgus monkeys. *Biological Psychiatry, 41,* 871–882.

Shorter, E. (1992). *From paralysis to fatigue: A history of psychosomatic illness in the modern era.* New York: Free Press.

Shorter, E. (1997). *A history of psychiatry: From the era of the asylum to the age of Prozac.* New York: Wiley.

Shugart, M. A., & Lopez, E. M. (2002). Depression in children and adolescents. *Postgraduate Medicine, 112,* 53–59.

Simon, R. W. (2002). Revisiting the relationship among gender, marital status, and mental health. *American Journal of Sociology, 107,* 1065–1096.

Skodol, A. E., & Spitzer, R. L. (1982). The development of reliable diagnostic criteria in psychiatry. *Annual Review of Medicine, 33,* 317–326.

Sloman, L., Gilbert, P., & Hasey, G. (2003). Evolved mechanisms in depression: The role and interaction of attachment and social rank in depression. *Journal of Affective Disorders, 74,* 107–121.

Smith, M. C. (1985). *A social history of the minor tranquillizers.* New York: Pharmaceutical Products Press.

Solomon, A. (2001). *The noonday demon: An atlas of depression.* New York: Scribner.

Soranus. (1950). *On acute diseases and on chronic diseases* (I. E. Drabkin, Ed. & Trans.). Chicago: University of Chicago Press.

Spiegel, A. (2005, January 3). The dictionary of disorder: How one man revolutionized psychiatry. *New Yorker,* 56–63.

Spijker, J., de Graaf, R., Bijl, R. V., Beekman, A. T. F., Ormel, J., & Nolen, W. A. (2003). Duration of major depressive episodes in the general population: Results from the Netherlands mental health survey and incidence study. *Acta Psychiatrica Scandinavica, 106,* 208–213.

Spitzer, R. L. (1975). On pseudoscience in science, logic in remission and psychiatric diagnosis: A critique of Rosenhan's "On being sane in insane places." *Journal of Abnormal Psychology, 84,* 442–452.

Spitzer, R. L. (1978). The data-oriented revolution in psychiatry. *Man and Medicine,* *3,* 193–194.

Spitzer, R. L. (1982). Feighner, et al., invisible colleges, and the Matthew Effect. *Schizophrenia Bulletin, 8,* 592.

Spitzer, R. L. (1999). Harmful dysfunction and the *DSM* definition of mental disorder. *Journal of Abnormal Psychology, 108,* 430–432.

Spitzer, R. L., Endicott, J., & Robins, E. (1975). Clinical criteria for psychiatric diagnosis and *DSM-III. American Journal of Psychiatry, 132,* 1187–1192.

Spitzer, R. L., Endicott, J., & Robins, E. (1978). Research Diagnostic Criteria: Rationale and reliability. *Archives of General Psychiatry 35,* 773–782.

Spitzer, R. L., & Fleiss, J. L. (1974). A re-analysis of the reliability of psychiatric diagnosis. *American Journal of Psychiatry, 125,* 341–347.

Spitzer, R. L., Kroenke, K., & Williams, J. B. W. (1999). Validation and utility of a self-report version of PRIME-MD. *Journal of the American Medical Association, 282,* 1737–1744.

Spitzer, R. L. & Williams, J. B. W. (1988). Having a dream: A research strategy for *DSM-IV. Archives of General Psychiatry, 45,* 871–874.

Spitzer, R. L., Williams, J. B. W., Kroenke, K., Linzer, M., deGruy, F. V., III, Hahn, S. R., et al. (1994). Utility of a new procedure for diagnosing mental disorders in primary care: The PRIME-MD 1000 study. *Journal of the American Medical Association, 272,* 1749–1756.

Spitzer, R. L., Williams, J. B. W., & Skodol, A. E. (1980). *DSM-III:* The major achievements and an overview. *American Journal of Psychiatry, 137,* 151–164.

Squier, S. (2004). The paradox of Prozac as an enhancement technology. In C. Elliott & T. Chambers (Eds.), *Prozac as a way of life* (pp. 143–163). Chapel Hill: University of North Carolina Press.

Srole, L., Langner, T. S., Michael, S. T., Kirkpatrick, P., Opler, M. K., & Rennie, T. A. C. (1978). *Mental health in the metropolis: The Midtown Manhattan study* (Rev. ed., enlarged). New York: McGraw Hill. (Original work published 1962)

Stevens, A., & Price, J. (2000). *Evolutionary psychiatry: A new beginning* (2nd ed.). London: Routledge.

Stroebe, W., & Stroebe, M. S. (1987). *Bereavement and health.* New York: Cambridge University Press.

Styron, W. (1991). *Darkness visible: A memoir of madness.* London: Cape.

Sullivan, P. F., Neale, M. C., & Kendler, K. S. (2000). Genetic epidemiology of major depression: Review and meta-analysis. *American Journal of Psychiatry, 157,* 1552–1562.

Suomi, S. J. (1991). Adolescent depression and depressive symptoms: Insights from longitudinal studies with Rhesus monkeys. *Journal of Youth and Adolescence, 20,* 273–287.

Surtees, P. G., Wainwright, N. W., Willis-Owen, S. A., Luben, R., Day, N., & Flint, J. (2006). Social adversity, the serotonin transporter (5-HTTLPR) polymorphism and depressive disorder. *Biological Psychiatry, 59,* 224–229.

Sweeney, M., & Horwitz, A. V. (2001). Infidelity, initiation, and the emotional climate of divorce: Are there implications for mental health? *Journal of Health and Social Behavior, 42,* 295–310.

Szasz, T. S. (1961). *The myth of mental illness*. New York: Hoeber-Harper.

Tausig, M., & Fenwick, R. (1999). Recession and well-being. *Journal of Health and Social Behavior, 40*, 1–17.

Temerlin, M. K. (1968). Suggestion effects in psychiatric diagnosis. *Journal of Nervous and Mental Disorders, 147*, 349–358.

Thomas, C. P., Conrad, P., Casler, R., & Goodman, E. (2006). Trends in the use of psychotropic medications among adolescents, 1994 to 2001. *Psychiatric Services, 57*, 63–69.

Tooby, J., & Cosmides, L. (1990). The past explains the present: Emotional adaptations and the structure of ancestral environments. *Ethology and Sociobiology, 11*, 375–424.

Treatment for Adolescents with Depression Study Team. (2004). Fluoxetine, cognitive-behavioral therapy, and their combination for adolescents with depression. *Journal of the American Medical Association, 292*, 807–820.

Tredgold, R. F. (1941). Depressive states in the soldier: Their symptoms, causation, and prognosis. *British Medical Journal, 2*, 109–112.

Trivedi, M. H., Rush, A. J., Wisniewski, S. R., Nierenberg, A. A., Warden, D., Ritz, L., et al. (2006). Evaluation of outcomes with Catalopram for depression using measurement-based care in STAR-D: Implications for clinical practice. *American Journal of Psychiatry, 163*, 26–40.

Tufts Health Plan. (2005). Clinical guidelines for the treatment of depression in the primary care setting. Retrieved Dec. 22, 2005, from http://www.tuftshealthplan.com/providers/pdf/clinicalguidelines_depression

Turner, J. B. (1995). Economic context and the health effects of unemployment. *Journal of Health and Social Behavior, 36*, 213–230.

Turner, J. (2000). *On the origins of human emotions: A sociological inquiry into the evolution of human affect*. Palo Alto, CA: Stanford University Press.

Turner, R. J. (1999). Social support and coping. In A. V. Horwitz & T. L. Scheid (Eds.), *A handbook for the study of mental health: Social contexts, theories, and systems* (pp. 198–210). New York: Cambridge University Press.

Turner, R. J. (2003). The pursuit of socially modifiable contingencies in mental health. *Journal of Health and Social Behavior, 44*, 1–18.

Turner, R. J., & Avison, W. R. (2003). Status variations in stress exposure. *Journal of Health and Social Behavior, 44*, 488–505.

Turner, R. J., & Lloyd, D. A. (1999). The stress process and the social distribution of depression. *Journal of Health and Social Behavior, 40*, 374–404.

Turner, R. J., Wheaton, B., & Lloyd, D. A. (1995). The epidemiology of stress. *American Sociological Review, 60*, 104–125.

Ullman, M. (1978). *Islamic medicine*. Edinburgh, UK: Edinburgh University Press.

Umberson, D., Wortman, C. B., & Kessler, R. C. (1992). Widowhood and depression: Explaining long-term gender differences in vulnerability. *Journal of Health and Social Behavior, 33*, 10–24.

U.S. Department of Health and Human Services. (1999). *Mental health: A report of the Surgeon General*. Rockville, MD: Author.

U.S. Department of Health and Human Services. (2001). *Mental health: Culture and ethnicity: A supplement to mental health: A report of the Surgeon General*. Rockville, MD: Author.

U.S. Preventive Services Task Force. (2002). Screening for depression: Recommendations and rationales. *Internal Medicine, 136,* 760–764.

Valenstein, E. S. (1998). *Blaming the brain.* New York: Free Press.

Van Elst, L., Ebert, D., & Trimble, M. R. (2001). Hippocampus and amygdala pathology in depression. *American Journal of Psychiatry, 158,* 652–653.

Vedantam, S. (2003, July 18). Variation in one gene linked to depression. *The Washington Post,* A1.

Videbech, P., & Ravnkilde, B. (2004). Hippocampal volume and depression: A meta-analysis of MRI studies. *American Journal of Psychiatry, 161,* 1957–1966.

Vitiello, B., & Swedo, S. (2004). Antidepressant medications in children. *New England Journal of Medicine, 350,* 1489–1491.

Von Knorring, A., Cloninger, C. R., Bohman, M., & Sigvardsson, S. (1983). An adoption study of depressive disorders and substance abuse. *Archives of General Psychiatry, 40,* 943–950.

Von Krafft-Ebing, R. (1904). *Text-book of insanity* (C. G. Chaddock, Trans.). Philadelphia: Davis.

Wade, T. J., & Pevalin, D. J. (2004). Marital transitions and mental health. *Journal of Health and Social Behavior, 45,* 155–170.

Waite, L. J. (1995). Does marriage matter? *Demography, 32,* 483–501.

Wakefield, J. C. (1992). The concept of mental disorder: On the boundary between biological facts and social values. *American Psychologist, 47,* 373–388.

Wakefield, J. C. (1999). The measurement of mental disorder. In A. V. Horwitz & T. L. Scheid (Eds.), *A handbook for the study of mental health: Social contexts, theories, and systems* (pp. 29–57). New York: Cambridge University Press.

Wakefield, J. C., Schmitz, M. F., First, M. B., & Horwitz, A. V. (2007). Extending the bereavement exclusion for major depression to other losses: Evidence from the National Comorbidity Survey. *Archives of General Psychiatry* (in press).

Wakefield, J. C., & Spitzer, R. L. (2002). Lowered estimates—but of what? *Archives of General Psychiatry, 59,* 129–130.

Wang, P. S., Lane, M., Olfson, M., Pincus, H. A., Wells, K. B., & Kessler, R. C. (2005). Twelve-month use of mental health services in the United States. *Archives of General Psychiatry, 62,* 629–640.

Watson, D. (2006). Rethinking the mood and anxiety disorders: A quantitative hierarchical model for DSM-V. *Journal of Abnormal Psychology, 114,* 522–536.

Watson, P. J., & Andrews, P. W. (2002). Toward a revised evolutionary adaptationist analysis of depression: The social navigation hypothesis. *Journal of Affective Disorders, 72,* 1–14.

Weissman, M. M., & Myers, J. K. (1978). Rates and risks of depressive symptoms in a United States urban community. *Acta Psychiatrica Scandinavica, 57,* 219–231.

Wells, K. B., Schoenbaum, M., Unutzer, J., Lagomasino, I. T., & Rubenstein, L. V. (1999). Quality of care for primary care patients with depression in managed care. *Archives of Family Medicine, 8,* 529–536.

Wells, K. B., Stewart, A., Hays, R. D., Burnam, M. A., Rogers, W., Danies, M., et al. (1989). The functioning and well-being of depressed patients: Results from the Medical Outcomes Study. *Journal of the American Medical Association, 262,* 914–919.

Wenegrat, B. (1995). *Illness and power: Women's mental disorders and the battle between the sexes.* New York: New York University Press.

Wethington, E., & Serido, J. (2004, May). *A case approach for coding and rating life events and difficulties using a standard survey interview.* Paper presented at the International Conference on Social Stress Research, Montreal, Quebec, Canada.

Wheaton, B. (1990). Life transitions, role histories, and mental health. *American Sociological Review, 55,* 209–223.

Wheaton, B. (1999). The nature of stressors. In A. V. Horwitz & T. L. Scheid (Eds.), *A handbook for the study of mental health: Social contexts, theories, and systems* (pp. 176–197). New York: Cambridge University Press.

Whittington, C. J., Kendall, T., Fonagy, P., Cottrell, D., Cotgrove, A., & Boddington, E. (2004). Selective serotonin reuptake inhibitors in childhood depression: Systematic review of published versus unpublished data. *Lancet, 363,* 1341–1345.

Whooley, M. A., Avins, A. L., Miranda, J., & Browner, W. S. (1997). Case-finding instruments for depression: Two questions are as good as many. *Journal of General Internal Medicine, 12,* 439–445.

Wikan, U. (1988). Bereavement and loss in two Muslim communities: Egypt and Bali compared. *Social Science and Medicine, 27,* 451–460.

Wikan, U. (1990). *Managing turbulent hearts: A Balinese formula for living.* Chicago: University of Chicago Press.

Williams, J. W., Jr., Rost, K., Dietrich, A. J., Ciotti, M. C., Zyzanski, S. J., & Cornell, J. (1999). Primary care physicians' approach to depressive disorders: Effects of physician specialty and practice structure. *Archives of Family Medicine, 8,* 58–67.

Willner, P. (1991). Animal models as research tools in depression. *International Journal of Geriatric Psychiatry, 6,* 469–476.

Wilson, M. (1993). *DSM-III* and the transformation of American psychiatry: A history. *American Journal of Psychiatry, 150,* 399–410.

Wittchen, H. (1994). Reliability and validity studies of the WHO-Composite International Diagnostic Interview (CIDI): A critical review. *Journal of Psychiatric Research, 28,* 57–84.

Wittchen, H., Ustun, T. B., & Kessler, R. C. (1999). Diagnosing mental disorders in the community. A difference that matters? *Psychological Medicine, 29,* 1021–1027.

Woodruff, R. A., Goodwin, D. W., & Guze, S. B. (1974). *Psychiatric diagnosis.* New York: Oxford University Press.

World Health Organization. (1998). *Info package: Mastering depression in primary care.* Frederiksborg, Denmark: WHO Regional Office for Europe, Psychiatric Research Unit.

World Health Organization. (2004). Prevalence, severity, and unmet need for treatment of mental disorders in the World Health Organization World Mental Health Surveys. *Journal of the American Medical Association, 291,* 2581–2590.

Wortman, C. B., & Silver, R. C. (1989). The myths of coping with loss. *Journal of Consulting and Clinical Psychology, 57,* 349–357.

Wortman, C. B., Silver, R. C., & Kessler, R. C. (1993). The meaning of loss and adjustment to bereavement. In M. S. Stroebe, W. Stroebe, & R. O. Hansson (Eds.), *Handbook of bereavement: Theory, research, and intervention* (pp. 349–366). New York: Cambridge University Press.

Wrosch, C., Scheier, M. F., Carver, C. S., & Schulz, R. (2003). The importance of goal disengagement in adaptive self-regulation: When giving up is beneficial. *Self and Identity, 2,* 1–20.

Wurtzel, E. (1995). *Prozac nation.* New York: Riverhead.

Young, A. (2003). Evolutionary narratives about mental disorders. *Anthropology and Medicine, 10,* 239–253.

Zaun, T. (2004, March 9). Head of farm in bird flu outbreak is found dead. *The New York Times,* W1.

Zimmerman, M. (1990). Is *DSM-IV* needed at all? *Archives of General Psychiatry, 47,* 974–976.

Zimmerman, M., Chelminski, I., & Young, D. (2004). On the threshold of disorder: A study of the impact of the *DSM-IV* clinical significance criterion on diagnosing depressive and anxiety disorders in clinical practice. *Journal of Clinical Psychiatry, 65,* 1400–1405.

Zimmerman, M., Coryell, W., & Pfohl, B. (1986). Melancholic subtyping: A qualitative or quantitative distinction? *American Journal of Psychiatry, 143,* 98–100.

Zimmerman, M., & Spitzer, R. L. (1989). Melancholia: From *DSM-III* to *DSM-III-R. American Journal of Psychiatry, 146,* 20–28.

Zisook, S., Paulus, M., Shuchter, S. R., & Judd, L. L. (1997). The many faces of depression following spousal bereavement. *Journal of Affective Disorders, 45,* 85–94.

Zisook, S., & Shuchter, S. R. (1991). Depression through the first year after the death of a spouse. *American Journal of Psychiatry, 148,* 1346–1352.

Zisook, S., Schuchter, S. R., Pedrelli, P., Sable, J., & Deaciuc, S. C. (2001). Bupropion sustained release for bereavement: Results of an open trial. *Journal of Clinical Psychiatry, 62,* 227–230.

Zuvekas, S. H. (2005). Prescription drugs and the changing patterns of treatment for mental disorders, 1996–2001. *Health Affairs, 24,* 195–205.

Index